DIAGNOSIS AND TREATMENT OF PARKINSON'S DISEASE

Edited by **Abdul Qayyum Rana**

Diagnosis and Treatment of Parkinson's Disease
Edited by Abdul Qayyum Rana

Published by InTech
Janeza Trdine 9, 51000 Rijeka, Croatia

Publishing Process Manager Silvia Vlase

Technical Editor Teodora Smiljanic

Cover Designer InTech Design Team

Additional hard copies can be obtained from orders@intechopen.com

Diagnosis and Treatment of Parkinson's Disease, Edited by Abdul Qayyum Rana
p. cm.
ISBN 978-953-307-465-8

For EU product safety concerns:
IN TECH d.o.o., Prolaz Marije Krucifikse Kozulić 3, 51000 Rijeka, Croatia,
info@intechopen.com or visit our website at intechopen.com.

Meet the editor

Dr. Abdul Qayyum Rana is a Canadian neurologist who specializes in the field of Parkinson's disease and Movement Disorders. He is a fellow of the Royal College of Physicians and Surgeons of Canada. After completing his neurology residency training, Dr. Rana undertook a clinical fellowship in Parkinson's disease and Movement Disorders at the University of Ottawa, Canada. He is currently the director of the Parkinson's Clinic of Eastern Toronto and Movement Disorders Centre located in Toronto, Canada. He is also founder of World Parkinson's Education Program. He is the author of "Frequently Asked Questions About Parkinson's Disease", which is a series of thirteen brochures about Parkinson's disease, translated in many languages and used in several countries around the world. Dr. Rana has also written the following books: "A Synopsis of Neurological Emergencies", "An Aid to Neuro-ophthalmology ", "An introduction to Essential Tremor", "50 Ways Parkinson's Could Affect You", and "What is Parkinson's disease in Arabic?".

Contents

Preface XI

Chapter 1 **Diagnosis and Differential Diagnosis of Parkinson's Disease 1**
Paul Lingor, Jan Liman, Kai Kallenberg, Carsten-Oliver Sahlmann and Mathias Bähr

Chapter 2 **Impact of Dopamine Transporter Scan in Parkinson´s Disease 21**
Jörg Spiegel

Chapter 3 **CFS Biomarkers in Parkinson's Disease 29**
Lucilla Parnetti, Anna Castrioto, Claudia De Carlo, Davide Chiasserini, Nicola Tambasco, Aroldo Rossi, Chiara Balducci, Tommaso Beccari and Paolo Calabresi

Chapter 4 **Neuropsychological Functions and SPECT Neuroimaging in Parkinson's Disease 49**
Lambros Messinis, Athanasios Papathanasiou, Epameinondas Lyros, George Gatzounis and Panagiotis Papathanasopoulos

Chapter 5 **Imaging Dyskinesias in Parkinson's Disease 69**
Marios Politis and Clare Loane

Chapter 6 **Combinations of Markers Provide Clues to the Underlying Neurodegenerative Disorder in REM Sleep Behavior Disorder 89**
Tomoyuki Miyamoto and Masayuki Miyamoto

Chapter 7 **Advances in Drug Therapy: Alternative Treatments for the Control of Motor Fluctuations and Dyskinesias 105**
José Matías Arbelo González and Rocío Malo de Molina Zamora

Chapter 8 **The Role of Feedback in Decision Making 117**
Magda Osman

Chapter 9 **Balance and Gait Rehabilitation in Patients with Parkinson's Disease 141**
Nicola Smania, Alessandro Picelli, Christian Geroin, Patrizia Ianes, Elisabetta La Marchina, Andrea Zenorini and Marialuisa Gandolfi

Chapter 10 **How to Stay Active with Parkinson's Disease 183**
Abu Qutubuddin

Chapter 11 **Invasive and Non-Invasive Stimulation in Parkinson's Disease 189**
Caspar Stephani

Chapter 12 **Mechanisms of High Frequency Stimulation of the Subthalamic Nucleus in Parkinson's Disease: From Local to Distal Effects on the Basal Ganglia Network 211**
Marc Savasta, Carole Carcenac and Sabrina Boulet

Chapter 13 **Thalamic Deep Brain Stimulation for Parkinson's Disease 233**
Ryoma Morigaki, Shinji Nagahiro, Ryuji Kaji and Satoshi Goto

Chapter 14 **Post-Operative Management of Parkinson Patients with Deep Brain Stimulation 253**
Niels Allert and Volker Arnd Coenen

Preface

Diagnosis of Parkinson's disease at times could be challenging even for the expert clinicians. Currently there are no laboratory investigations available for the definite diagnosis of this complicated condition; however some progress is being made to develop tools which may aid in the diagnosis of Parkinson's disease. A summary of current knowledge about biomarkers and various imaging techniques which may be helpful in diagnosis of Parkinson's disease is given in various chapters of this book. A discussion about the differential diagnosis of Parkinson's disease has been generated.

As Parkinson's disease advances, both motor and non-motor symptoms also progress, the management of which becomes challenging for the treating physician. This book provides an up to date account of all available treatments of Parkinson's disease. Various modes of treatment such as pharmacotherapy, physical therapy have discussed in detail in addition to the latest developments on the surgical treatments of Parkinson's disease. A chapter on postoperative care of patients has also been included in this text. Not only clinicians dealing with day to day problems caused by Parkinson's disease can use this book as a guideline, but other health care workers may find useful information in this book.

Clinical information presented in this book is considered generally accepted practice; however the authors, editor, and publisher are not responsible for any errors, omissions, or consequences from the application of this information. Every effort has been made to present correct and up to date information in this book but medicine is a field with ongoing research and development, therefore readers may use other sources if the content of this book is found to be insufficient.

Dr. Abdul Qayyum Rana
Parkinson's Clinic of Eastern Toronto & Movement Disorders Center
Toronto, Canada

1

Diagnosis and Differential Diagnosis of Parkinson's Disease

Paul Lingor[1], Jan Liman[1], Kai Kallenberg[2],
Carsten-Oliver Sahlmann[3] and Mathias Bähr[1]
[1]*University Medicine Göttingen, Departments of Neurology,*
[2]*Neuroradiology,*
[3]*Nuclear Medicine,*
Germany

1. Introduction

Parkinsonian syndromes are a heterogeneous entity of movement disorders, which can be subdivided into idiopathic Parkinson's disease, rare genetic forms of Parkinson's disease as well as symptomatic and atypical parkinsonian syndromes. In addition, a number of other neurodegenerative disorders may show clinical signs of Parkinsonism. The etiology, histopathology, clinical manifestation and disease course varies significantly among these disorders. A correct and early differential diagnosis therefore is essential for proper prognostic estimation and consultancy of the patient as well as a prerequisite for inclusion in clinical studies.

This chapter will summarize diagnostic criteria mainly focussing on the diagnosis of idiopathic Parkinson's disease (iPD) and delineate specific factors to differentiate this disorder from other disease entities.

2. Clinical signs

Idiopathic Parkinson's disease is a progressive, neurodegenerative movement disorder, which in its most classical manifestation is characterized by the triad of bradykinesia, muscular rigidity and tremor. IPD is the most frequent neurodegenerative movement disorder with a mean prevalence of ~150/100.000 (Errea et al., 1999; Walker et al., 2010). A definite diagnosis has to be based on histopathological analysis and requires cell loss in the substantia nigra, the presence of Lewy bodies, which stain for alpha-synuclein and ubiquitin, and usually can be obtained only post mortem. In addition, the histology has to exclude histopathological features of other disorders, which could mimick clinical PD, such as atypical parkinsonian syndromes (Gelb et al., 1999). While these criteria are useful for post mortem classification, several attempts have been made to define clinical diagnostic criteria, e.g. by the UK Parkinson's Disease Society Brain Bank (UKPDSBB) (Hughes et al., 1992) or the National Institute of Neurological Disorders and Stroke (NINDS) (Gelb et al., 1999). For clinical practice, the implementation of modified UKPDSBB criteria has proven useful: here, the diagnosis is based on (1) the identification of parkinsonian symptoms, (2) the absence of exclusion criteria and (3) the presence of prospective positive criteria (Table 1). However, it has to be kept in mind, that even if these criteria are verified by expert neurologists, the diagnostic certainty is only between 75 - 90 % when compared with the results of the autopsy (Hughes et al., 2001; Dickson et al., 2009).

Step 1 Diagnosis of Parkinsonian syndrome
- Bradykinesia (slowness of initiation of voluntary movement with progressive reduction in speed and amplitude of repetitive actions)
- and at least one of the following:
- muscular rigidity
- 4-6 Hz rest tremor
- postural instability not caused by primary visual, vestibular, cerebellar, or proprioceptive dysfunction
Step 2 Exclusion criteria for idiopathic Parkinson's disease
- Repeated strokes with stepwise progression of parkinsonian features
- Repeated head injury
- History of definite encephalitis
- Oculogyric crises
- Neuroleptic treatment at onset of symptoms
- More than one affected relative
- Sustained remission
- Strictly unilateral features after 3 years
- Supranuclear gaze palsy
- Cerebellar signs
- Early severe autonomic involvement
- Early severe dementia with disturbances of memory, language, and praxis
- Babinski sign
- Presence of cerebral tumour or communicating hydrocephalus on CT scan
- Negative response to large doses of levodopa (if malabsorption excluded)
- MPTP exposure
Step 3 Supportive prospective positive criteria for idiopathic Parkinson's disease (Three or more required for diagnosis of definite Parkinson's disease)
- Unilateral onset
- Rest tremor present
- Progressive disorder
- Persistent asymmetry affecting side of onset most
- Excellent response (70-100%) to levodopa
- Severe levodopa-induced chorea
- Levodopa response for 5 years or more
- Clinical course of 10 years or more

Table 1. UK Parkinson's Disease Society Brain Bank (UKPDSBB) clinical diagnostic criteria for idiopathic Parkinson's disease (from (Hughes et al., 1992).

Although numerous supplementary technical exams are available, which may increase diagnostic certainty, the initial diagnosis remains a clinical one and can be based purely on medical history and clinical examination. Motor symptoms in iPD are clinically most striking, but a number of less prominent non-motor symptoms may already be present at

onset. These non-motor symptoms (such as olfactory dysfunction or altered sleep behaviour) have not yet been sufficiently recognized in structured diagnostic criteria, but are likely to be included in the future. The importance of non-motor symptoms is further underlined by recent studies suggesting a premotor phase ranging from 5 - 20 years before the onset of motor symptoms (Savica et al., 2010). Even more importantly, when patients were asked about the impact of symptoms on health-related quality of life autonomic dysfunction, psychiatric complications, pain, fatigue, and sleep problems were mainly correlated with a negative impact (Gallagher et al., 2010).
IPD has been observed in all age groups, but about 75 % of all cases show first motor symptoms after an age of 60. Age is the single most consistent risk factor for developing iPD and should be considered in the differential diagnosis (Hindle, 2010). Only ~ 5 % of all PD cases begin before the age of 40 and these are likely to be caused by genetic mutations (Wickremaratchi et al., 2009).

2.1 Motor symptoms

The initial presentation may vary, with tremor beeing the most common motor symptom in patients, in which the diagnosis of iPD has been verified post-mortem (Hughes et al., 1993). A recent community-based study in 358 patients identified tremor as initially leading symptom in approximately half of the patients. Some 44 % showed an akinetic-rigid phenotype and only 7 % presented with a leading gait disturbance. Interestingly, the akinetic-rigid presentation was more pronounced in younger patients, while tremor and gait disturbance as initial symptoms increase with the age at presentation (Wickremaratchi et al., 2011).

2.1.1 Bradykinesia

Slowness of initiation and execution of voluntary movements, such as limb movements, facial expression or gait, characterizes bradykinesia. Diadochokinesis (the ability to perform rapid alternating movements) is usually slowed (Haaxma et al., 2010). Micrographia with a characteristic decrease of character size towards the end of the line, the shuffling gait with a diminished gait quadrangle and reduced arm swing, and hypomimia with a progressive loss of facial expression are classical manifestations of bradykinesia. Because of the severe hypomimia with a lack to adequately support emotional expression, PD patients may wrongly be considered depressive. At the same time, one has to keep in mind that depression is a common concomitant disorder, which may occur in up to ~ 20 % of PD patients (Brown et al., 2011).

2.1.2 Tremor

The characteristic tremor is a low-frequency (4-6 Hz) resting tremor, but other tremor forms, such as an action tremor or a postural tremor may occur as the disease progresses (Jankovic et al., 1999). Other tremor entities, most importantly essential tremor (ET), have to be considered in the differential diagnosis and tremor frequency is a major differentiation criterion (see part 4.4). Therefore, a tremor analysis may be a helpful additional examination to quantify the characteristics of the tremor presented. There is evidence to suggest that there is an association and even histopathological overlap in some cases of ET and iPD, but the case is not yet closed on this issue (Raethjen and Deuschl, 2009). Like most symptoms in iPD, the tremor manifests with a unilateral preference. In the course of the disease, tremor intensity may diminish and give way to the bradykinetic symptoms. Very importantly one has to note, that about one of four of all iPD patients does not develop a characteristic tremor during the entire course of the disease (Hughes et al., 1993).

2.1.3 Rigidity

Rigidity becomes apparent at the clinical examination, when the passive movement of a limb is impaired by a wax-like resistance. In combination with the tremor frequency this results in the cogwheel phenomenon upon passive movement in a joint. Many patients with iPD initially complain of unilateral back and/or shoulder pain as a consequence of the asymetric muscular tone, which may result in the consultation of an orthopedic specialist before final referral to a neurologist (Madden and Hall, 2010).

2.1.4 Postural instability

Postural instability regularly appears in the course of the disease, most often in more advanced stages (Coelho et al., 2010). In progressive disease it may be considered as important diagnostic feature and supports the initial diagnosis (Hughes et al., 1992). However, pronounced postural instability at the initial presentation may be an indicator for progressive supranuclear palsy (PSP) instead of iPD (Litvan et al., 1996) and therefore has to be carefully set into context with other motor features.
Usually the motor symptoms are asymetrically distributed and in cases with a strict bilateral presentation one should consider the differential diagnosis of a symptomatic or atypical parkinsonian syndrome.

2.2 Non-motor symptoms

Since the landmark studies of Braak and colleagues the picture of iPD as a mainly nigrostriatal disorder is no longer sustainable. In fact, these analyses suggest that the pathoanatomical changes, such as the presence of Lewy bodies and Lewy neurites appear first in the medulla oblongata, the pons and the olfactory bulb, then spread to the midbrain and lastly affect the neocortex (Braak et al., 2003). It is no surprise thus, that symptoms deriving from dysfunction of these brain regions may precede motor symptoms and other non-motor symptoms may develop in late stage disease.

2.2.1 Olfactory dysfunction

Olfactory dysfunction has been recognized to be an early clinical sign in patients with iPD and bedside testing can be easily performed by standardized odour test batteries (see part 3.3.1). Approximately 70 - 90 % of all iPD patients present with a significant lack of odour discrimination and it seems to be present well before the onset of motor symptoms (Doty et al., 1988; Kranick and Duda, 2008), which could result in a future use of olfactory testing in combination with other parameters as a biomarker in putative neuroprotective therapies. A recent study evaluating brain glucose metabolism suggests that hyposmia is related to cognitive imparment due to cortical dysfunction in iPD patients and that the cognitive deficit in olfactory perception is at least partially responsible for diminished smell differentiation. Altered metabolism in the amygdala and the piriform cortex could be responsible for this sensory deficiency (Baba et al., 2011).

2.2.2 Dysautonomia

Dysautonomic features, such as seborrhoea, orthostatic hypotension, gastrointestinal or urinary dysfunction may occur before or after the onset of motor symptoms (Bassetti, 2010). Their early presence (especially urinary dysfunction, orthostatic hypotension) should however always challenge the diagnosis of iPD and lead to consideration of the differential diagnosis of atypical parkinsonian syndromes, such as multisystem atrophy (MSA) or progressive supranuclear palsy (PSP) (Colosimo et al., 2010).

Urinary dysfunction is especially debilitating for the patient and usually manifests as overactive bladder syndrome, which has been attributed to the degeneration of central serotonergic projections. It correlates with disease severity (measured by the UPDRS-III score) and patient age (Iacovelli et al., 2010).

Gastrointestinal symptoms are present in more than half of iPD patients and may comprise constipation, dysphagia, nausea, vomiting, incomplete bowel emptying or incontinence. As for other dysautonomic symptoms, the prevalence in atypical parkinsonian syndromes, such as MSA or PSP, but also in DLB is much higher (Colosimo et al., 2010).

Symptomatic postural hypotension is less frequent in iPD, but ~20 % of the patients show a drop in systolic blood pressure of more than 20 mmHg associated with postural events (Senard et al., 1997). If orthostatic hypotension is prominent at initial presentation, the diagnosis of MSA should be considered.

While above-mentioned symptoms are likely to be verbalized by the patients, sexual dysfunction is not. Patients may not even be aware of the fact that erectile dysfunction and loss of libido are part of the non-motory symptom complex observed in iPD and these symptoms are therefore likely to be underreported. Nevertheless, a recent study analyzing the most bothersome symptoms reported by iPD patients in early stage disease (up to 6 years disease duration) listed sexual dysfunction at place 12 of 24 and this was similar in late stage disease patients (Politis et al., 2010).

2.2.3 Depression and anxiety

Neuropsychiatric disorders, such as depression and anxiety are frequently found alongside with motor symptoms - approximately 40 % of all iPD patients show anxiety-related, depressive or combined psychopathology (Brown et al., 2011). A recently published analysis demonstrates a positive correlation between depression and higher UPDRS/Hoehn and Yahr stages. Also, other non-motor symptoms, such as anxiety, hallucinations and sleep disturbances were more frequently observed in depressed iPD patients (Dissanayaka et al., 2011). Disease severity in iPD has also been shown to be positively correlated with anxiety and patients with young onset, gait dysfunction and postural instability were especially prone to develop an anxiety disorder (Dissanayaka et al., 2010)

2.2.4 Cognitive decline and dementia

About 40 % of all patients initially diagnosed with iPD will develop cognitive decline with dementia in the course of the disease (Aarsland et al., 2001). According to the current diagnostic criteria, the occurence of cognitive dysfunction in patients with parkinsonian symptoms later than 12 months after the first presentation of motor symptoms is considered as Parkinson's disease dementia. When cognitive decline occurs before or within the first year of motor symptom onset, dementia with Lewy-bodies (DLB) has to be diagnosed rather then iPD (McKeith et al., 1996). Because of their histopathological similarities, it is likely that iPD and DLB are not separate entities, but different manifestations within the spectrum of disorders, which are defined by the presence of pathologic alpha-synuclein aggregates, so-called alpha-synucleinopathies. The neuropsychological examination for Parkinson's disease dementia should include specific scales which should be powered to detect cortical dysfunction. For example, the Scales for Outcomes of Parkinson's disease-Cognition (SCOPA-COG), Parkinson's Disease-Cognitive Rating Scale (PD-CRS), and Parkinson Neuropsychometric Dementia Assessment (PANDA) are likely to yield a more precise assessment of the patient's cognitive dysfunction than general dementia assessments (Kulisevsky and Pagonabarraga, 2009).

2.2.5 REM-sleep behaviour disorder

REM-sleep behaviour disorder (RBD) is an especially interesting feature of iPD patients, because it can appear many years before the diagnosis of the disease based on classical motor symptoms (Claassen et al., 2010) and is observed in up to 25 % of all iPD patients (Gjerstad et al., 2008 JNNP). RBD is characterized by increased motor activity during REM sleep, which may result in vocalization and vigorous limb movements. Patients usually also describe a vivid and sometimes terrifying dreaming experience. Sleep disturbances as well as restless legs are ranked high in the list of most bothersome symptoms for early and even more late stage iPD patients (Politis et al., 2010). In addition, up to 50 % of iPD patients complain of excessive daytime sleepiness, which also can precede the manifestation of motor symptoms by many years (Abbott et al., 2005).

Autonomic failure
- Gastrointestinal dysfunction
- Urinary dysfunction
- Sexual dysfunction
- Orthostatic hypotension
Neuropsychiatric and sleep disturbances
- Depression
- Anxiety
- Panic attacks
- Impulse control disorder
- Hallucinations
- Psychosis
- Dementia
- REM sleep behavior disorder and insomnia
- Excessive daytime sleepiness and fatigue
Sensory deficits
- Olfactory dysfunction
- Pain

Table 2. Non-motor features which may occur in idiopathic Parkinson's disease.

3. Additional exams

Although the diagnosis of iPD can be made based purely on clinical examination, additional technical exams can help to differentiate other degenerative disorders, most importantly secondary or atypical parkinsonian syndromes.

3.1 Imaging approaches

3.1.1 MRI

There are currently no MRI-criteria in clinical use for the verification of a putative iPD diagnosis. No single morphological marker could be identified permitting the diagnosis of iPD, even though several parameters exist, which help to differentiate iPD from atypical parkinsonian syndromes. Recent approaches combining different magnetic resonance parameters (such as R_2* value, mean diffusivity and fractional anisotropy) have been shown to achieve a high accuracy for the discrimination of iPD patients and controls (Péran et al.,

2010). It remains to be seen whether similar techniques find application in the clinical practice and whether they will be able to separate other entities from iPD.
Nevertheless, conventional CT and MRI imaging has its place in the diagnostic workup for suspected iPD and is widely used to exclude common differential diagnoses, such as vascular PD, Wilson's disease, or atypical parkinsonian syndromes (see section 4).

3.1.2 SPECT imaging

Imaging with radiolabeled ligands has markedly improved the functional diagnostics of Parkinson's disease. PET and SPECT techniques permit to visualize the pre- and postsynaptic compartment of the nigrostriatal projections and thus draw a semiquantitative picture about functionality of these pathways. In clinical use, they are mostly used for the differentiation of iPD from atypical parkinsonian syndromes or from essential tremor (ET).
The dopaminergic deficit can be quantified by a DAT-SPECT (DaTSCAN®) using [^{123}I]-FP-CIT and is a measure for the presynaptic dopamine transporter in the striatal dopaminergic synapse (Booij et al., 1997). The DaTSCAN should be used, if the dopaminergic deficit itself is clinically unclear, i.e. too subtle, or if tremor is the prominent symptom, which makes the discrimination between iPD and ET difficult (Benamer et al., 2000). The DaTSCAN also correlates with the rate of dopaminergic degeneration in the course of the disease (Winogrodzka et al., 2001) and, similarly to the clinical presentation, the signal reduction is usually found with a unilateral preference. With further progression and degeneration in later disease stages signal reduction appears bilaterally (Fig. 1a). According to a study of 122 patients with iPD, the DaTSCAN shows different patterns in tremor-dominant versus akinetic-rigid iPD (Eggers et al., 2011). Unfortunately, the [^{123}I]-FP-CIT SPECT does not reliably distinguish iPD from atypical parkinsonian syndromes, such as MSA, PSP, CBD and a similar nigrostriatal deficit is also detected in LBD (Pirker et al., 2000; Kägi et al., 2010). Other imaging techniques focussing on the D2-receptor expression are more useful to answer this question.
As mentioned earlier, autonomic denervation is an early phenomenon in iPD and [^{123}I]-MIBG scintigraphy is a mean to visualize the postganglionic, presynaptic sympathetic terminals.

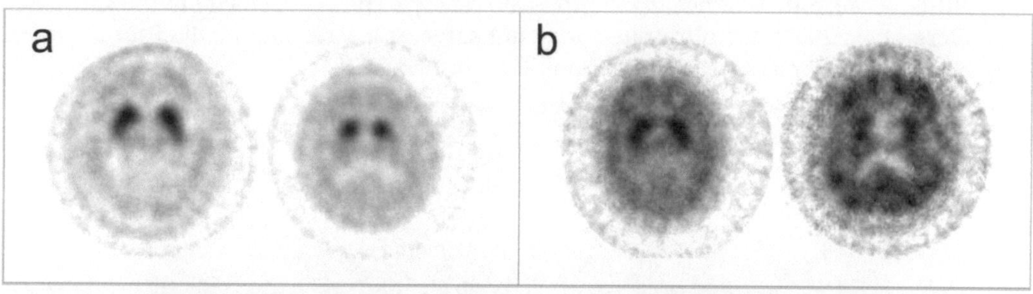

Fig. 1. **a:** DAT-SPECT; transversal section; 3 h after injection of 220 MBq [^{123}I]-FP-CIT (DaTSCAN®). Left: normal dopamine transporter labeling. Right: reduced putaminal dopamine transporter labeling suggestive of a nigrostriatal deficit (e.g. IPD, LBD, MSA).
b: D2-receptor-SPECT; transversal section; 1,5 h after injection of 185 MBq [^{123}I]-IBZM. Left: normal D2-receptor expression with good contrast in the basal ganglia relative to cortex. Right: reduced D2-receptor expression with low contrast of basal ganglia relative to cortex (e.g.: MSA).

Reduced tracer uptake by nerve terminals in the heart is observed in iPD already in the beginning of the disease and it remains fairly stable in later stages even though it does not seem to correlate significantly with clinical symptoms of autonomic dysfunction (Matsui et

al., 2006). Due to better sensitivity and the correlation to clinical progression the DaTSCAN currently may be more suitable in the early diagnosis of iPD than [^{123}I]-MIBG scintigraphy.
SPECT imaging also allows quantifying the postsynaptic dopamine receptor status, which can be helpful in the differentiation of iPD and atypical parkinsonian syndromes. D2 receptors can be imaged by application of [^{123}I]-IBZM or [^{123}I]-IBF and are decreased in atypical parkinsonian syndromes, such as MSA or PSP, but normal or even upregulated in early iPD (Kim et al., 2002) (Fig. 1b). Imaging techniques aiming at the visualization of cerebral blood flow, such as [^{99m}Tc]-ECD (so-called Neurolite) or FDG, can help in the identification of corticobasal degeneration, where an asymmetrical reduction of perfusion in cortical areas can be revealed (Hossain et al., 2003) and discriminate towards PSP (Zhang et al., 2001).
Non-dopaminergic functions are also accessible to PET and SPECT imaging, although these examinations are not performed routinely. For example, the ^{11}C-WAY100635 PET can visualize reduced serotonin receptor expression in iPD, which has been suggested to play a role in iPD-associated depression, and evaluation of ^{11}C-PK11195 binding by PET examination reflects microglial activation associated with iPD (Brooks, 2007).

3.1.3 Transcranial ultrasound

Transcranial ultrasound has meanwhile become a standard exam for the initial bedside diagnostics in suspected iPD. Since the first description of hyperechogenicity in the substantia nigra in iPD patients (Becker et al., 1995) a large number of studies confirmed these findings demonstrating that these alterations occur in more than two thirds of all iPD patients and that substantia nigra hyperechogenicity is detectable in a very early stage of disease (Fig. 2). Although the histopathological correlate of this alteration is still a matter of debate, there is evidence to suggest that increased iron deposition and/or microglial activation is responsible for this phenomenon. As in each ultrasound examination, the quantification and quality of the readout depends highly on the skill of the examiner, but as recent studies have shown, reproducibility in experienced sonographers is high (van de Loo et al., 2010). Because 10 % of healthy controls also show hyperechogenicity in the substantia nigra (Berg et al., 2001), the ultrasound may not serve as a screening method for a general population, but rather as a supporting exam in suspected iPD.

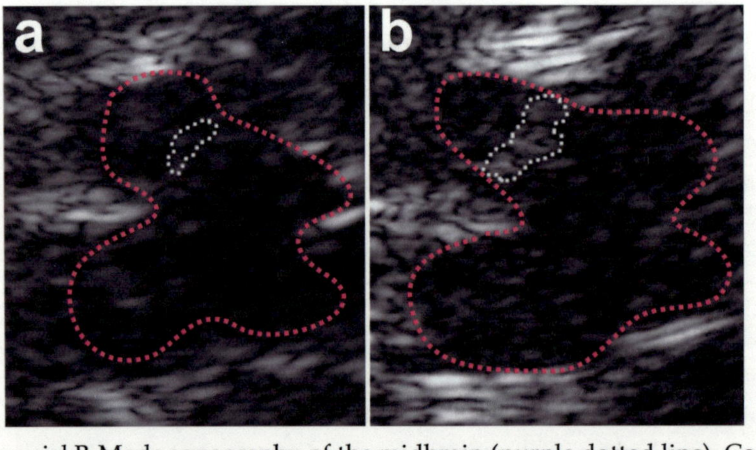

Fig. 2. Transcranial B-Mode sonography of the midbrain (purple dotted line). Controls show little to no hyperechogenicity (white dotted line) in the substantia nigra (**a**) as compared to markedly increased hyperechogenicity in iPD patients (**b**).

3.2 Laboratory analysis

Up to now, no laboratory test is available for the diagnosis of iPD and no single marker has been identified so far (see section 5). There is no routine workup, but assessment of serum copper and ceruloplasmin as well as urine copper may be indicated especially in patients with young onset PD, if Wilson's disease is suspected.

3.3 Other technical exams

3.3.1 Olfactory testing

Olfactory testing is an inexpensive, but useful supplementary exam and should be performed in each patient presenting with suspected iPD. Commercial kits are available, where different odorants, including trigeminal irritants and controls, are presented to the patient (e.g. Sniffin' Sticks®, (Wolfensberger and Schnieper, 1999). Most patients (90 %) with iPD show olfactory dysfunction early in the disease course (Katzenschlager and Lees, 2004). There are therefore reasons to suggest olfactory testing as an early clinical biomarker for iPD (Morley and Duda, 2010). Olfaction can also be impaired in patients with MSA, but it seems to be mostly unaffected in PSP or CBD (Wenning et al., 1995; Müller et al., 2002). Therefore, olfactory testing can be a useful additional tool in the differentiation between iPD and atypical parkinsonian syndromes.

3.3.2 Genetic testing

If a family history of Parkinson's disease exists or if disease manifestation occurs at a young age, patients may benefit from genetic counselling. Up to now, at least 6 PD susceptibility loci have been identified and at least 11 other genes are known to cause genetic Parkinson's disease (reviewed in (Shulman et al., 2010). A recently published study identified individuals with an age of onset of 30 years or younger (50 years or younger in patients with Jewish or Hispanic ancestry) or those with a history of Parkinson's disease in a first-degree relative as most likely to bear a mutation in a iPD-associated gene (Alcalay et al., 2010). These patients may undergo genetic testing after thorough information about possible consequences of the test results for family members, familial planning and prognostic considerations.

3.3.3 Dopaminergic response test

The histopathologically prominent nigrostriatal degeneration and the consecutive depletion of dopamine in the striatum can be identified as the pathoanatomical and biochemical correlate of the motor symptoms in iPD, most importantly of the bradykinetic symptoms. Thus, it is not surprising that dopamine replacement therapy initially results in transient, but marked amelioration of these symptoms, an effect which patients often experience as the "honeymoon-phase" due to the dramatic symptom reduction. Responsiveness to dopaminomimetic therapy is an important supportive factor for the confirmation of the diagnosis of idiopathic Parkinson's disease and a lacking improvement of motor symptoms suggests the presence of an atypical parkinsonian syndrome, such as PSP, MSA or CBD.

Clinical testing for dopaminergic response can be performed with levodopa (e.g. 200/50 mg levodopa/dopadecarboxylase inhibitor) by oral application or with apomorphine, a dopaminergic drug requiring subcutaneous administration. The test is usually considered positive, if the patient improves by at least 30 % in the UPDRS – a number which may be too ambitious in patients presenting only with mild symptoms (Reichmann, 2010).

It has to be considered though, that even atypical parkinsonian syndromes may show an initial response to L-DOPA therapy, which usually is transient and less pronounced than in iPD (Srulijes et al., 2011). Also, tremor is the symptom, which is most resistant to dopaminergic therapy and therefore may result only in an insufficient response.

4. Differential diagnosis

In the following part of this chapter, a number of clinically relevant differential diagnoses are discussed. The main clinical differences are presented along with the appropriate diagnostic tools for the discrimination against iPD.

4.1 Progressive supranuclear palsy (PSP)

As one of the most frequent atypical parkinsonian syndroms, PSP belongs to the group of so-called tauopathies, disorders which are characterized by pathological processing of the tau protein. Compared to iPD, PSP is still quite rare (1-6/100.000 inhabitants) (Schrag et al., 1999; Nath et al., 2001). Clinically, at least two distinct variants can be differentiated: PSP-parkinsonism (PSP-P) and the Richardson's syndrome (RS). While PSP-P initially may present with typical iPD-features, such as tremor, bradykinesia, rigidity and even a temporary response to dopaminergic medication, other symptoms, such as the supranuclear vertical gaze palsy, postural instability and cognitive decline take center place in the later course of the disease (Litvan et al., 1996). In RS (the original syndrome described by Richardson in 1963) these additional symptoms are present in the very beginning of the disease (Richardson et al., 1963). The protracted appearance of these additional symptoms in PSP-P may complicate the diagnosis and it's no surprise that less than 50 % of pathologically verified PSP-cases are not diagnosed correctly at their first visit (Osaki et al., 2004).

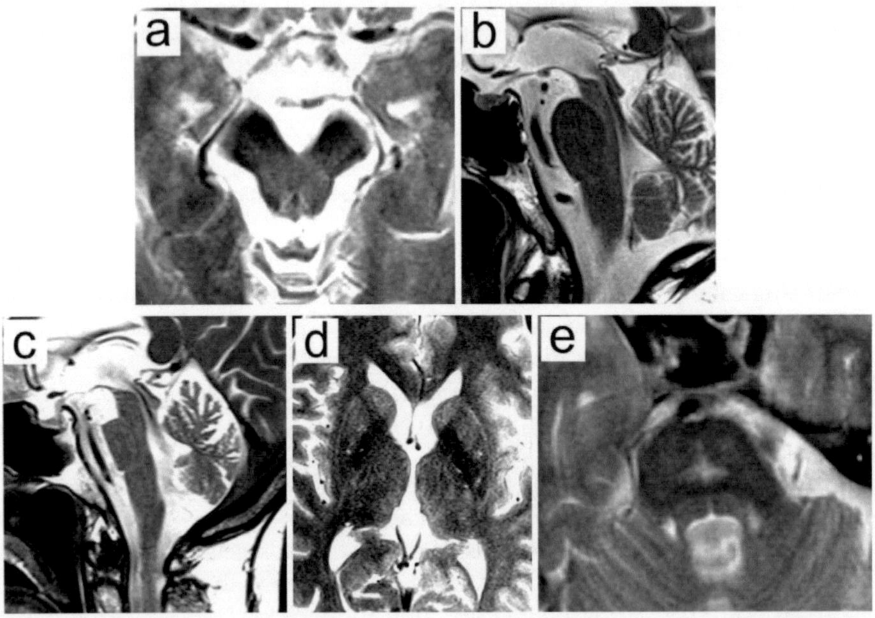

Fig. 3. Characteristic MRI findings in PSP and MSA. Thinning of cerebral peduncles ("Mickey mouse sign") (**a**) and mesencephalic atrophy ("hummingbird sign") (**b**) on T2-weighted images in PSP. Cerebellar and pontine atrophy (**c**), hyperintense putaminal rim (**d**) and degeneration of pontocerebellar projections ("hot cross bun sign") (**e**) as observed on T2-weighted images in patients with MSA.

In clinical differentiation, the symmetrical and mostly axial presentation of bradykinesia, frequent falls and an initially pathological pull test for postural instability should direct attention towards possible PSP. A positive "applause sign" (a tendency to continue applauding after having been instructed to clap three times) may be useful in the differential diagnosis between iPD and PSP, but it has been recently recognized to be even more specific for CBD patients (Dubois et al., 2005; Wu et al., 2008). Pathological tracer distribution in the [^{123}I]-IBZM-SPECT may also be found in PSP (see 3.1.2). On MRI examination patients with PSP may display a mesencephalic atrophy, which can appear as so-called "penguin sign" or "hummingbird sign" in the mid-sagittal section (Oba et al., 2005). On axial T2-weighted sections, the anteroposterior diameter of the midbrain is reduced and, together with a thinning of the cerebral peduncles, may result in the so-called "mickey mouse sign" (Fig. 3a). The reduction of a-p diameter below 14 mm seems to specifically differentiate patients with PSP from iPD (Warmuth-Metz et al., 2001).

4.2 Multiple system atrophy (MSA)

As an atypical parkinsonian syndrome multiple system atrophy (MSA) has a slightly lower prevalence than PSP. Similar to iPD, MSA is an alpha-synucleinopathy, but here inclusions are found in oligodendrocytes instead of neurons (Tu et al., 1998). Because patients can present with a primarily parkinsonian or a primarily cerebellar phenotype a differentiation into MSA-P and MSA-C is clinically used. MSA-P patients can initially show typical signs of iPD, but additional signs, such as orthostatic hypotension, urinary incontinence and erectile dysfunction should be regarded as red flags for the diagnosis of MSA. Cerebellar dysfunction with ataxic gait and limb movements, dysarthria and sustained gaze-evoked nystagmus may initially lead in MSA-C patients, but may also be present or appear in the course of the disease in patients presenting with MSA-P. Some patients may also show positive corticospinal tract signs (Gilman et al., 1999). Response to dopaminergic medication can be initially positive, but the effects are mostly transient (Hughes et al., 1992).
SPECT imaging using [^{123}I]-IBZM may show decreased D2 receptor binding in MSA, but measurements of the striatal regional apparent diffusion coefficients (rADC) by diffusion-weighted images on MRI scans (MRI-DWI) may be even more sensitive in differentiating MSA from iPD (Seppi et al., 2004). Conventional MRI in MSA-P can show a hyperintense putaminal rim on T2-weighted images. Cerebellar and pontine atrophy as well as a cross-like hyperintensity on T2-weighted images (so-called "hot-cross-bun"-sign reflecting the degeneration of pontocerebellar projections) can also be observed in MSA-C (Fig. 3b-d)(Lee et al., 2004).

4.3 Corticobasal degeneration (CBD)

This rare tauopathy may have more common features with frontotemporal dementia (Pick's disease) or PSP than with iPD, but an initial appearance with unilateral bradykinesia and tremor may evoke the latter differential diagnosis. Red flags for the presence of CBD are a slowly progressive unilateral apraxia together with dystonia and jerky movements mostly in the upper limb as well as a visual-tactile neglect. The so-called "alien-limb sign", indicating the loss of voluntary control over one extremity, is present in about half of the patients. Signs of corticospinal tract degeneration, dysarthria, gait difficulties and supranuclear opthalmoplegia can be found in the later disease course (Rinne et al., 1994). Cognitive decline with development of dementia is frequent (Grimes et al., 1999).

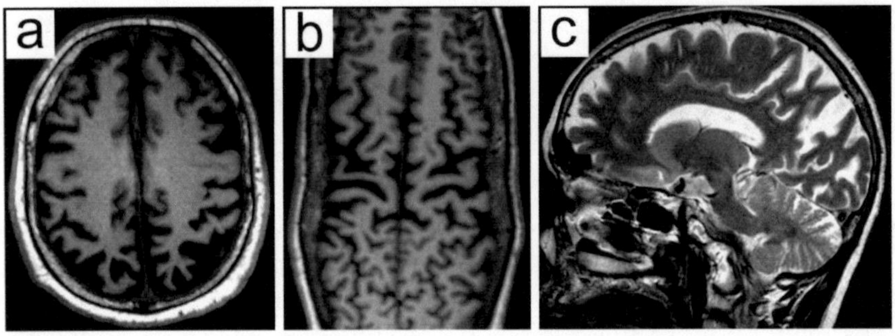

Fig. 4. Characteristic MRI findings in CBD. Asymmetric frontoparietal cortical atrophy with an emphasis on the central region in a conventional T1-weighted axial section (**a**), curved planar reformation or "pancake" representation of the cortex (**b**) or paramedian sagittal T2-weighted image (**c**).

Focal or asymmetric cortical atrophy with a frontoparietal preference may be present on MRI (Fig. 4) and a corresponding hypoperfusion/hypometabolism may be detected by SPECT/PET (see section 3.1.2).

4.4 Essential tremor (ET)

A positive family history, clinical responsivity to beta-blockers and small doses of alcohol suggests the presence of ET. Rest tremor is unusual in ET and the manifestation is mostly as a symmetrical, postural and kinetic tremor (Bain et al., 2000). Since tremor may be one of the first and sometimes solitary symptoms at initial presentation of iPD, differential diagnosis may be difficult.

DaTSCAN analysis should usually be able to differentiate versus iPD by exclusion of a striatal dopaminergic deficit, but a clinical overlap has been suggested and it is still controversial whether at least a subgroup of ET patients may develop iPD and vice versa (Quinn et al., 2010).

4.5 Lewy-body dementia (LBD)

Histopathology suggests that LBD and iPD may indeed be very similar disorders and probably can be considered as a neuropathological spectrum of an alpha-synucleinopathy with Lewy bodies (Jellinger, 2009). As the name suggests, cognitive decline is the primary feature in LBD and - per definition - must be present before the onset of motor dysfunctions, which most frequently present as bradykinesia and rigidity. The clinical challenge is the separation from Parkinson's disease dementia, which may occur in up to 40 % of all iPD patients (see section 2.2.4). The term Parkinson's disease dementia should only be used when dementia occurs at least 12 months after onset of motor symptoms in iPD, which however is an arbitrary cut-off. According to consensus criteria, LBD patients show also pronounced fluctuations in cognition and attention. Also, optical hallucinations can occur and patients can display a marked sensitivity to neuroleptic treatment (McKeith et al., 1996; McKeith et al., 2005).

4.6 Vascular parkinsonism

It is now widely acknowledged that white matter changes observed in arteriosclerotic disease, e.g. due to long history of arterial hypertension, may be associated with the presentation of parkinsonian-like features. However, there are no commonly-accepted diagnostic criteria,

which may be due to the heterogeneity of this disorder as well as a possible coincidence of vascular changes and iPD. Clinically, patients may present with a slowly progressive difficulty of gait, while the upper extremities usually are less affected - thus the term "lower-body parkinsonism". Tremor is less frequent, but patients may show a multitude of additional symptoms, such as corticospinal tract signs, pseudobulbar palsy, dementia or incontinence, depending on the distribution of the microvascular alterations (systematically reviewed in (Kalra et al., 2010). Rarely, symptoms occur abruptly after an ischemic incidence (Alarcón et al., 2004). Response to dopaminergic therapy usually is limited.
In contrast to iPD, the native CT scan and the MRI may be helpful in the identification of vascular lesions and a history of arteriosclerosis, hypertension and other cardiovascular risk factors may be indicative.

4.7 Normal pressure hydrocephalus (NPH)

Because of the therapeutic consequences arising from the diagnosis of NPH and its relatively high prevalence, it is of high clinical relevance to differentiate this disorder from iPD. Recent estimates of the prevalence with ~22/100.000 inhabitants are very likely understated (Brean and Eide, 2008). Cognitive decline up to dementia as well as urinary incontinence in combination with a gait disturbance build the classical triad of symptoms initially described by Hakim and Adams (Hakim and Adams, 1965). Not all patients, however, present with all three symptoms at the initial visit, which may delay diagnosis. In addition, the slow, shuffling and broad-based gait shows striking similarities to the one observed in iPD (Bugalho and Guimarães, 2007).
Enlarged ventricles can be observed on CT or MRI scans (Fig. 5) and the diagnostics should be followed by a large-volume lumbar puncture. Structured analysis of gait and cognitive function has to be performed before and after taking CSF. An improvement, which is most likely to occur in the gait analysis, favours the diagnosis of NPH and permits to identify patients, who will benefit of ventriculoperitoneal shunting (Bergsneider et al., 2005).

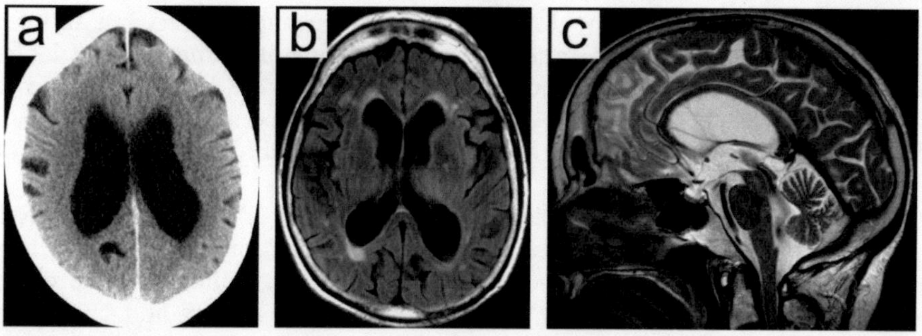

Fig. 5. Characteristic findings in NPH. Enlarged ventricles without pronounced global atrophy on CT scan (**a**), axial MRI T1-weighted (**b**) or sagittal T2-weighted images (**c**).

4.8 Drug-induced Parkinsonism

Different medications can result in a clinically apparent parkinsonism. The symptoms are usually symmetric and tremor is less frequent in contrast to iPD (reviewed in (Susatia and Fernandez, 2009). Most importantly, dopamine receptor blockers (e.g. neuroleptics or antiemetics) and other dopamine-depleting drugs have to be considered (Ebadi and Srinivasan, 1995). However, valproic acid, lithium, flunarizine as well as some SSRIs have also been reported to cause extrapyramidal symptoms (Susatia and Fernandez, 2009).

The prognosis of drug-induced Parkinsonism is rather good as most patients recover after discontinuation of medication. If parkinsonian symptoms are not reversible, one should consider the presence of iPD, which has been unmasked by the anti-dopaminergic medication.

4.9 Other differential diagnoses

In addition to the above-mentioned disorders, there are a number of less frequent causes for parkinsonian syndromes. Because basically any kind of lesion to the extrapyramidal system can potentially result in a parkinsonian presentation, the list of possible etiologies cannot be complete. Some of them have been listed as exclusion criterion in the UKPDSBB clinical diagnostic criteria, for example repeated head trauma, history of encephalitis, cerebral tumour or MPTP exposure (see Table 1). Other neurodegenerative (Huntington's disease, spinocerebellar ataxia, frontotemporal dementia), neurometabolic (Wilson's disease, Fahr's disease, hypoxia) or toxin-induced (occupational manganese exposure, carbon monoxide intoxication) disorders can also present with signs of parkinsonism, even though usually other symptoms are additionally present (reviewed in (Tolosa et al., 2006)).

5. Strategies to improve diagnostic security and early diagnosis

The need to establish an early and reliable diagnosis resulted in a vast ongoing research activity to identify early biomarkers for iPD. Numerous studies focussed on serum or CSF samples, because these fluids can be easily collected and are readily available for large-scale examinations. Numerous publications document the effort to analyze levels of candidate proteins as putative biomarkers, i.e. alpha-synuclein, oligomeric alpha-synuclein, tau, abeta, DJ-1 and combinations thereof, just to name a few (Tokuda et al., 2006; Borroni et al., 2008; Waragai et al., 2010; Tokuda et al., 2010). A recently published large cohort study could show reduced alpha-synuclein levels in synucleinopathies (DLB, iPD and MSA), but was not able to discriminate between these different entities (Mollenhauer et al., 2011). Levels of dopamine metabolites (Lunardi et al., 2009), transition metals (Jiménez-Jiménez et al., 1998) or neurotrophic factors (Pålhagen et al., 2010) have also been quantified, but at the moment there is no clinically helpful single biomarker or combination of biomarkers available.

Novel imaging techniques mainly based on MRI algorithms could move the field forward, but an automated analysis of several parameters appears to be mandatory and has not yet reached clinical practice (Jubault et al., 2009; Vaillancourt et al., 2009; Boelmans et al., 2010; Jubault et al., 2011).

Next to imaging and laboratory analysis the identification of clinical markers may be even more important, since preclinical symptoms precede the onset of motor symptoms significantly. A combined strategy taking into account a cumulative score involving premotor symptoms, such as olfactory dysfunction, sleep disorders and neuropsychiatric disorders could be a promising approach and will have to be evaluated for its prognostic value (reviewed in (Wu et al., 2011).

6. Summary

The diagnosis of idiopathic Parkinson's disease is mainly based on clinical criteria of motor symptoms, such as bradykinesia, tremor and rigidity.

If these are met, other signs of atypical and secondary parkinsonian syndromes, for example MSA, PSP, CBD, vascular parkinsonism, NPH or LBD have to be excluded. In addition to clinical signs typical of these disorders, auxiliary exams, including olfactory testing, MRI and SPECT imaging can help to identify these entities.

Finally, the diagnosis of iPD is supported by prospective criteria, which have to be met during the course of the disease, such as levodopa response, asymmetric symptoms and disease progression.
There is no single reliable biomarker for iPD available yet and a definite diagnosis currently can be made only by histology.

7. References

Aarsland D, Andersen K, Larsen JP, Lolk A, Nielsen H, Kragh-Sørensen P (2001) Risk of dementia in Parkinson's disease: a community-based, prospective study. Neurology 56:730-6

Abbott RD, Ross GW, White LR, Tanner CM, Masaki KH, Nelson JS, Curb JD, Petrovitch H (2005) Excessive daytime sleepiness and subsequent development of Parkinson disease. Neurology 65:1442-6

Alarcón F, Zijlmans JCM, Dueñas G, Cevallos N (2004) Post-stroke movement disorders: report of 56 patients. Journal of neurology, neurosurgery, and psychiatry 75:1568-74

Alcalay RN et al. (2010) Frequency of known mutations in early-onset Parkinson disease: implication for genetic counseling: the consortium on risk for early onset Parkinson disease study. Archives of neurology 67:1116-22

Baba T, Takeda A, Kikuchi A, Nishio Y, Hosokai Y, Hirayama K, Hasegawa T, Sugeno N, Suzuki K, Mori E, Takahashi S, Fukuda H, Itoyama Y (2011) Association of olfactory dysfunction and brain. Metabolism in Parkinson's disease. Movement disorders : official journal of the Movement Disorder Society

Bain P, Brin M, Deuschl G, Elble R, Jankovic J, Findley L, Koller WC, Pahwa R (2000) Criteria for the diagnosis of essential tremor. Neurology 54:S7

Bassetti CL (2010) Nonmotor Disturbances in Parkinson's Disease. Neuro-degenerative diseases

Becker G, Seufert J, Bogdahn U, Reichmann H, Reiners K (1995) Degeneration of substantia nigra in chronic Parkinson's disease visualized by transcranial color-coded real-time sonography. Neurology 45:182-4

Benamer TS et al. (2000) Accurate differentiation of parkinsonism and essential tremor using visual assessment of [123I]-FP-CIT SPECT imaging: the [123I]-FP-CIT study group. Movement disorders : official journal of the Movement Disorder Society 15:503-10

Berg D, Siefker C, Becker G (2001) Echogenicity of the substantia nigra in Parkinson's disease and its relation to clinical findings. Journal of neurology 248:684-9

Bergsneider M, Black PM, Klinge P, Marmarou A, Relkin N (2005) Surgical management of idiopathic normal-pressure hydrocephalus. Neurosurgery 57:S29-39; discussion ii-v

Boelmans K, Bodammer NC, Suchorska B, Kaufmann J, Ebersbach G, Heinze H-J, Niehaus L (2010) Diffusion tensor imaging of the corpus callosum differentiates corticobasal syndrome from Parkinson's disease. Parkinsonism & related disorders 16:498-502

Booij J, Tissingh G, Winogrodzka A, Boer GJ, Stoof JC, Wolters EC, Royen EA van (1997) Practical benefit of [123I]FP-CIT SPET in the demonstration of the dopaminergic deficit in Parkinson's disease. European journal of nuclear medicine 24:68-71

Borroni B, Malinverno M, Gardoni F, Alberici A, Parnetti L, Premi E, Bonuccelli U, Grassi M, Perani D, Calabresi P, Di Luca M, Padovani A (2008) Tau forms in CSF as a reliable biomarker for progressive supranuclear palsy. Neurology 71:1796-803

Braak H, Tredici KD, Vos RAID, Steur ENHJ, Braak E (2003) Staging of brain pathology related to sporadic Parkinson's disease. Neurobiology of Aging 24:197-211

Brean A, Eide PK (2008) Prevalence of probable idiopathic normal pressure hydrocephalus in a Norwegian population. Acta neurologica Scandinavica 118:48-53

Brooks DJ (2007) Imaging non-dopaminergic function in Parkinson's disease. Molecular imaging and biology 9:217-22

Brown RG, Landau S, Hindle JV, Playfer J, Samuel M, Wilson KC, Hurt CS, Anderson RJ, Carnell J, Dickinson L, Gibson G, Schaick RV, Sellwood K, Thomas BA, Burn DJ, Group P-pd S (2011) Depression and anxiety related subtypes in Parkinson ' s disease. Journal of neurology, neurosurgery, and psychiatry

Bugalho P, Guimarães J (2007) Gait disturbance in normal pressure hydrocephalus: a clinical study. Parkinsonism & related disorders 13:434-7

Claassen DO, Josephs KA, Ahlskog JE, Silber MH, Tippmann-Peikert M, Boeve BF (2010) REM sleep behavior disorder preceding other aspects of synucleinopathies by up to half a century. Neurology 75:494-9

Coelho M, Marti MJ, Tolosa E, Ferreira JJ, Valldeoriola F, Rosa M, Sampaio C (2010) Late-stage Parkinson's disease: the Barcelona and Lisbon cohort. Journal of neurology 257:1524-32

Colosimo C et al. (2010) Non-motor symptoms in atypical and secondary parkinsonism: the PRIAMO study. Journal of neurology 257:5-14

Dickson DW, Braak H, Duda JE, Duyckaerts C, Gasser T, Halliday GM, Hardy J, Leverenz JB, Del Tredici K, Wszolek ZK (2009) Neuropathological assessment of Parkinson's disease: refining the diagnostic criteria. The Lancet Neurology 8:1150-1157

Dissanayaka NNW, Sellbach A, Matheson S, O'Sullivan JD, Silburn PA, Byrne GJ, Marsh R, Mellick GD (2010) Anxiety disorders in Parkinson's disease: prevalence and risk factors. Movement disorders : official journal of the Movement Disorder Society 25:838-45

Dissanayaka NNW, Sellbach A, Silburn PA, O'Sullivan JD, Marsh R, Mellick GD (2011) Factors associated with depression in Parkinson's disease. Journal of affective disorders

Doty RL, Deems DA, Stellar S (1988) Olfactory dysfunction in parkinsonism: a general deficit unrelated to neurologic signs, disease stage, or disease duration. Neurology 38:1237-44

Dubois B, Slachevsky A, Pillon B, Beato R, Villalponda JM, Litvan I (2005) "Applause sign" helps to discriminate PSP from FTD and PD. Neurology 64:2132-3

Ebadi M, Srinivasan SK (1995) Pathogenesis, prevention, and treatment of neuroleptic-induced movement disorders. Pharmacological reviews 47:575-604

Eggers C, Kahraman D, Fink GR, Schmidt M, Timmermann L (2011) Akinetic-rigid and tremor-dominant Parkinson's disease patients show different patterns of FP-CIT Single photon emission computed tomography. Movement disorders : official journal of the Movement Disorder Society

Errea JM, Ara JR, Aibar C, Pedro-Cuesta J de (1999) Prevalence of Parkinson's disease in lower Aragon, Spain. Movement disorders : official journal of the Movement Disorder Society 14:596-604

Gallagher DA, Lees AJ, Schrag A (2010) What are the most important nonmotor symptoms in patients with Parkinson's disease and are we missing them? Movement disorders : official journal of the Movement Disorder Society 25:2493-500

Gelb DJ, Oliver E, Gilman S (1999) Diagnostic criteria for Parkinson disease. Archives of neurology 56:33-9

Gilman S, Low PA, Quinn N, Albanese A, Ben-Shlomo Y, Fowler CJ, Kaufmann H, Klockgether T, Lang AE, Lantos PL, Litvan I, Mathias CJ, Oliver E, Robertson D,

Schatz I, Wenning GK (1999) Consensus statement on the diagnosis of multiple system atrophy. Journal of the neurological sciences 163:94-8
Grimes DA, Lang AE, Bergeron CB (1999) Dementia as the most common presentation of cortical-basal ganglionic degeneration. Neurology 53:1969-74
Haaxma CA, Bloem BR, Overeem S, Borm GF, Horstink MWIM (2010) Timed motor tests can detect subtle motor dysfunction in early Parkinson's disease. Movement disorders : official journal of the Movement Disorder Society 25:1150-6
Hakim S, Adams RD (1965) The special clinical problem of symptomatic hydrocephalus with normal cerebrospinal fluid pressure. Observations on cerebrospinal fluid hydrodynamics. Journal of the neurological sciences 2:307-27
Hindle JV (2010) Ageing, neurodegeneration and Parkinson's disease. Age and ageing 39:156-61
Hossain AKMM, Murata Y, Zhang L, Taura S-ichi, Saitoh Y, Mizusawa H, Oda K, Matsushima E, Okubo Y, Shibuya H (2003) Brain perfusion SPECT in patients with corticobasal degeneration: analysis using statistical parametric mapping. Movement disorders: official journal of the Movement Disorder Society 18:697-703
Hughes AJ, Daniel SE, Blankson S, Lees AJ (1993) A clinicopathologic study of 100 cases of Parkinson's disease. Archives of neurology 50:140-8
Hughes AJ, Daniel SE, Kilford L, Lees AJ (1992) Accuracy of clinical diagnosis of idiopathic Parkinson's disease: a clinico-pathological study of 100 cases. J. Neurol. Neurosurg. Psychiatry 55:181-184
Hughes AJ, Daniel SE, Lees AJ (2001) Improved accuracy of clinical diagnosis of Lewy body Parkinson ' s disease. Neurology
Iacovelli E, Gilio F, Meco G, Fattapposta F, Vanacore N, Brusa L, Giacomelli E, Gabriele M, Rubino A, Locuratolo N, Iani C, Pichiorri F, Colosimo C, Carbone A, Palleschi G, Inghilleri M (2010) Bladder symptoms assessed with overactive bladder questionnaire in Parkinson's disease. Movement disorders : official journal of the Movement Disorder Society 25:1203-9
Jankovic J, Schwartz KS, Ondo W (1999) Re-emergent tremor of Parkinson's disease. Journal of neurology, neurosurgery, and psychiatry 67:646-50
Jellinger KA (2009) Formation and development of Lewy pathology: a critical update. Journal of neurology 256 Suppl:270-9
Jiménez-Jiménez FJ, Molina JA, Aguilar MV, Meseguer I, Mateos-Vega CJ, González-Muñoz MJ, Bustos F de, Martínez-Salio A, Ortí-Pareja M, Zurdo M, Martínez-Para MC (1998) Cerebrospinal fluid levels of transition metals in patients with Parkinson's disease. Journal of neural transmission (Vienna, Austria : 1996) 105:497-505
Jubault T, Brambati SM, Degroot C, Kullmann B, Strafella AP, Lafontaine A-L, Chouinard S, Monchi O (2009) Regional brain stem atrophy in idiopathic Parkinson's disease detected by anatomical MRI. PloS one 4:e8247
Jubault T, Gagnon J-F, Karama S, Ptito A, Lafontaine A-L, Evans AC, Monchi O (2011) Patterns of cortical thickness and surface area in early Parkinson's disease. NeuroImage 55:462-7
Kalra S, Grosset DG, Benamer HTS (2010) Differentiating vascular parkinsonism from idiopathic Parkinson's disease: a systematic review. Movement disorders : official journal of the Movement Disorder Society 25:149-56
Katzenschlager R, Lees AJ (2004) Olfaction and Parkinson's syndromes: its role in differential diagnosis. Current opinion in neurology 17:417-23
Kim YJ, Ichise M, Ballinger JR, Vines D, Erami SS, Tatschida T, Lang AE (2002) Combination of dopamine transporter and D2 receptor SPECT in the diagnostic evaluation of

PD, MSA, and PSP. Movement disorders : official journal of the Movement Disorder Society 17:303-12

Kranick SM, Duda JE (2008) Olfactory dysfunction in Parkinson's disease. Neuro-Signals 16:35-40

Kulisevsky J, Pagonabarraga J (2009) Cognitive impairment in Parkinson's disease: tools for diagnosis and assessment. Movement disorders : official journal of the Movement Disorder Society 24:1103-10

Kägi G, Bhatia KP, Tolosa E (2010) The role of DAT-SPECT in movement disorders. Journal of neurology, neurosurgery, and psychiatry 81:5-12

Lee EA, Cho HI, Kim SS, Lee WY (2004) Comparison of magnetic resonance imaging in subtypes of multiple system atrophy. Parkinsonism & related disorders 10:363-8

Litvan I, Agid Y, Calne D, Campbell G, Dubois B, Duvoisin RC, Goetz CG, Golbe LI, Grafman J, Growdon JH, Hallett M, Jankovic J, Quinn NP, Tolosa E, Zee DS (1996) Clinical research criteria for the diagnosis of progressive supranuclear palsy (Steele-Richardson-Olszewski syndrome): report of the NINDS-SPSP international workshop. Neurology 47:1-9

Loo S van de, Walter U, Behnke S, Hagenah J, Lorenz M, Sitzer M, Hilker R, Berg D (2010) Reproducibility and diagnostic accuracy of substantia nigra sonography for the diagnosis of Parkinson's disease. Journal of neurology, neurosurgery, and psychiatry 81:1087-92

Lunardi G, Galati S, Tropepi D, Moschella V, Brusa L, Pierantozzi M, Stefani A, Rossi S, Fornai F, Fedele E, Stanzione P, Hainsworth AH, Pisani A (2009) Correlation between changes in CSF dopamine turnover and development of dyskinesia in Parkinson's disease. Parkinsonism & related disorders 15:383-9

Madden MB, Hall DA (2010) Shoulder pain in Parkinson's disease: a case-control study. Movement disorders : official journal of the Movement Disorder Society 25:1105-6

Matsui H, Nishinaka K, Oda M, Komatsu K, Kubori T, Udaka F (2006) Does cardiac metaiodobenzylguanidine (MIBG) uptake in Parkinson's disease correlate with major autonomic symptoms? Parkinsonism & related disorders 12:284-8

McKeith IG et al. (2005) Diagnosis and management of dementia with Lewy bodies: third report of the DLB Consortium. Neurology 65:1863-72

McKeith IG et al. (1996) Consensus guidelines for the clinical and pathologic diagnosis of dementia with Lewy bodies (DLB): report of the consortium on DLB international workshop. Neurology 47:1113-24

Mollenhauer B, Locascio JJ, Schulz-Schaeffer W, Sixel-Döring F, Trenkwalder C, Schlossmacher MG (2011) α-Synuclein and tau concentrations in cerebrospinal fluid of patients presenting with parkinsonism: a cohort study. Lancet neurology 10:230-40

Morley JF, Duda JE (2010) Olfaction as a biomarker in Parkinson's disease. Biomarkers in medicine 4:661-70

Müller A, Müngersdorf M, Reichmann H, Strehle G, Hummel T (2002) Olfactory function in Parkinsonian syndromes. Journal of clinical neuroscience : official journal of the Neurosurgical Society of Australasia 9:521-4

Nath U, Ben-Shlomo Y, Thomson RG, Morris HR, Wood NW, Lees AJ, Burn DJ (2001) The prevalence of progressive supranuclear palsy (Steele-Richardson-Olszewski syndrome) in the UK. Brain : a journal of neurology 124:1438-49

Oba H, Yagishita A, Terada H, Barkovich AJ, Kutomi K, Yamauchi T, Furui S, Shimizu T, Uchigata M, Matsumura K, Sonoo M, Sakai M, Takada K, Harasawa A, Takeshita K, Kohtake H, Tanaka H, Suzuki S (2005) New and reliable MRI diagnosis for progressive supranuclear palsy. Neurology 64:2050-5

Osaki Y, Ben-Shlomo Y, Lees AJ, Daniel SE, Colosimo C, Wenning G, Quinn N (2004) Accuracy of clinical diagnosis of progressive supranuclear palsy. Movement disorders : official journal of the Movement Disorder Society 19:181-9

Pirker W, Asenbaum S, Bencsits G, Prayer D, Gerschlager W, Deecke L, Brücke T (2000) [123I]beta-CIT SPECT in multiple system atrophy, progressive supranuclear palsy, and corticobasal degeneration. Movement disorders : official journal of the Movement Disorder Society 15:1158-67

Politis M, Wu K, Molloy S, G Bain P, Chaudhuri KR, Piccini P (2010) Parkinson's disease symptoms: the patient's perspective. Movement disorders : official journal of the Movement Disorder Society 25:1646-51

Pålhagen S, Qi H, Mårtensson B, Wålinder J, Granérus A-K, Svenningsson P (2010) Monoamines, BDNF, IL-6 and corticosterone in CSF in patients with Parkinson's disease and major depression. Journal of neurology 257:524-32

Péran P, Cherubini A, Assogna F, Piras F, Quattrocchi C, Peppe A, Celsis P, Rascol O, Démonet J-F, Stefani A, Pierantozzi M, Pontieri FE, Caltagirone C, Spalletta G, Sabatini U (2010) Magnetic resonance imaging markers of Parkinson's disease nigrostriatal signature. Brain : a journal of neurology 133:3423-33

Quinn NP, Schneider SA, Schwingenschuh P, Bhatia KP (2010) Tremor-some controversial aspects. Movement disorders : official journal of the Movement Disorder Society

Raethjen J, Deuschl G (2009) Tremor. Current opinion in neurology 22:400-5

Reichmann H (2010) Clinical criteria for the diagnosis of Parkinson's disease. Neuro-degenerative diseases 7:284-90

Richardson JC, Steele J, Olszewski J (1963) SUPRANUCLEAR OPHTHALMOPLEGIA, PSEUDOBULBAR PALSY, NUCHAL DYSTONIA AND DEMENTIA. A CLINICAL REPORT ON EIGHT CASES OF "HETEROGENOUS SYSTEM DEGENERATION". Transactions of the American Neurological Association 88:25-9

Rinne JO, Lee MS, Thompson PD, Marsden CD (1994) Corticobasal degeneration. A clinical study of 36 cases. Brain : a journal of neurology 117 (Pt 5:1183-96

Savica R, Rocca WA, Ahlskog JE (2010) When does Parkinson disease start? Archives of neurology 67:798-801

Schrag A, Ben-Shlomo Y, Quinn NP (1999) Prevalence of progressive supranuclear palsy and multiple system atrophy: a cross-sectional study. Lancet 354:1771-5

Senard JM, Raï S, Lapeyre-Mestre M, Brefel C, Rascol O, Rascol A, Montastruc JL (1997) Prevalence of orthostatic hypotension in Parkinson's disease. Journal of neurology, neurosurgery, and psychiatry 63:584-9

Seppi K, Schocke MFH, Donnemiller E, Esterhammer R, Kremser C, Scherfler C, Diem A, Jaschke W, Wenning GK, Poewe W (2004) Comparison of diffusion-weighted imaging and [123I]IBZM-SPECT for the differentiation of patients with the Parkinson variant of multiple system atrophy from those with Parkinson's disease. Movement disorders : official journal of the Movement Disorder Society 19:1438-45

Shulman JM, De Jager PL, Feany MB (2010) Parkinson's Disease: Genetics and Pathogenesis. Annual review of pathology 6:193-222

Srulijes K, Mallien G, Bauer S, Dietzel E, Gröger A, Ebersbach G, Berg D, Maetzler W (2011) In vivo comparison of Richardson's syndrome and progressive supranuclear palsy-parkinsonism. Journal of neural transmission (Vienna, Austria : 1996)

Susatia F, Fernandez HH (2009) Drug-induced parkinsonism. Current treatment options in neurology 11:162-9

Tokuda T, Qureshi MM, Ardah MT, Varghese S, Shehab SAS, Kasai T, Ishigami N, Tamaoka A, Nakagawa M, El-Agnaf OMA (2010) Detection of elevated levels of {alpha}-

synuclein oligomers in CSF from patients with Parkinson disease. Neurology 75:1766-72

Tokuda T, Salem SA, Allsop D, Mizuno T, Nakagawa M, Qureshi MM, Locascio JJ, Schlossmacher MG, El-Agnaf OMA (2006) Decreased alpha-synuclein in cerebrospinal fluid of aged individuals and subjects with Parkinson's disease. Biochemical and biophysical research communications 349:162-6

Tolosa E, Wenning G, Poewe W (2006) The diagnosis of Parkinson's disease. Review Literature And Arts Of The Americas:75-86

Tu PH, Galvin JE, Baba M, Giasson B, Tomita T, Leight S, Nakajo S, Iwatsubo T, Trojanowski JQ, Lee VM (1998) Glial cytoplasmic inclusions in white matter oligodendrocytes of multiple system atrophy brains contain insoluble alpha-synuclein. Annals of neurology 44:415-22

Vaillancourt DE, Spraker MB, Prodoehl J, Abraham I, Corcos DM, Zhou XJ, Comella CL, Little DM (2009) High-resolution diffusion tensor imaging in the substantia nigra of de novo Parkinson disease. Neurology 72:1378-84

Walker RW, Hand A, Jones C, Wood BH, Gray WK (2010) The prevalence of Parkinson's disease in a rural area of North-East England. Parkinsonism & related disorders 16:572-5

Waragai M, Sekiyama K, Sekigawa A, Takamatsu Y, Fujita M, Hashimoto M (2010) α-Synuclein and DJ-1 as Potential Biological Fluid Biomarkers for Parkinson's Disease. International journal of molecular sciences 11:4257-66

Warmuth-Metz M, Naumann M, Csoti I, Solymosi L (2001) Measurement of the midbrain diameter on routine magnetic resonance imaging: a simple and accurate method of differentiating between Parkinson disease and progressive supranuclear palsy. Archives of neurology 58:1076-9

Wenning GK, Shephard B, Hawkes C, Petruckevitch A, Lees A, Quinn N (1995) Olfactory function in atypical parkinsonian syndromes. Acta neurologica Scandinavica 91:247-50

Wickremaratchi MM, Ben-Shlomo Y, Morris HR (2009) The effect of onset age on the clinical features of Parkinson's disease. European journal of neurology: the official journal of the European Federation of Neurological Societies 16:450-6

Wickremaratchi MM, Knipe MDW, Sastry BSD, Morgan E, Jones A, Salmon R, Weiser R, Moran M, Davies D, Ebenezer L, Raha S, Robertson NP, Butler CC, Ben-Shlomo Y, Morris HR (2011) The motor phenotype of Parkinson's disease in relation to age at Onset. Movement disorders: official journal of the Movement Disorder Society

Winogrodzka A, Bergmans P, Booij J, Royen EA van, Janssen AG, Wolters EC (2001) [123I]FP-CIT SPECT is a useful method to monitor the rate of dopaminergic degeneration in early-stage Parkinson's disease. Journal of neural transmission (Vienna, Austria : 1996) 108:1011-9

Wolfensberger M, Schnieper I (1999) [Sniffin'Sticks: a new system for olfactory assessment in routine clinical practice]. HNO 47:629-36

Wu LJC, Sitburana O, Davidson A, Jankovic J (2008) Applause sign in Parkinsonian disorders and Huntington's disease. Movement disorders : official journal of the Movement Disorder Society 23:2307-11

Wu Y, Le W, Jankovic J (2011) Preclinical biomarkers of Parkinson disease. Archives of neurology 68:22-30

Zhang L, Murata Y, Ishida R, Saitoh Y, Mizusawa H, Shibuya H (2001) Differentiating between progressive supranuclear palsy and corticobasal degeneration by brain perfusion SPET. Nuclear medicine communications 22:767-72

2

Impact of Dopamine Transporter Scan in Parkinson's Disease

Jörg Spiegel
Department of Neurology, Saarland University, Germany

1. Introduction

1.1 Technique of nigrostriatal FP-CIT SPECT

The density of the presynaptic dopamine reuptake transporters (DAT) can be quantified with [^{123}I]FP-CIT SPECT. The tracer Fluorpropyl-Carbomethoxy-Iodophenyl-Tropan (FP-CIT), marked by radioactive ^{123}iodine [^{123}I] (therefore the name [^{123}I]FP-CIT), binds reversibly to the DAT on the presynaptic membrane. Before application of FP-CIT, the iodine uptake of the thyroid gland is blocked with sodium perchlorate. Then the radioactive tracer [^{123}I]FP-CIT (110 - 185 MBq, specific activity: 580 - 1040 GBq/mg) is injected intravenously. 3 – 6 hours following the intravenous tracer injection, cerebral SPECT images are obtained by a gamma camera. At the moment, FP-CIT is the preferred tracer to visualize DAT due to its pharmacokinetic properties including fast (3 - 6 hours after intravenous injection) and highly affine binding (K_i = 3.1 nM) at DAT (4, 22). The exposure to radiation at the examination of an individual with a body weight of 70 kilograms amounts to 4.35 milli-Sievert (mSv). For comparison: the average effective exposure to natural background radiation in middle Europe at sea level runs up to 2.4 mSv.

Due to the similarity between dopamine reuptake transporters and serotonin reuptake transporters, serotonin reuptake inhibitors, widely used as antidepressants, must not be taken in the last two weeks before FP-CIT SPECT examination (fluoxetine for a period of six weeks). Furthermore therapy with selegiline should be discontinued to avoid interaction of its metabolites with FP-CIT at the dopamine transporter (19). Further anti-parkinsonian medication may be continued during SPECT examination, since present data (11, 16, 19, 21) do not show any effect of antiparkinsonian drugs on dopamine transporter binding.

Beyond FP-CIT-SPECT there exist further nuclear medicine methods to quantify the nigrostriatal presynaptic DAT density: [^{123}I]-beta-CIT SPECT (2beta-Carbomethoxy-Iodophenyl-Tropan; late SPECT after application of beta-CIT; [9, 15, 16]) and TRODAT SPECT (6, 23).

2. Evaluation of nigrostriatal FP-CIT SPECT

Registration and semiquantitative analysis are performed on a workstation. The caudate nucleus, putamen and occipital lobe binding of [^{123}I]FP-CIT is assessed semiquantitatively by a regions of interest (ROI) technique. The work station performs an automatic fitting of the studies to a model database. This fitting is controlled by an experienced nuclear medicine physician and if necessary manually adjusted. The special binding ratios of *caudate nucleus / occipital lobe* and *putamen / occipital lobe* are calculated. The quotients *[caudate nucleus binding / occipital lobe binding]* and *[putamen binding / occipital lobe binding]* for both sides are calculated. The occipital lobe serves as reference region. In healthy people these quotients amount to 3 up to 4.

FP-CIT SPECT has to be considered as pathological, if 1) absolute FP-CIT binding into putamen or caudate nucleus remains below a lower norm value or 2) side-to-side difference (right versus left or vice versa) exceeds an upper norm value. The norm values of the department of Nuclear Medicine of the Saarland University were obtained in healthy volunteers without any present or previous neurological or psychiatric disease (age 38 - 76 years, 59 ± 11 years, mean ± SD). In these volunteers the ratio *putamen / occipital lobe binding* was 3.44 ± 0.35 (resulting norm value = mean – 2 SD: ≥ 2.74) for the right putamen and 3.52 ± 0.36 (norm value ≥ 2.80) for the left putamen. The ratio *caudate nucleus / occipital lobe binding* was 3.67 ± 0.36 (norm value ≥ 2.95) for the right caudate nucleus and 3.67 ± 0.37 (norm value ≥ 2.93) for the left caudate nucleus. The norm value for the side-to-side difference (affected versus unaffected striatal area) is ≤ Δ0.15 (mean + 2 SD; [25]).

3. Clinical impact of FP-CIT SPECT

With reference to the definite post-mortem histopathological diagnosis of PD, the UK Brain Bank criteria (13) disclose a predictive value for PD of 90%. However, 10% of real PD patients ("real" means: with regard to the definite post-mortem histopathological diagnosis) 1) are not diagnosed as having PD or 2) make the differential diagnostic difficult even for experienced neurologists (13, 14). Therefore additional apparative measurements are necessary that support the clinical PD diagnosis. At the moment, the nuclear medicine measurement of DAT density, which is reduced in PD, represents one of the best apparative methods to clarify the PD diagnosis. Primarily the [^{123}I]FP-CIT SPECT represents an established method to quantify the nigrostriatal DAT density.

Motor symptoms of PD are based on a functional loss of the presynaptic dopaminergic nigrostriatal neuron. This functional loss correlates inversely with the DAT density on the membrane of the presynaptic neuron. Thus, a reduced nigrostriatal DAT density is typical for PD (Figures 1 and 2). FP-CIT SPECT correlates significantly with the extent of motor PD symptoms (2, 5, 25). At all PD stages presynaptic dopaminergic degeneration is more advanced in the putamen than that in the caudate nucleus (10, 25). The test-retest reliability of FP-CIT SPECT in PD patients is very high (26).

The prognostic validity of FP-CIT concerning the clinical progression of PD is unclear. Djaldetti et al. (8) applied FP-CIT SPECT in 19 patients with early PD and observed the following 12-15 months: striatal [123-I]FP-CIT uptake correlated significantly with the progression of motor symptoms (= difference [*motor symptom* at follow-up visit] – [*motor symptom* at baseline visit]) within these 12 – 15 months. These results suggest that a single SPECT may predict the disease severity over a period of 12 – 15 months. In contrast, another study (12) reported that the FP-CIT SPECT does not allow forecasting the progress of motor symptoms of PD over a longer time period of 3-7 years.

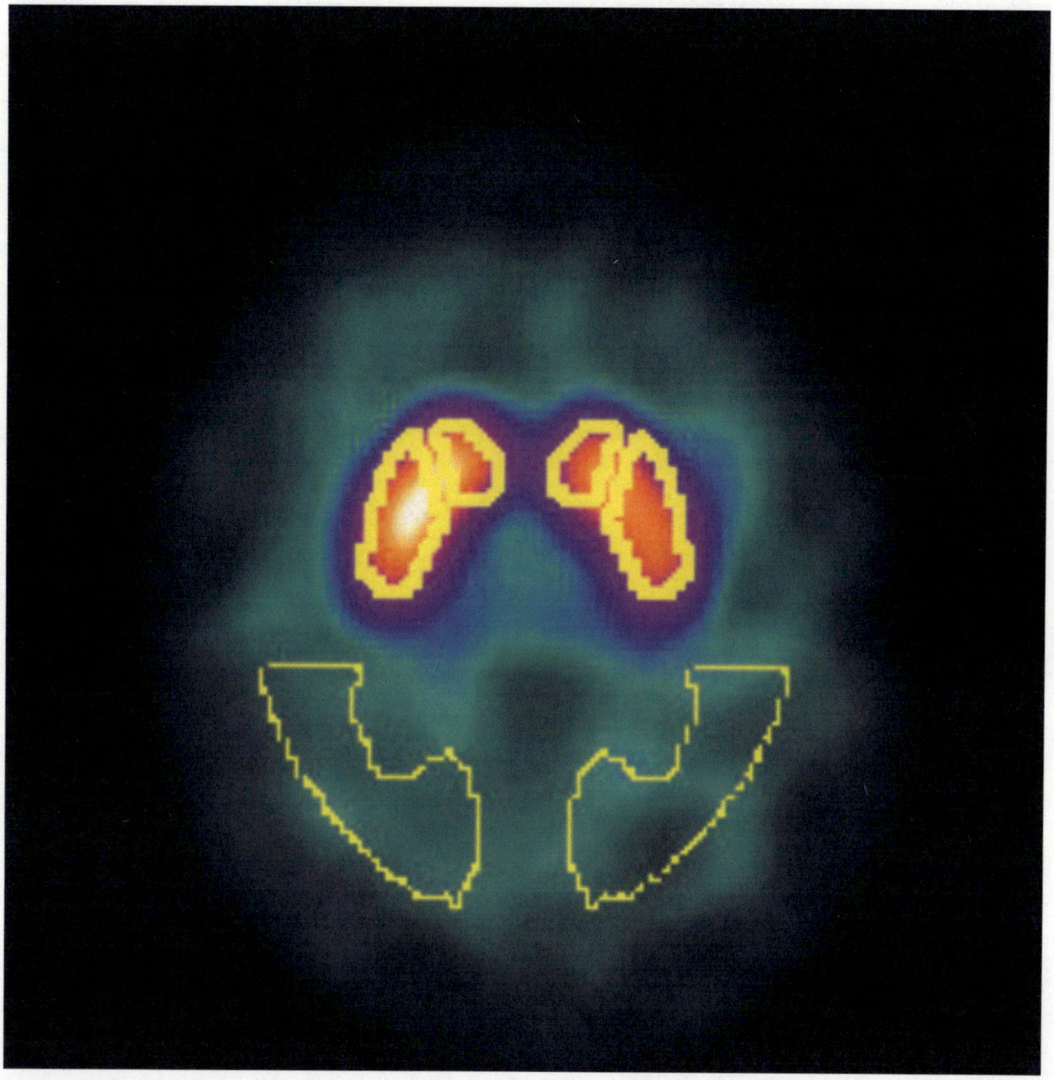

Fig. 1. FP-CIT SPECT in a patient with PD of the tremor dominant type. The striatal FP-CIT uptake is reduced bilaterally.

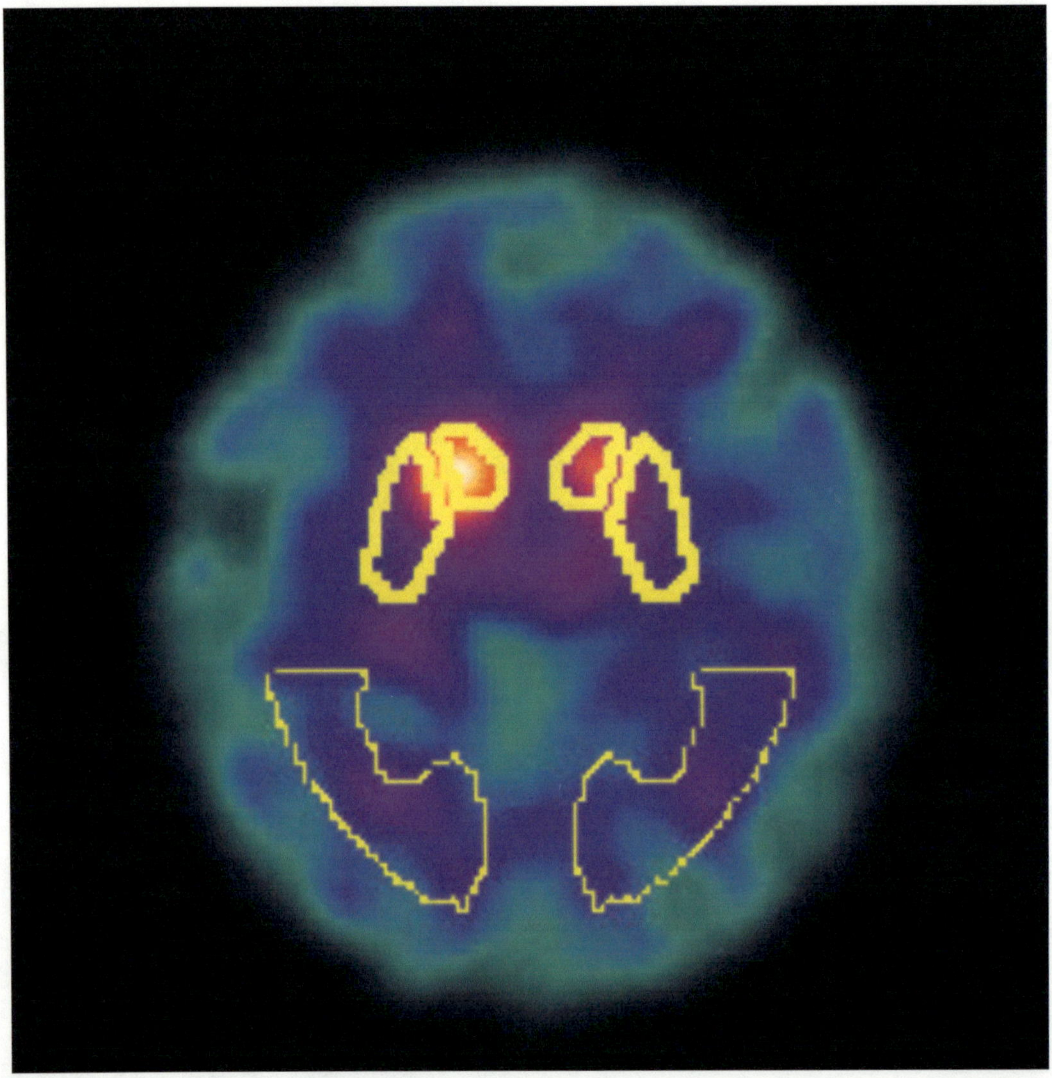

Fig. 2. FP-CIT SPECT in a patient with PD of the hypokinetic rigid type. The striatal FP-CIT uptake is bilaterally more reduced than in Figure 1.

4. Sensitivity, specificity and predictive value of FP-CIT SPECT

A multicenter study with 158 PD patients, 27 patients with essential tremor and 35 healthy volunteers reported a sensitivity of FP-CIT SPECT concerning PD of 95% (2, 3). Already in the earliest stage of PD, the sensitivity of the FP-CIT SPECT reaches between 95% and 100% (10, 18, 25) and amounts to nearly 100% in the more advanced stages of PD (24).

The differentiation between PD and essential tremor represents the main clinical indication for the FP-CIT SPECT. The specificity of FP-CIT SPECT concerning PD versus essential tremor is high (100%, [3]). In contrast to this, specificity of FP-CIT SPECT against atypical parkinsonian syndromes is very low. The term "atypical parkinsonian syndromes" (APS) denotes idiopathic neurodegenerative disorders, clinically characterized by a combination of an akinetic rigid symptoms with additional symptoms, which are different from those in PD. The group of APS includes the multiple system atrophy, the corticobasal degeneration and the progressive supranuclear palsy. In contrast to PD, which is induced by a presynaptic nigrostriatal dopaminergic degeneration, the APS are based on a postsynaptic nigrostriatal dopaminergic degeneration. This postsynaptic degeneration in the APS is followed by a secondarily reduced density of presynaptic DAT. Since the DAT density is secondarily impaired in the APS, the FP-CIT SPECT cannot sufficiently differentiate between APS and PD (1, 17, 20).

5. Scientific impact of FP-CIT SPECT

As explained above, FP-CIT SPECT measures the density of presynaptic dopamine reuptake transporters. This means that FP-CIT SPECT reflects exactly the underlying pathophysiology of PD. This allows further insights into the pathophysiological processes of PD. In the following we present some of these insights.

Recent studies found that the reduction of dopaminergic function - quantified by FP-CIT SPECT - correlates significantly with the extent of parkinsonian cardinal symptoms bradykinesia and rigidity but not with the extent of tremor in PD (2, 25). PD patients with tremor dominant type show a significantly higher striatal FP-CIT uptake than patients with akinetic rigid or equivalence type at the same stage of disease (Figure 1 and 2, [25]). These findings correlate with the clinical observation that bradykinesia and rigidity respond better to levodopa or dopamine agonists than tremor (7). The missing correlation between striatal FP-CIT uptake and tremor suggests, that further systems besides the nigrostriatal dopaminergic system may contribute to generation of parkinsonian tremor.

In addition, the FP-CIT SPECT may play an important role in the diagnosis of preclinical stage of PD (preclinical means: before first motor symptoms occur). Booij et al. (5) applied FP-CIT SPECT in 33 patients with suspected beginning Parkinsonism and performed a clinical follow-up of these patients 2-4 years after SPECT imaging. In nine of these 33 patients, SPECT was pathological; all these nine patients developed PD in the clinical follow-up. None of the 24 subjects without normal SPECT developed PD in the clinical follow-up. These data suggest a high positive predictive value of the FP-CIT SPECT. A study of Filippi et al. (10) involved 29 de-novo PD patients with one-sided clinical symptoms and 18 gender- and age-matched controls. In the PD patients, both ipsilateral and contralateral putamen and caudate nucleus showed a significantly reduced FP-CIT uptake. The pathological ipsilateral FP-CIT SPECT indicates that a pathological FP-CIT SPECT precedes clinical symptoms at the not affected body side.

6. References

Antonini A, Benti R, De Notaris R, Tesei S, Zecchinelli A, Sacilotto G, et al. 123I-Ioflupane/SPECT binding to striatal dopamine transporter (DAT) uptake in patients with Parkinson's disease, multiple system atrophy, and progressive supranuclear palsy. Neurol Sci 2003; 24: 149-150.

Benamer HT, Patterson J, Wyper DJ, Hadley DM, Macphee GJ, Grosset DG. Correlation of Parkinson's disease severity and duration with 123I-FP-CIT SPECT striatal uptake. Mov Disord 2000a; 15: 692-698.

Benamer TS, Patterson J, Grosset DG, Booij J, de Bruin K, van Royen E, et al. Accurate differentiation of parkinsonian and essential tremor using visual assessment of [123I]-FP-CIT-SPECT imaging: the [123I]-FP-CIT study group. Mov Disord 2000b; 15: 503-510.

Booij J, Sokole EB, Stabin MG, Janssen AGM, de Bruin K, van Royen EA. Human biodistribution and dosimetry of [^{123}I]FP-CIT: a potent radioligand for imaging of dopamine transporters. Eur J Nucl Med 1998; 25: 24-30.

Booij J, Speelman JD, Horstink MW, Wolters EC. The clinical benefit of imaging striatal dopamine transporters with [^{123}I]FP-CIT SPECT in differentiating patients with presynaptic Parkinson from those with other forms of parkinsonism. Eur J Nucl Med 2001; 28: 266-272.

Chou KL, Hurtig HI, Stern MB, Colcher A, Ravina B, Newberg A, Mozley PD, Siderowf A. Diagnostic accuracy of [99mTc]TRODAT-1 SPECT imaging in early Parkinson's disease. Parkinsonism Relat Disord 2004; 10: 375-379.

Deuschl G, Krack P. Morbus Parkinson, Bd. 2. In: Hopf HC, Deuschl G, Diener HC, Reichmann H: Neurologie in Praxis und Klinik, 3. Auflage 1999, Georg Thieme Verlag Stuttgart New York, pp. 49-69.

Djaldetti R, Treves TA, Ziv I, Melamed E, Lampl Y, Lorberboym M: Use of a single [(123)I]-FP-CIT SPECT to predict the severity of clinical symptoms of Parkinson disease. Neurol Sci 2009; 30:301-305.

Eerola J, Tienari PJ, Kaakkola S, Nikkinen P, Launes J. How useful is [123I]beta-CIT SPECT in clinical practice? J Neurol Neurosurg Psychiatry 2005; 76:1211-1216.

Filippi L, Manni C, Pierantozzi M, Brusa L, Danieli R, Stanzione P, Schillaci O. 123I-FP-CIT semi-quantitative SPECT detects preclinical bilateral dopaminergic deficit in early Parkinson's disease with unilateral symptoms. Nucl Med Commun 2005; 26: 421-426.

Guttman M, Stewart D, Hussey D, Wilson A, Houle S, Kish S. Influence of L-dopa and pramipexole on striatal dopamine transporter in early PD. Neurology 2001; 56: 1559-1564.

Hubbuch M, Farmakis G, Schaefer A, Behnke S, Schneider S, Hellwig D, Fassbender K, Kirsch CM, Dillmann U, Spiegel J. FP-CIT SPECT does not predict the progression of motor symptoms in Parkinson´s disease. Eur Neurol 2011; 65: 187-192.

Hughes A, Daniel SE, Kilford L, Lees AJ. Accuracy of clinical diagnosis of idiopathic Parkinson´s disease: a clinico-pathological study of 100 cases. J Neurol Neurosurg Psychiatry 1992a; 55: 181-184.

Hughes AJ, Ben-Shlomo Y, Daniel SE, Lees AJ. What features improve the accuracy of clinical diagnosis in Parkinson's disease: a clinicopathologic study. Neurology. 1992 Jun; 42(6):1142-6. Erratum in: Neurology 1992b; 42: 1142-1146.

Ichise M, Kim YJ, Ballinger JR, Vines D, Erami SS, Tanaka F, Lang AE (1999) SPECT imaging of pre- and postsynaptic dopaminergic alterations in L-dopa untreated Parkinson´s disease. Neurology 52: 1206-1214.

Innis RB, Marek KL, Sheff K, Zoghbi S, Castronuovo J, Feigin A, Seibyl JP. Effect of treatment with L-dopa/carbidopa or L-selegiline on striatal dopamine transporter SPECT imaging with [123I]beta-CIT. Mov Disord 1999; 14: 436-442.

Kim YJ, Ichise M, Ballinger JR, Vines D, Erami SS, Tatschita T, et al. Combination of dopamine transporter and D2 receptor SPECT in the diagnostic evaluation of PD, MSA und PSP. Mov Disord 2002; 17: 303-312.

Van Laere K, De Ceuninck L, Dom R, Van den Eynden J, Vanbilloen H, Cleynhens J, et al. Dopamine transporter SPECT using fast kinetic ligands: 123I-FP-beta-CIT versus 99mTc-TRODAT-1. Eur J Nucl Med Mol Imaging 2004; 31:1119-1127.

Laruelle M, Baldwin RM, Malison RT, Zea-Ponce Y, Zogbhi SS, Al-Tikriti MS, et al. SPECT imaging of dopamine and serotonin transporters with [123I]ß-CIT: pharmacological characterization of brain uptake in non-human primates. Synapse 1993; 13: 295-309.

Plotkin M, Amthauer H, Klaffke S, Kühn A, Lüdemann L, Arnold G, et al. Combined 123I-FP-CIT and 123I-IBZM SPECT for the diagnosis of parkinsonian syndromes: study on 72 patients. J Neural Transm 2005; 112: 677-692.

Schillaci O, Pierantozzi M, Filippi L, Manni C, Brusa L, Danieli R, et al. The effect of levodopa therapy on dopamine transporter SPECT imaging with(123)I-FP-CIT in patients with Parkinson's disease. Eur J Nucl Med Mol Imaging 2005; 32: 1452-1456.

Seibyl JP, Marek K, Sheff K, Zoghbi S, Baldwin RM, Charney DS, et al. Iodine-123-beta-CIT and iodine-123-FPCIT-SPECT measurement of dopamine transporters in healthy subjects and Parkinson´s patients. J Nucl Med 1998; 39: 1500-1508.

Siderowf A, Newberg A, Chou KL, Lloyd M, Colcher A, Hurtig HI, et al. [99mTc]TRODAT-1 SPECT imaging correlates with odor identification in early Parkinson disease. Neurology 2005; 64: 1716-1720.

Spiegel J, Möllers MO, Behnke S, Hellwig D, Jost WH, Samnick S, Dillmann U, Becker G, Kirsch CM: Transcranial sonography and [I-123]FP-CIT SPECT disclose complementary aspects of Parkinson's disease. Brain 2006; 129: 1188-1193.

Spiegel J, Hellwig D, Samnick S, Jost WH, Möllers MO, Fassbender K, Kirsch CM, Dillmann U. Striatal FP-CIT uptake differs in the subtypes of early Parkinson's disease. J Neural Transm. 2007; 114: 331-335.

Tsuchida T, Ballinger JR, Vines D, Kim YJ, Utsunomiya K, Lang AE, Ichise M. Reproducibility of dopamine transporter density measured with 123I-FPCIT SPECT in normal control and Parkinson's disease patients. Ann Nucl Med 2004; 18: 609-616.

3

CSF Biomarkers in Parkinson's Disease

Lucilla Parnetti[1]*, Anna Castrioto[1]* et al.,
[1]*Clinica Neurologica, Ospedale S. Maria della Misericordia, Università degli Studi di Perugia,*
[2]*Department of SEEA, University of Perugia, Italy*

1. Introduction

1.1 Do we need biological markers for Parkinson's disease?

In the recent years increasing attention on biomarkers for neurodegenerative diseases, including Parkinson's disease (PD), has been paid.

The reasons of this growing tendency are several:

(i) PD is one of the most common neurodegenerative diseases, affecting approximately 1% of people over 60 years of age (Samii et al., 2004). Diagnosis of PD is based on clinical criteria, relying on motor features: rigidity, bradykinesia, resting tremor and in the late stages postural instability (Hughes et al., 1992). However, clinical diagnosis especially in the early stages of disease can be challenging owing to the difficult differential diagnosis with essential tremor and atypical parkinsonism, namely multiple system atrophy (MSA), progressive sopranuclear palsy (PSP), and corticobasal degeneration (CBD). Although in movement disorder specialized settings the diagnostic accuracy is satisfactory (≥80%), almost one third of the clinical diagnoses in patients with parkinsonism is revised in the first five years of disease (Hughes et al., 2002). Diagnostic accuracy in the early stages of disease is important, in view of forthcoming disease-modifying therapies (Olanow et al., 2008). In this perspective, diagnostic biomarkers are urgently needed. (ii) Also, there is the need for progression biomarkers, ie, parameters reflecting a feature associated with disease- severity (Maetzler et al., 2009). (iii) Finally, PD per se is a heterogeneous disease, with different clinical phenotypes (the akinetic-rigid type vs. the tremor dominant variant) and different etiologies (genetic vs. sporadic form), which might have different progression rate, prognosis, thus requiring different therapeutic approaches. PD is not merely a motor disorder.

Recently, great attention has been drawn to non-motor symptoms, namely cognitive decline, behavioural changes, sleep disorders and autonomic dysfunction, due to their relevant impact on quality of life of parkinsonian patients (Chaudhuri et al., 2006). Both in early and in advanced stages, these symptoms represent a challenge in the clinical management of PD

---

* The Authors equally contributed to the preparation of this chapter.
Claudia De Carlo[1], Davide Chiasserini[1], Nicola Tambasco[1], Aroldo Rossi[1], Chiara Balducci[2], Tommaso Beccari[2] and Paolo Calabresi[1]

patients. Among non-motor features, i.e. hyposmia and R.E.M. sleep behavior disorders (RBD), cognitive decline dramatically changes the prognosis of disease. In this perspective, a biomarker distinguishing parkinsonian patients who will develop cognitive decline from those who will not, would have a great impact. Moreover, cognitive performances are impaired not only in PD but also in other parkinsonism, such as PSP or dementia with Lewy bodies (DLB), and again a biomarker differentiating these neurodegenerative diseases is required.

In order to develop a specific and successful treatment, the tendency to group together parkinsonism solely on a clinical ground should be replaced by the systematic use of reliable and validated biomarkers as the peripheral expression of the underlying pathogenetic mechanisms (Schlossmacher and Mollenhauer, 2010). In medicine biomarkers have different purposes: to identify subjects at risk of developing a certain disease (marker of trait); to identify the manifestation of disease (marker of state); to reflect the progression of disease (progression marker); to predict the onset of disease (marker of fate) (Schlossmacher and Mollenhauer, 2010). In this perspective, biomarkers are needed in order to reach an early and accurate PD diagnosis, also allowing a differential diagnosis between PD and other parkinsonism; to differentiate PD with dementia from Alzheimer's disease (AD), DLB and other dementias; to differentiate between variants of PD; to monitor disease progression and treatment response (Nyhlén et al., 2010).

An ideal biomarker should be sensitive, reproducible, closely associated to the disease process, easy to measure, inexpensive, non-invasive and thoroughly validated (Michell et al., 2004; van Dijk et al., 2010). Unfortunately such a marker is not available yet in PD.

Potential biomarkers in PD include imaging markers, such as striatal dopamine transporter binding measured with single photon emission computed tomography (Isaias and Antonini, 2010), transcranial ultrasound (Berg and Becker, 2002), or body fluid markers. Although many efforts have been made to detect reliable biomarkers in blood and urine, the most promising source of biomarkers is cerebrospinal fluid (CSF). The main advantage of CSF is its direct contact with brain so that it is thought that biochemical alterations in the brain are reflected in CSF. This is one of the reasons why CSF is the main source of biomarkers also in other neurodegenerative diseases, such as Alzheimer's disease, where it has become of support in early diagnosis (Dubois et al., 2007; Dubois et al., 2010).

This chapter will be dedicated to candidate CSF biomarkers in PD. However, some considerations should be taken in account while reviewing CSF studies in neurodegenerative disease and specifically in PD. CSF proteins pool is formed by a main part of blood-derived proteins and a minor part of brain tissue protein (Mollenhauer and Trenkwalder, 2009; van Dijk et al., 2010). Special attention should be driven on technical aspects in the collection of CSF, particularly to avoid blood contamination during lumbar puncture, which can enormously increase CSF content of protein owing to the high concentration of proteins in blood (Hong et al., 2010), and to limit circadian fluctuations of protein concentrations (Nilsson et al., 1992).

In this section we will consider α-synuclein, the main component of Lewy bodies; molecules expressing mitochondrial dysfunction and oxidative stress, such as DJ-1, and other oxidative stress related proteins; molecules reflecting impaired protein degradation, protein aggregation and LBs formation, such as protein tissue transglutaminase, osteopontine, and neurofilaments; molecules reflecting inflammation, glial activation, apoptosis and cell death. Also, classical CSF AD biomarkers - β-amyloid$_{1-42}$ (Aβ$_{1-42}$) , total tau, hyperphosphorylated tau – and their correlation with cognitive impairment in PD will be discussed.

2. Alpha-synuclein as disease-state marker

The neuropathological hallmarks of PD are the loss of pigmented neurons in the substantia nigra pars compacta (SNpc) and the Lewy bodies, LBs (Braak et al., 2003). LBs are intraneuronal spherical inclusions, which appear eosinophilic with a dense core surrounded by a halo at hematoxylin/eosin staining (Shults, 2006). LBs' main component is α-synuclein (α-syn), a 140-amino acids protein mainly located in the presynaptic terminals of most neurons. It is a member of a highly conserved family of proteins consisting of α-, β-, and γ-syn (Spillantini et al., 1997, Eriksen et al., 2003). Alpha-syn consists of: i) the N-terminal region, which contains a number of imperfect repeats, with the consensus motif KTKEGV; ii) the central hydrophobic region, called NAC (non-amyloid component), suggested to be responsible for the aggregation process (Giasson et al., 2001); and iii) the acidic C-terminal region involved in the regulation of fibril formation (Murray et al., 2003). Several studies suggest that α-syn exists in equilibrium between a cytosolic unfolded conformation and a membrane-bound, alpha-helical structure (Cole et al., 2002; McLean et al., 2000). Although its physiological function is still unknown, its localization and ability to interact with membranes suggest that α-syn might play a role in vesicle dynamics and trafficking at the presynaptic terminal and in brain lipid metabolism (Willingham et al. 2003; Darios et al., 2010).

Inclusions of α-syn are neuropathological features also in other neurodegenerative diseases that, together with PD, form the spectrum of synucleinopathies. They include multiple system atrophy (MSA), an oligodendrogliopathy, and DLB, the most frequent cause of degenerative dementia after AD (Spillantini & Goedert, 2000; Galvin et al., 2001). The discovery of missense mutations (Polymeropoulos et al., 1997; Kruger et al., 1998; Zarranz et al., 2004) and multiplications (duplications and triplications) (Chartier-Harlin et al., 2004; Singleton et al., 2003) within the gene encoding α-syn (*SNCA*) in familial case of PD has further increased the interest on this protein implicated in the etiopathogenesis of PD. More recently, *SNCA* polymorphisms have been associated with increased risk of sporadic PD and MSA, reinforcing the hypothesis of its implication in the etiopathogenesis of synucleinopathies (Simón-Sánchez et al., 2009; Satake et al., 2009; Scholz et al., 2009). Despite these evidences of a direct implication of α-syn in the pathogenesis of PD, the mechanisms through which this happens are not so clear. The lack of pathological phenotype associated to α-syn knock-out mice (Chandra et al., 2004) together with the observation of familial PD cases related to duplications/triplications of α-syn, as well as the presence of α-syn aggregates in PD brains, suggest for α–syn a gain-of-function pathogenetic mechanism. In line with this view, it has been shown that α-syn tends to aggregate into amyloid-like, beta-sheet fibrils (Bisaglia et al., 2009) and fibrillization is increased in the presence of mutations or elevated protein levels (Conway et al., 2001; Li et al., 2001; Shtilerman et al., 2002).

In PD and other synucleinopathies, α-syn in its monomeric form tends to aggregate into insoluble fibrils. Soluble oligomers and α-syn protofibrils, the intermediate stages in the development of these aggregates, are considered to be the toxic forms of α-syn (El-Agnaf et al., 2003a). Several factors such as phosphorylation at Ser129, decrease in pH, temperature increase, presence of metal ions and small charged molecules influence fibril formation and aggregation (Uverski 2007). Aggregation of α-syn can be promoted also by the protein tissue transglutaminase, which induces crosslinkings (Junn et al., 2003).

Alpha-syn degradation is mediated mainly through proteasomal system and autophagy pathway via lysosomes. Self-digestion of protein via lysosomes activity can occur in a chaperon-dependent or -independent way (Cuervo et al., 2004; Shin et al., 2005; Lee et al., 2005).

3. Is CSF alpha-syn a diagnostic marker of PD and other synucleynopathies?

Several studies have detected α-syn in human biological fluids, including plasma and CSF (El-Agnaf et al., 2003b; Lee et al., 2005; Mollenhauer et al., 2008; Mollenhauer et al., 2010). More recently attention has been focused on CSF α-syn as potential biomarker (see table 1).
The presence of α-syn in the CSF was first reported in 2000 using an immunoprecipitation and immunoblotting approach with the limit of low specificity (Borghi et al. 2000). In another study CSF collected at autopsy was analyzed, thus raising the concern of a possible increase of α-syn due to autolysis (El-Agnaf et al., 2003b). Finally the proof of the presence of α-syn in CSF was provided using affinity enrichment of CSF followed by mass spectrometry (Mollenhauer et al., 2008). In the last years, several studies on CSF α-syn as potential biomarker of synucleinopathy have been published, but the results have remained so far inconclusive, mainly owing to differences in sample handling and in measurement methods. The wide range of absolute concentration reported even in the same group of patients has been a hindrance to the interpretation of results (Mollenhauer et al., 2010). Another concern is the possible contamination of CSF sample with blood during lumbar puncture. Indeed, since levels of α-syn stored in human blood cells are much higher than in CSF, minimal contamination of CSF with blood may increase CSF α-syn concentration (Hong et al., 2010). Neither rostrocaudal gradient nor diurnal fluctuations of α-syn CSF concentrations have been found so far (Hong et al., 2010; Mollenhauer et al., 2010). Other possible confounders in CSF α-syn levels are age and total CSF protein content. These parameters have been only partially investigated. Some studies have shown some negative correlation of α-syn with age (Mollenhauer et al., 2008; Tokuda et al., 2006; Ohrfelt et al., 2009; Noguchi-Shinohara et al., 2009; Parnetti et al., 2011), whereas one study (Hong et al., 2010) reported an opposite trend. In some studies reduced levels of α-syn in CSF from PD and DLB have been detected compared to controls or AD (Tokuda et al., 2006; Mollenhauer et al., 2008; Tokuda et al., 2010; Kasuga et al., 2010; Hong et al., 2010; Parnetti et al., 2011). Conversely, in other studies no significant difference between groups was observed (Öhrfelt et al., 2009; Noguchi-Shinohara et al., 2009; Spies et al., 2009).
Recently we investigated CSF concentration of α-syn and classical CSF biomarkers - Aβ1-42, total tau, phosphorylated tau - in patients with PD (n. 38), DLB (n. 32), AD (n. 48), frontotemporal dementia (n. 31) and in age-matched controls (n. 32). Results show that α-syn are significantly lower in all pathological groups as compared to controls, whereas the total tau/α-syn and phosphorylated tau/α-syn ratios were significantly lower only in PD. Our study supports that α-syn alone has a low specificity for PD, but a better performance can be achieved with the ratio total tau/α-syn (Parnetti et al., 2011). This finding strengthens the need of measuring different biomarkers in order to better know the neurochemical profile of neurodegenerative diseases.
To shed further light into this complex scenario a large study including 721 patients has been recently published (Mollenhauer et al., 2011). In this study CSF α-syn and tau levels were measured in both synucleinopathies (PD, DLB, MSA) and tauopathies (AD, PSP). The study has been conducted in three cohorts of patients: a "training set" from the collaboration of three centres; a validation cohort; and an-autopsy-confirmed group of AD, DLB and controls (table 1). This work confirms that synucleinopathies are characterized by lower concentrations of CSF α-syn. However, since the specificity of α-syn alone is low, the combination of CSF α-syn and tau increases the discriminative power for differentiating PD

Study	Patients	Quantification methods	Capturing Ab (binding site)	Reading Ab (binding site)	CSF α -syn
Tokuda et al., 2006	33 PD, 38 controls	Direct sandwich ELISA	mAb 211 (aa 121-125)	pAb FL-140 (full length)	↓ in PD (correlation with age and with H&Y stage)
Mollenhauer et al., 2008	8 PD, 38 DLB, 13 AD, 8 CJD, 13 controls	Direct sandwich ELISA (384-well plates)	pAb mSA-1 (full length)	mAb Syn1 (aa 84-96)	↓ in PD and DLB, ↓ in CJD
Ohrfelt et al., 2009	15 DP, 15 DLB, 66 AD, 55 healthy controls	Indirect and amplified sandwich ELISA	mAb Syn1 (aa 84-96)	Syn 5d (aa 127-140)	↓ in AD (correlation with MMSE)
Noguchi-Shinohara et al., 2009	16 DLB, 21 AD	Direct sandwich ELISA	mAb 211 (aa 121-125)	pAb FL-140 (full length)	↓ in DLB (not significant)
Spies et al., 2009	40 DLB, 131 AD, 28 VaD, 39 FTD	Direct sandwich ELISA	mAb 211 (aa 121-125)	pAb FL-140 (full length)	no significant differences, tendencies to lower levels in DLB/AD. Similar profile thar tau
Hong et al., 2010	117 PD, 50 AD, 132 healthy controls	xMAP analysis	mAb LB 509 (aa 115-124)	mAb 211 (aa 121-125)	↓ in PD (no correlation with disease duration)
Kasuga et al., 2010	34 DLB, 31 AD, 21 other dementias, 2 SNCA duplication	Direct sandwich ELISA	mAb Syn1 (aa 84-96)	pAb FL-140 (full length)	↓ in DLB. ↓ in subjects with SNCA
Tokuda et al., 2010	32 PD, 18 control & 25 PD, 35 AD, 18 PSP, 43 controls	Direct sandwich ELISA (for α-syn oligomers ELISA 384-well plate)	mAb 211 (aa 121-125)	pAb FL-140 (full length)	↓ in PD. α-syn oligomers ↓ in PD (no correlations with age, disease duration or H&Y stage)
Parnettin et al., 2011	38 PD, 32 DLB, 48 AD, 31 FTD, 32 neurological controls	Direct sandwich ELISA	mAb 211 (aa 121-125)	pAb FL-140 (full length)	↓ in pathological group than i controls. total tau/ α-syn ratio significantly ↓ only in PD
Mollenhauer et al., 2011	721 pts from 3 cohorts: (a) 62 AD, 76 controls, 55 DLB, 51 PD, 29 AD; (b) 23 controls, 22 NPH, 8 PSP, 66 DLB, 273 PD, 15 MSA; (c) 21 AD, 7 controls, 13 DLB	Direct sandwich ELISA (384-well plates)	mAb Syn1-BB	pAb mSA-1 (full length)	↓ in PD, DLB, MSA. Combination of α-syn and taı provide the best discrimination of synucleinopathies from other groups.

Table 1. Overview of the studies published on CSF determination of total alpha-synuclein.

from the other neurodegenerative diseases. The major merits of the study by Mollenhauer and colleagues are the large sample size and the completeness of the range of synucleinopathies assessed, allowing us to be more confident of the interpretation of the results obtained by the measurement of total CSF α-synuclein. It also confirms the reliability of the assay, fixing the cutoff value at 1.6 pg/μL—ie, lower levels strongly suggest the presence of a synucleinopathy. This achievement is likely to be fundamental to the systematic use of α-synuclein as a biomarker in a clinical setting (Parnetti, 2011).

Another perspective, which highlights the direction toward a combination of biomarkers rather than toward a single marker, is the combination of CSF total α-syn and α-syn oligomers, with the latter found increased in PD in two recent papers (Paleologou et al., 2009; Tokuda et al., 2010). Whether α-syn is a marker of trait or a marker of progression is under investigation. According to the knowledge so far collected no clear-cut correlation with disease duration or disease severity (Hong et al., 2010; Parnetti et al., 2011) has been highlighted, suggesting that decrease of CSF α-syn is a marker of trait in synucleinopathies.

4. Other possible CSF biomarkers of PD: CSF proteins reflecting PD pathogenesis

Beyond α-syn, several other proteins and molecules have been investigated as potential biomarkers in PD. Most of them reflect PD pathogenesis and are classified upon different pathogenetic mechanisms.

4.1 Molecules expressing mitochondrial dysfunction and oxidative stress

The evidences for the implication of mitochondrial dysfunction and increased oxidative stress in the pathogenesis of PD are several (Schapira, 2008; Van Dijk et al., 2010): (i) mitochondrial complex I activity is reduced in the substantia nigra (Schapira et al., 1989); (ii) MPTP and rotenone toxicity is mediated via mitochondrial complex I inhibition (Tipton & Singer, 1993; Betarbet et al., 2003); (iii) mitochondrial-related proteins, such as prohibitin, ATP synthase and superoxide dismutase (SOD2), are altered in the nigra and frontal cortex of PD patients (Ferrer et al., 2007); and (iv) some monogenic forms of PD are caused by mutations of DJ-1 (Bonifati et al., 2003), PINK-1 (Valente et al., 2004), LRRK2 (Paisán-Ruíz et al., 2004; Zimprich et al., 2004), all implicated in the mitochondrial function and oxidative stress (Lin & Beal, 2006).

Thus, attention has been focused on markers linked to the mitochondrial dysfunction and oxidative stress.

4.1.2 DJ-1

CSF DJ-1 levels have been investigated in two studies, yielding opposite results (Waragai et al., 2006; Hong et al., 2010). Waragai et al. (2006) found increased CSF DJ-1 levels (assessed by means of western blotting) in PD-patients (n. 40) as compared to controls (n. 38). More recently, in a larger study involving PD (n. 117), controls (n. 132) and AD (n. 50), using a multiplex technology, CSF DJ-1 concentrations were found to be decreased in the PD group (Hong et al., 2010). Similarly for what found for α-syn, DJ-1 levels were influenced by blood contamination. Also CSF levels were correlated with age and not with disease severity (Hong et al., 2010). Divergent results in the two studies might be mostly due to different methods.

4.1.3 Other oxidative stress related proteins

Other oxidative stress related proteins have been investigated in the CSF of PD patients, with the limits of single observations, small sample size, inconclusive results and lack of disease specificity.

Increased CSF concentration of nitrated manganese superoxide dismutase (Mn-SOD) in PD, AD and amyotrophic lateral sclerosis (ALS) have been reported (Aoyama et al., 2000). Another study investigating oxidative stress in PD, AD, ALS and Huntington's disease (HD) found decreased Cu/Zn-dependent superoxide dismutase (SOD1) activity in all these diseases (Boll et al., 2008); also, an increase of modified forms of Cu/Zn-dependent SOD has been published (Guo et al., 2009). Other studies found reduced CSF concentration of ceruloplasmin and ferroxidase activity, the enzyme that catalyzes the conversion of Fe^{2+} in Fe^{3} (Boll et al., 1999; Boll et al., 2008; Abdi et al. 2006), whereas CSF transferrin levels where unchanged in PD (Loeffler et al., 1994; van Kamp et al., 1995).

4.2 Impaired protein degradation

Impaired protein degradation, leading to aggregation of misfolded, mutant and toxic variant of proteins, plays a key role in the pathogenesis of PD and neurodegenerative diseases. Two main systems are implicated in protein degradation, namely the lysosomal and the ubiquitin-proteasome systems. Autophagy is a crucial pathway for the degradation of α-syn (Cuervo et al., 2004; Shin et al., 2005; Lee et al., 2005). In recent years a strong link between mutations in glucocerebrosidase gene (GBA), the gene implicated in Gaucher disease (GD), and PD has been discovered supporting the link between lysosomal system and pathogenesis of PD (DePaolo et al., 2009; Velayaty et al., 2010). GD is an autosomal recessive lipidosis resulting from a deficiency of glucocerebrosidase enzyme. The observation of patients with GD and parkinsonism (Tayebi et al., 2003, Goker-Alpan et al., 2008), the increased rate of GBA mutations and polymorphism in PD patients (Sidransky et al., 2009) along with neuropathological findings in brain of GD patients with parkinsonism similar to PD and DLB, all strengthening this hypothesis. The deficit in GBA might act through an impaired degradation of proteins via lysosomes leading to abnormal protein aggregates and Lewy bodies formation. Moving from these observations, in the last years we studied the activities of CSF beta-glucocerebrosidase and others lysosomal enzymes, finding that alpha-mannosidase, beta-mannosidase, and more evidently glucorebrosidase, were significantly reduced in PD (Balducci et al., 2007) and, even more markedly, in DLB patients (Parnetti et al., 2009).

4.3 Protein aggregation and Lewy body formation

One of the neuropathological hallmarks of PD is inclusions of misfolded, mutant, and damaged proteins and the formation of Lewy bodies (LBs) and Lewy neurites (LN) (Shults, 2006). The main component of LBs is α-synuclein (α-syn). As described previously, α-syn tends to aggregate into toxic oligomers and α-syn protofibrils, the intermediate stages of insoluble fibrils (El-Agnaf et al., 2003a). The aggregation of α-syn is modulated by several factors and promoted by the protein tissue transglutaminase, a regulator of apoptosis that appears to modulate α-syn oligomerization promoting crosslinkings. A study investigating CSF tissue transglutaminase levels in 54 PD-patients and in 34 controls found increased levels only in PD (Vermes et al., 2004).

Several other proteins are present in Lewy bodies, such as osteopontin and neurofilaments.

Osteopontin is a protein involved in apoptosis and oxidative stress, identified in several neurodegenerative diseases, including AD (Simonsen et al., 2007) and shown to be increased in CSF of PD patients as compared to controls (Maetzler et al., 2007).

Neurofilaments are component of the cytoskeleton. In PD both light and heavy chain neurofilaments have been shown to be unchanged compared to controls, whereas they have been found to be elevated in other parkisonism, including MSA and progressive sopranuclear palsy (PSP) (Abdo et al., 2007; Holmberg et al., 1998). These observations have suggested that neurofilaments might be a promising marker in the differential diagnosis of parkinsonism.

4.4 Inflammation and glial activation

Among the several molecular and cellular changes leading to cellular death in PD, neuroinflammatory mechanisms seem to play an important contribution (Hirsch & Hunot, 2009). Post-mortem studies have shown microglial activation, astrogliosis, and lymphocytic infiltration in the nigra of PD patients (Mc Geer et al., 1988; Damier et al., 1993). Increased concentrations of TNF-α, β2-microglobulin, epidermal growth factor (EGF), transforming growth factor α (TGF-α), TGF-β1, and interleukins 1β, 6 and 2 have been detected in the striatum of PD (Mogi et al., 1994a; Mogi et al., 1994b; Mogi et al., 1995a; Mogi et al., 1995b; Mogi et al., 1996a). Some CSF studies have tried to investigate the involvement of inflammatory mechanisms in PD. Increased levels of interleukins, including interleukin 1β, interleukin-8 and 6, and decreased levels of components of complement have been detected in CSF of PD patients (Mogi et al., 1995a; Blum-Degen et al., 1995; Muller et al., 1998; Finehout et a., 2005; Guo et al., 2009). However, it is still unclear whether these changes are the cause or the consequence of neuronal degeneration (Hirsch & Hunot, 2009). Moreover, these changes are not disease specific, being shared by many neurodegenerative diseases. A recent study, carried out in a large cohort including PD (n. 126), MSA (n. 32), AD (n. 50), and controls (n. 137), showed significantly lower CSF levels of the cytokine Flt3 ligand in MSA patients as compared to PD subjects (Shi et al., 2011).

4.5 Apoptosis and cell death

Apoptosis is an important mechanism of cell death in neurodegenerative diseases, including PD, as supported by a neuropathological study showing apoptotic process in 8 out of 11 midbrains from PD patients (Mochizuki et al., 1996). Moreover, the anti-apoptotic protein bcl-2, the apoptosis-signaling receptor Fas, and the Annexin V have been found to be increased in the substantia nigra of PD (Mogi et al. 1996b; Mogi et al., 1996c; Werner et al., 2008). A CSF study showed lower levels of Annexin V in PD as compared to controls. This result was interpreted as the consequence of the consumption of this protein during neuronal apoptosis in PD (Vermes et al., 1999). CSF study targeting bcl2 and Fas have failed, since neither bcl2 nor Fas are measurable in CSF (Mogi et al. 1996b; Mogi et al. 1996c).

5. Classical CSF biomarkers and risk of cognitive impairment in PD

The prevalence of cognitive impairment in PD-patients is higher compared to general population (30%) even in early PD (Aarsland et al., 2009; Aarsland & Kurz 2010), and the risk of dementia dramatically increases over the course of disease occurring in up to 80% of patients after 20 years of follow-up (Hely et al., 2008). Cognitive impairment and dementia represent one of the most disabling non-motor symptoms in PD, with a relevant impact on quality of life of patients and caregivers. The spreading of Lewy body pathology to neocortical regions altogether with AD-type pathology in terms of β-amyloid deposits, have been implicated in the pathogenesis of cognitive decline in PD (Braak et al., 2005; Ballard et al., 2006), suggesting an interplay between synucleinopathies and tauopathies. Recently, a growing amount of investigations in PD has focused on CSF biomarkers traditionally used in AD, namely β-amyloid$_{1-42}$ (Aβ $_{1-42}$), total tau, hyperphosphorylated tau, in order to improve the ability to detect risk for cognitive impairment and dementia (Sjögren et al., 2002; Mollenhauer et al., 2006; Parnetti et al., 2008; Compta et al., 2009; Alves et al., 2010; Siderowf et al., 2010; Montine et al., 2010; Leverenz et al., 2011) (table 2). Tau protein, a microtubule associated protein, in its phosphorylated form represents the major component of the neurofibrillary tangles (Grundke-Iqbal et al., 1986). Increased CSF levels of tau and phosphorylated tau have been found to be specific markers for AD (Blennow et al., 1995). The different enzymatic cleavage of the 120kDa transmembrane amyloid precursor protein (APP) by three different secretases produces different β-amyloid peptides (Glenner et al., 1984). Beta-amyloid$_{1-42}$ peptide (Aβ $_{1-42}$), the main component of amyloid plaques in the brain of patients with AD and DLB, has been shown to be decreased in the CSF of AD patients for the first time in 1995 (Motter et al, 1995). These findings have lead to a revision of the National Institute of Neurological Disorders and Stroke-Alzheimer Disease and Related Disorders (NINCDS-ADRDA) criteria for the diagnosis of AD including CSF biomarkers (Dubois et al., 2007). Studies report normal CSF levels of tau and phosphorylated tau in PD (Blennow et al., 1995; Parnetti et al., 2008; Alves et al., 2010; Shi et al., 2010), whereas unchanged or slightly decreased levels of Aβ $_{1-42}$ have been reported (Sjögren et al., 2002; Mollenhauer et al., 2006; Bibl et al., 2006; Parnetti et al., 2008; Compta et al., 2009; Alves et al., 2010; Siderowf et al., 2010; Montine et al., 2010; Leverenz et al., 2011; Shi et al., 2011). More recently, several studies have been published reporting a possible association between low Aβ $_{1-42}$ levels and cognitive impairment in PD (Compta et al., 2009; Alves et al., 2010; Siderowf et al., 2010; Montine et al., 2010; Leverenz et al., 2011). Lower levels of CSF Aβ $_{1-42}$ were found in 20 PD-patients with dementia compared to 20 PD-patients and 30 controls, whereas higher concentrations of CSF tau and phosphorylated tau were associated with impaired memory and naming, suggesting an underlying AD pathology in PDD (Compta et al., 2009). A recent study compared CSF concentrations of Aβ$_{1-42}$, Aβ$_{1-40}$, Aβ $_{1-38}$, total tau and phosphorylated tau in a large cohort of de novo and untreated PD-patients (n. 109), recruited from the Norwegian ParkWest study, with those of 36 age-matched controls and 20 mild AD patients (Alves et al., 2010). In PD patients reduced levels of Aβ $_{1-42}$, Aβ $_{1-40}$, Aβ $_{1-38}$ compared to controls were found. Authors showed also a significant association between CSF levels of Aβ $_{1-42}$, Aβ $_{1-40}$, Aβ $_{1-38}$ and memory impairment. A recent prospective study in a cohort of 45 PD patients with 1-year follow-up showed that lower levels of Aβ $_{1-42}$ at baseline were associated with a more rapid cognitive decline (Siderowf et al., 2010). Another recent study reported an association between low levels of Aβ $_{1-42}$ levels in 22 non-demented PD patients and worse performance at Digit Symbol test (Leverenz et al., 2011). Although the limitations of these studies, including the small sample size, the heterogeneity of clinical features of patients, the lack of a group of control, the results are interesting and support the role of amyloid plaques in the pathogenesis of dementia in PD patients, in line with a recent report of altered in vivo amyloid imaging in 2 autopsy-confirmed PDD patients (Burack et al., 2010).

Study	Patients	CSF Aβ42	CSF T-tau	CSF P-tau	Relationship with cognitive impairment
Parnetti et al., 2008	20 PD, 18 PDD, 19DLB, 20 controls	CTRL>PD> PDD>DLB	CTRL=PD DLB>PDD> PD	CTRL=PD, PDD,DLB	↓ Aβ42 associated with ↓ performance at Word Fluency and Prose Memory tests
Compta et al., 2009	20 PD, 20 PDD, 30 controls	CTRL>PD> PDD	CTRL=PD PDD>PD	CTRL=PD PDD>PD	↓ Aβ42 in patients with ↓ performance at Verbal Fluency test
Siderowf et al., 2010	45 PD, no controls	= = =	= = =	= = =	↓ baseline Aβ42 associated with faster cognitive decline (↓Aβ42 independent predictor of cognitive decline)
Alves et al., 2010	109 de novo PD, 36 controls	PD<CTRL	CTRL=PD	CTRL=PD	↓ Aβ42 associated with poorer performances on memory tests
Leverenz et al., 2011	22 PD, no controls	= = =	= = =	Not measured	Association between ↓Aβ42 and/or Aβ42/T-tau and ↓ performance at Digit Symbol and Category Fluency tests

Table 2. CSF Aβ42 and cognitive impairment in PD.

6. Conclusions and perspectives

Neurodegenerative diseases, including PD, are common and become more common with increasing age. At present, diagnosis substantially relies on clinical criteria, which makes it difficult to achieve an accurate early diagnosis. Moreover, it is not rare that in an elderly patient two or more neurodegenerative diseases, as well as cerebrovascular changes, coexist (Nyhlen et al., 2010). It is also possible that conceptually distinct disease processes may reinforce or modify each other. For example, α-syn aggregation may promote Ab aggregation and *vice versa;* also, tau has been shown to interact with α-syn, promoting its fibrillization. It can be claimed that PD- and AD-like changes often occur simultaneously, contribute to the clinical symptoms and make it difficult to identify the underlying pathology based only on clinical phenotype changes. In this context, the systematic assessment of CSF biomarkers may be of help, also suggesting the possibility to adopt a different nomenclature for identifying distinct disease-associated processes rather than the single disease.

In view of available disease-modifying drugs able to directly interfere with the etiopathogenetic events – ie, anti-amyloid agents; inhibitors of tau or α-syn phosphorylation, etc. - early diagnosis is mandatory for all neurodegenerative diseases. This concept is even more important when considering clinically heterogeneous disorders as PD is. At present, we have promising candidate biomarkers, which also guarantee to reliably exclude other diagnoses than PD.

7. References

Aarsland, D., Brønnick, K., Larsen, J.P., Tysnes, O.B., Alves, G.; Norwegian ParkWest Study Group. (2009). Cognitive impairment in incident, untreated Parkinson disease: the Norwegian ParkWest study. *Neurology* 72:1121-1126.

Aarsland, D. & Kurz, M.W. (2010). The epidemiology of dementia associated with Parkinson disease. *J Neurol Sci* 289:18-22.

Abdi, F., Quinn, J.F., Jankovic, J., McIntosh, M., Leverenz, J.B., Peskind, E., Nixon, R., Nutt, J., Chung, K., Zabetian, C., Samii, A., Lin, M., Hattan, S., Pan, C., Wang, Y., Jin, J., Zhu, D., Li, G.J., Liu, Y., Waichunas, D., Montine, T.J., Zhang, J. (2006). Detection of biomarkers with a multiplex quantitative proteomic platform in cerebrospinal fluid of patients with neurodegenerative disorders. *J Alzheimers Dis* 9:293-348.

Abdo, W.F., Bloem, B.R., Van Geel, W.J., Esselink, R.A., Verbeek, M.M. (2007) CSF neurofilament light chain and tau differentiate multiple system atrophy from Parkinson's disease. *Neurobiol Aging* 28:742-747.

Alves, G., Brønnick, K., Aarsland, D., Blennow, K., Zetterberg, H., Ballard, C., Kurz, M.W., Andreasson, U., Tysnes, O.B., Larsen, J.P., Mulugeta, E. CSF amyloid-beta and tau proteins, and cognitive performance, in early and untreated Parkinson's disease: the Norwegian ParkWest study. (2010). *J Neurol Neurosurg Psychiatry* 81:1080-1086.

Aoyama, K., Matsubara, K., Fujikawa, Y., Nagahiro, Y., Shimizu, K., Umegae, N., Hayase, N., Shiono, H., Kobayashi, S.Nitration of manganese superoxide dismutase in cerebrospinal fluids is a marker for peroxynitrite-mediated oxidative stress in neurodegenerative diseases. *Ann Neurol* 47:524-527.

Balducci, C., Pierguidi, L., Persichetti, E., Parnetti, L., Sbaragli, M., Tassi, C., Orlacchio, A., Calabresi, P., Beccari, T., Rossi, A. (2007). Lysosomal hydrolases in cerebrospinal fluid from subjects with Parkinson's disease. *Mov Disord* 22:1481-1484.

Ballard, C., Ziabreva, I., Perry, R., Larsen, J.P., O'Brien, J., McKeith, I., Perry, E., Aarsland, D. (2006). Differences in neuropathologic characteristics across the Lewy body dementia spectrum. *Neurology* 67:1931-1934.

Berg, D., Becker, G. (2002). Perspectives of B-mode transcranial ultrasound. *Neuroimage* 15: 463-473.

Betarbet, R., Sherer, T.B., MacKenzie, G., Garcia-Osuna, M., Panov, A.V., Greenamyre, J.T. (2000). Chronic systemic pesticide exposure reproduces features of Parkinson's disease. *Nat Neurosci* 3:1301-1306.

Bibl, M., Mollenhauer, B., Esselmann, H., Lewczuk, P., Klafki, H.W., Sparbier, K., Smirnov, A., Cepek, L., Trenkwalder, C., Rüther, E., Kornhuber, J., Otto, M., Wiltfang, J. (2006). CSF amyloid-beta-peptides in Alzheimer's disease, dementia with Lewy bodies and Parkinson's disease dementia. *Brain* 129:1177-1187.

Bisaglia, M., Mammi, S., Bubacco, L. (2009). Structural insights on physiological functions and pathological effects of alpha-synuclein. *Faseb J* 23:329–340.

Blennow, K., Wallin, A., Agren, H., Spenger, C., Siegfried, J., Vanmechelen, E. (1995) Tau protein in cerebrospinal fluid: a biochemical marker for axonal degeneration in Alzheimer disease? *Mol Chem Neuropathol* 26:231-245.

Blum-Degen, D., Muller, T., Kuhn, W., Gerlach, M., Przuntek, H., Riederer, P. (1995). Interleukin-1 beta and interleukin-6 are elevated in the cerebrospinal fluid of Alzheimer's and de novo Parkinson's disease patients. *Neurosci Lett* 202: 17–20.

Boll, M.C., Sotelo, J., Otero, E., Alcaraz-Zubeldia, M., Rios, C. (1999). Reduced ferroxidase activity in the cerebrospinal fluid from patients with Parkinson's disease. *Neurosci Lett* 265:155-158.

Boll, M.C., Alcaraz-Zubeldia, M., Montes, S., Rios, C. (2008) Free copper, ferroxidase and SOD1 activities, lipid peroxidation and NO(x) content in the CSF. A different marker profile in four neurodegenerative diseases. *Neurochem Res* 33:1717-1723.

Bonifati, V., Rizzu, P., van Baren, M.J., Schaap, O., Breedveld, G.J., Krieger, E., Dekker, M.C., Squitieri, F., Ibanez, P., Joosse, M., van Dongen, J.W., Vanacore, N., van Swieten, J.C., Brice, A., Meco, G., van Duijn, C.M., Oostra, B.A., Heutink, P. (2003). Mutations in the DJ-1 gene associated with autosomal recessive early-onset parkinsonism. *Science* 299:256-269.

Borghi, R., Marchese, R., Negro, A., Marinelli, L., Forloni, G., Zaccheo, D., Abbruzzese, G., Tabaton, M. (2000). Full length alpha-synuclein is present in cerebrospinal fluid from Parkinson's disease and normal subjects. *Neurosci Lett* 287:65-67.

Braak, H., Del Tredici, K., Rub, U., de Vos, R.A., Jansen Steur, E.N., Braak, E. (2003). Staging brain pathology related to sporadic Parkinson's disease. *Neurobiol Aging* 24:197-211.

Braak, H., Rüb, U., Jansen Steur, E.N., Del Tredici, K., de Vos, R.A. (2005). Cognitive status correlates with neuropathologic stage in Parkinson disease. *Neurology* 64:1404-1410.

Burack, M.A., Hartlein, J., Flores, H.P., Taylor-Reinwald, L., Perlmutter, J.S., Cairns, N.J. (2010). In vivo amyloid imaging in autopsy-confirmed Parkinson disease with dementia. *Neurology* 74:77-84.

Chandra, S., Fornai, F., Kwon, H.B., Yazdani, U., Atasoy, D., Liu, X., Hammer, R.E., Battaglia, G., German, D.C., Castillo, P.E., Südhof, T.C. (2004). Double-knockout mice for alpha- and beta-synucleins: effect on synaptic functions. *Proc Natl Acad Sci USA* 101:14966–14971.

Chartier-Harlin, M.C., Kachergus, J., Roumier, C., Mouroux, V., Douay, X., Lincoln, S., Levecque, C., Larvor, L., Andrieux, J., Hulihan, M., Waucquier, N., Defebvre, L., Amouyel, P., Farrer, M., Destée, A. (2004) Alpha-synuclein locus duplication as a cause of familial Parkinson's disease. *Lancet* 364:1167-1169.

Chaudhuri, K.R., Healy, D.G., Schapira, A.H.V. (2006). Non-motor symptoms of Parkinson's disease: diagnosis and management. *Lancet Neurol* 5:235-245.

Cole, N.B., Murphy, D.D., Grider, T., Rueter, S., Brasaemle, D., Nussbaum, R.L. (2002). Lipid droplet binding and oligomerization properties of the Parkinson's disease protein alpha-synuclein. *J Biol Chem* 277:6344–6352

Compta, Y., Martí, M.J., Ibarretxe-Bilbao, N., Junqué, C., Valldeoriola, F., Muñoz, E., Ezquerra, M., Ríos, J., Tolosa, E. (2009). Cerebrospinal tau, phospho-tau, and beta-amyloid and neuropsychological functions in Parkinson's disease. *Mov Disord* 24:2203-2210.

Conway, K.A., Harper, J.D., Lansbury, P.T. (1998). Accelerated in vitro fibril formation by a mutant alpha-synuclein linked to early-onset Parkinson disease. *Nat Med* 4:1318–1320.

Cuervo, A.M., Stefanis, L., Fredenburg, R., Lansbury, P.T., Sulzer, D. (2004). Impaired degradation off mutant alpha-synuclein by chaperone-mediated autophagy. *Science* 305:1292-1295.

Damier, P., Hirsch, E.C., Zhang, P., Agid, Y., Javoy-Agid, F. (1993). Glutathione peroxidase, glial cells and Parkinson's disease. *Neuroscience* 52: 1–6.

Darios, F., Ruiperez, V., Lopez, I., Villanueva, J., Gutierrez, L.M., Davletov, B. (2010). Alpha-synuclein sequesters arachidonic acid to modulate SNARE-mediated exocytosis. *EMBO Rep* 11:528–533.

DePaolo, J., Goker-Alpan, O., Samaddar, T., Lopez, G., Sidransky, E. (2009). The association between mutations in the lysosomal protein glucocerebrosidase and parkinsonism. *Mov Disord* 24:1571-1578.

Dubois, B., Feldman, H.H., Jacova, C., Dekosky, S.T., Barberger-Gateau, P., Cummings, J., Delacourte, A., Galasko, D., Gauthier, S., Jicha, G., Meguro, K., O'brien, J., Pasquier, F., Robert, P., Rossor, M., Salloway, S., Stern, Y., Visser, P.J., Scheltens, P. (2007). Research criteria for the diagnosis of Alzheimer's disease: revising the NINCDS-ADRDA criteria. *Lancet Neurol* 6:734-746.

Dubois, B., Feldman, H.H., Jacova, C., Cummings, J.L., Dekosky, S.T., Barberger-Gateau, P., Delacourte, A., Frisoni, G., Fox, N.C., Galasko, D., Gauthier, S., Hampel, H., Jicha, G.A., Meguro, K., O'Brien, J., Pasquier, F., Robert, P., Rossor, M., Salloway, S., Sarazin, M., de Souza, L.C., Stern, Y., Visser, P.J., Scheltens, P. (2010). Revising the definition of Alzheimer's disease: a new lexicon. *Lancet Neurol* 9:1118-1127.

El-Agnaf, O.M., Walsh, D.M., Allsop, D. (2003a). Soluble oligomers for the diagnosis of neurodegenerative diseases. *Lancet Neurol* 2:461-462.

El-Agnaf, O.M., Salem, S.A., Paleologou, K.E., Cooper, L.J., Fullwood, N.J., Gibson, M.J., Curran, M.D., Court, J.A., Mann, D.M., Ikeda, S., Cookson, M.R., Hardy, J., Allsop, D. (2003b). Alpha-synuclein implicated in Parkinson's disease is present in extracellular biological fluids, including human plasma. *FASEB J* 17:1945-1947.

Eriksen, J.L., Dawson, T.M., Dickson, D.W., Petrucelli, L. (2003). Caught in the act: alpha-synuclein is the culprit in Parkinson's disease. *Neuron* 40:453-456.

Ferrer, I., Perez, E., Dalfó, E., Barrachina, M. (2007).Abnormal levels of prohibitin and ATP synthase in the substantia nigra and frontal cortex in Parkinson's disease. *Neurosci Lett* 415:205-209.

Finehout, E.J., Franck, Z., Lee, K.H. (2005). Complement protein isoforms in CSF as possible biomarkers for neurodegenerative disease. *Dis Markers* 21:93-101.

Galvin, J.E., Lee, V.M., Trojanowski, J.Q. (2001). Synucleinopathies: clinical and pathological implications. *Arch Neurol* 58:186-190.

Giasson, B.I., Murray, I.V., Trojanowski, J.Q., Lee, V.M. (2001). A hydrophobic stretch of 12 amino acid residues in the middle of alpha-synuclein is essential for filament assembly. *J Biol Chem* 276:2380-2386.

Glenner, G.G., Wong, C.W., Quaranta, V., Eanes, E.D. (1984). The amyloid deposits in Alzheimer's disease: their nature and pathogenesis. *Appl Pathol* 2:357-369.

Goedert, M. (1997). Alpha-synuclein in Lewy bodies. *Nature* 388: 839-840.

Goker-Alpan, O., Lopez, G., Vithayathil, J., Davis, J., Hallett, M., Sidransky, E. (2008). The spectrum of parkinsonian manifestations associated with glucocerebrosidase mutations. *Arch Neurol* 65:1353-1357.

Grundke-Iqbal, I., Iqbal, K., Tung, Y.C., Quinlan, M., Wisniewski, H.M., Binder, L.I. (1986). Abnormal phosphorylation of the microtubule-associated protein tau (tau) in Alzheimer cytoskeletal pathology. *Proc Natl Acad Sci U S A* 83:4913-4917.

Guo, J., Sun, Z., Xiao, S., Liu, D., Jin, G., Wang, E., Zhou, J., Zhou, J. (2009). Proteomic analysis of the cerebrospinal fluid of Parkinson's disease patients. *Cell Res* 19:1401-1403.

Hely, M.A., Reid, W.G., Adena, M.A., Halliday, G.M., Morris, J.G. (2008). The Sydney multicenter study of Parkinson's disease: the inevitability of dementia at 20 years. *Mov Disord* 23:837-844.

Hirsch, E.C., Hunot, S. (2009). Neuroinflammation in Parkinson' disease: a target for neuroprotection? *Lancet Neurol* 8:382-397.

Holmberg, B., Rosengren, L., Karlsson, J.E., Johnels, B. (1998). Increased cerebrospinal fluid levels of neurofilament protein in progressive supranuclear palsy and multiple-system atrophy compared with Parkinson's disease. *Mov Disord* 13:70-77.

Hong, Z., Shi, M., Chung, K.A., Quinn, J.F., Peskind, E.R., Galasko, D., Jankovic, J., Zabetian, C.P., Leverenz, J.B., Baird, G., Montine, T.J., Hancock, A.M., Hwang, H., Pan, C., Bradner, J., Kang, U.J., Jensen, P.H., Zhang, J. (2010). DJ-1 and alpha-synuclein in human cerebrospinal fluid as biomarkers of Parkinson's disease. *Brain* 133:713-726.

Hughes, A.J., Daniel, S.E., Kilford, L., Lees, A.J. (1992). Accuracy of clinical diagnosis of idiopathic Parkinson's disease: a clinico-pathological study of 100 cases. *J Neurol Neurosurg Psychiatry* 55:181-184.

Hughes, A.J., Daniel, S.E., Ben-Shlomo, Y., Lees, A.J. (2002). The accuracy of diagnosis of parkinsonian syndromes in a specialist movement disorder service. *Brain* 125: 861-870.

Isaias, I.U., Antonini, A. (2010). Single-photon emission computed tomography in diagnosis and differential diagnosis of Parkinson's disease. *Neurodegener Dis* 7:319-329.

Junn, E., Ronchetti, R.D., Quezado, M.M., Kim, S.Y., Mouradian, M.M. (2003). Tissue transglutaminase-induced aggregation of alpha-synuclein: Implications for Lewy body formation in Parkinson's disease and dementia with Lewy bodies. *Proc Natl Acad Sci U S A* 100:2047-2052

Kasuga, K., Tokutake, T., Ishikawa, A., Uchiyama, T., Tokuda, T., Onodera, O., Nishizawa, M., Ikeuchi, T. (2010). Differential levels of alpha-synuclein, beta-amyloid42 and tau in CSF between patients with dementia with Lewy bodies and Alzheimer's disease. *J Neurol Neurosurg Psychiatry* 81:608-610.

Krüger, R., Kuhn, W., Müller, T., Woitalla, D., Graeber, M., Kösel, S., Przuntek, H., Epplen, J.T., Schöls, L., Riess, O. (1998). Ala30Pro mutation in the gene encoding alpha-synuclein in Parkinson's disease. *Nat Genet* 18:106-108.

Lee, H.J., Patel, S., Lee S.J. (2005). Intravescicular localization and exocytosis of alpha-synuclein and its aggregates. *J Neurosci* 25: 6016-6024.

Leverenz, J.B., Watson, G.S., Shofer, J., Zabetian, C.P., Zhang, J., Montine, T.J. (2011). Cerebrospinal fluid biomarkers and cognitive performance in non-demented patients with Parkinson's disease. *Parkinsonism Relat Disord* 17:61-64.

Li, J., Uversky, V.N., Fink, A.L. (2001). Effect of familial Parkinson's disease point mutations A30P and A53T on the structural properties, aggregation, and fibrillation of human alpha-synuclein. *Biochemistry* 40:11604–11613.

Lin, M.T. & Beal, M.F. (2006). Mitochondrial dysfunction and oxidative stress in neurodegenerative diseases. *Nature* 443:787-795.

Loeffler, D.A., DeMaggio, A.J., Juneau, P.L., Brickman, C.M., Mashour, G.A., Finkelman, J.H., Pomara, N., LeWitt, P.A. (1994). Ceruloplasmin is increased in cerebrospinal fluid in Alzheimer's disease but not Parkinson's disease. *Alzheimer Dis Assoc Disord* 8:190-197.

Maetzler, W., Berg, D., Schalamberidze, N., Melms, A., Schott, K., Mueller, J.C., Liaw, L., Gasser, T., Nitsch, C. (2007). Osteopontin is elevated in Parkinson's disease and its absence leads to reduced neurodegeneration in the MPTP model. *Neurobiol Dis* 25:473-482.

Maetzler, W., Liepelt, I., Berg, D. (2009). Progression of Parkinson's disease in the clinical phase: potential biomarkers. *Lancet Neurol* 8: 1158-1171.

McLean, P.J., Kawamata, H., Ribich, S., Hyman, B.T. (2000). Membrane association and protein conformation of alpha-synuclein in intact neurons. Effect of Parkinson's disease-linked mutations. J Biol Chem 275:8812–8816.

McGeer, P.L., Itagaki, S., Boyes, B.E., McGeer, E.G. (1988). Reactive microglia are positive for HLA-DR in the substantia nigra of Parkinson's and Alzheimer's disease brains. *Neurology* 38: 1285–1291.

Michell, A.W., Lewis,S.J., Foltynie, T., Barker, R.A. (2004). Biomarkers and Parkinson's disease. *Brain* 127:1693-1705.

Mochizuki, H., Goto, K., Mori, H., Mizuno, Y. (1996). Histochemical detection of apoptosis in Parkinson's disease. *J Neurol Sci* 137:120-123.

Mogi, M., Harada, M., Riederer, P., Narabayashi, H., Fujita, K., Nagatsu, T. (1994a). Tumor necrosis factor-alpha (TNF-alpha) increases both in the brain and in the cerebrospinal fluid from parkinsonian patients. *Neurosci Lett* 165: 208–210.

Mogi, M., Harada, M., Kondo, J., Riederer, P., Inagaki, H., Minami, M., Nagatsu, T. (1994b). Interleukin-1 beta, interleukin-6, epidermal growth factor and transforming growth factor-alpha are elevated in the brain from parkinsonian patients. *Neurosci Lett* 180:147–150.

Mogi, M., Harada, M., Kondo, T., Narabayashi, H., Riederer, P., Nagatsu, T. (1995a). Transforming growth factor-beta 1 levels are elevated in the striatum and in ventricular cerebrospinal fluid in Parkinson's disease. *Neurosci Lett* 193:129–132.

Mogi, M., Harada, M., Kondo, T., Riederer, P., Nagatsu, T. (1995b). Brain beta 2-microglobulin levels are elevated in the striatum in Parkinson's disease. *J Neural Transm Park Dis Dement Sect* 9: 87–92.

Mogi, M., Harada, M., Kondo, T., Riederer, P., Nagatsu, T. (1996a). Interleukin-2 but not basic fibroblast growth factor is elevated in parkinsonian brain. *J Neural Transm;* 103: 1077–1081.

Mogi, M., Harada, M., Kondo, T., Mizuno, Y., Narabayashi, H., Riederer, P., Nagatsu, T. (1996b). bcl-2 protein is increased in the brain from parkinsonian patients. *Neurosci Lett* 215:137-139.

Mogi, M., Harada, M., Kondo, T., Mizuno, Y., Narabayashi, H., Riederer, P., Nagatsu, T. (1996c). The soluble form of Fas molecule is elevated in parkinsonian brain tissues. *Neurosci Lett* 220:195-198.

Mollenhauer, B., Trenkwalder, C., von Ahsen, N., Bibl, M., Steinacker, P., Brechlin, P., Schindehuette, J., Poser, S., Wiltfang, J., Otto, M. (2006). Beta-amlyoid 1-42 and tau-protein in cerebrospinal fluid of patients with Parkinson's disease dementia. *Dement Geriatr Cogn Disord* 22:200-208.

Mollenhauer, B., Cullen, V., Kahn, I., Krastins, B., Outeiro, T.F., Pepivani, I., Ng, J., Schulz-Schaeffer, W., Kretzschmar, H.A., McLean, P.J., Trenkwalder, C., Sarracino, D.A., Vonsattel, J.P., Locascio, J.J., El-Agnaf, O.M., Schlossmacher, M.G. (2008). Direct quantification of CSF alpha-synuclein by ELISA and first cross-sectional study in patients with neurodegeneration. *Exp Neurol* 213:315-325.

Mollenhauer, B. & Trenkwalder, C. (2009). Neurochemical biomarkers in the differential diagnosis of movement disorders. *Mov Disord* 24: 1411-1426.

Mollenhauer, B., El-Agnaf, O.M., Marcus, K., Trenkwalder, C., Schlossmacher, M.G. (2010). Quantification of α-synuclein in cerebrospinal fluid as a biomarker candidate: review of the literature and considerations for future studies. *Biomark Med* 4:683-699.

Mollenhauer, B., Locascio, J.J., Schulz-Schaeffer, W., Sixel-Döring, F., Trenkwalder, C., Schlossmacher, M.G. (2011). Alpha-synuclein and tau concentrations in cerebrospinal fluid of patients presenting with parkinsonism: a cohort study. *Lancet Neurol* 10:230-240.

Montine, T.J., Shi, M., Quinn, J.F., Peskind, E.R., Craft, S., Ginghina, C., Chung, K.A., Kim, H., Galasko, D.R., Jankovic, J., Zabetian, C.P., Leverenz, J.B., Zhang, J. (2010). CSF Aβ(42) and tau in Parkinson's disease with cognitive impairment. *Mov Disord* 25:2682-2685.

Motter, R., Vigo-Pelfrey, C., Kholodenko, D., Barbour, R., Johnson-Wood, K., Galasko, D., Chang, L., Miller, B., Clark, C., Green, R., et al. (1995). Reduction of beta-amyloid peptide42 in the cerebrospinal fluid of patients with Alzheimer's disease. *Ann Neurol* 38:643-648.

Muller, T., Blum-Degen, D., Przuntek, H., Kuhn, W. (1998). Interleukin-6 levels in cerebrospinal fl uid inversely correlate to severity of Parkinson's disease. *Acta Neurol Scand* 98:142–144.

Murray, I.V., Giasson, B.I., Quinn, S.M., Koppaka, V., Axelsen, P.H., Ischiropoulos, H., Trojanowski, J.Q., Lee, V.M. (2003). Role of alpha-synuclein carboxy-terminus on fibril formation in vitro. *Biochemistry* 42:8530-8540.

Nilsson, C., Ståhlberg, F., Thomsen, C., Henriksen, O., Herning, M., Owman, C. (1992). Circadian variation in human cerebrospinal fluid production measured by magnetic resonance imaging. *Am J Physiol* 262:R20-R24.

Noguchi-Shinohara, M., Tokuda, T., Yoshita, M., Kasai, T., Ono, K., Nakagawa, M., El-Agnaf, O.M., Yamada, M. (2009) CSF alpha-synuclein levels in dementia with Lewy bodies and Alzheimer's disease. *Brain Res* 1251:1-6.

Nyhlén, J., Constantinescu, R., Zetterberg, H. (2010). Problems associated with fluid biomarkers for Parkinson's disease. *Biomarkers Med* 4:671-681.

Olanow, W., Kieburtz, K., Schapira, A.V.H. (2008). Why have we failed to achieve neuroprotection in Parkinson's disease. *Ann Neurol* 64 (suppl): S101-S110.

Ohrfelt, A., Grognet, P., Andreasen, N., Wallin, A., Vanmechelen, E., Blennow, K., Zetterberg, H. (2009). Cerebrospinal fluid alpha-synuclein in neurodegenerative disorders-a marker of synapse loss? *Neurosci Lett* 450:332-335.

Paisán-Ruíz, C., Jain, S., Evans, E.W., Gilks, W.P., Simón, J., van der Brug, M., López de Munain, A., Aparicio, S., Gil, A.M., Khan, N., Johnson, J., Martinez, J.R., Nicholl, D.,

Carrera, I.M., Pena, A.S., de Silva, R., Lees, A., Martí-Massó, J.F., Pérez-Tur, J., Wood, N.W., Singleton, A.B. (2004). Cloning of the gene containing mutations that cause PARK8-linked Parkinson's disease. *Neuron* 44:595-600.

Paleologou, K.E., Kragh, C.L., Mann, D.M., Salem, S.A., Al-Shami, R., Allsop, D., Hassan, A.H., Jensen, P.H., El-Agnaf, O.M. (2009). Detection of elevated levels of soluble alpha-synuclein oligomers in post-mortem brain extracts from patients with dementia with Lewy bodies. *Brain* 132:1093-1101.

Parnetti, L., Tiraboschi, P., Lanari, A., Peducci, M., Padiglioni, C., D'Amore, C., Pierguidi, L., Tambasco, N., Rossi, A., Calabresi, P. (2008). Cerebrospinal fluid biomarkers in Parkinson's disease with dementia and dementia with Lewy bodies. *Biol Psychiatry* 64:850-855.

Parnetti, L., Balducci, C., Pierguidi, L., De Carlo, C., Peducci, M., D'Amore, C., Padiglioni, C., Mastrocola, S., Persichetti, E., Paciotti, S., Bellomo, G., Tambasco, N., Rossi, A., Beccari, T., Calabresi, P. (2009). Cerebrospinal fluid beta-glucocerebrosidase activity is reduced in Dementia with Lewy Bodies. *Neurobiol Dis* 34:484-6.

Parnetti, L. (2011). Biochemical diagnosis of neurodegenerative diseases gets closer. *Lancet Neurol* 10:203-205.

Parnetti, L., Chiasserini, D., Bellomo, G., Giannandrea, D., De Carlo, C., Qureshi, M.M., Ardah, M.T., Varghese, S., Bonanni, L., Borroni, B., Tambasco, N., Eusebi, P., Rossi, A., Onofrj, M., Padovani, A., Calabresi, P., El-Agnaf, O. (2011). Cerebrospinal fluid tau/alpha-synuclein ratio in Parkinson's disease and degenerative dementias. *Mov Disord* Apr 5. doi: 10.1002/mds.23670. [Epub ahead of print]

Polymeropoulos, M.H., Lavedan, C., Leroy, E., Ide, S.E., Dehejia, A., Dutra, A., Pike, B., Root, H., Rubenstein, J., Boyer, R., Stenroos, E.S., Chandrasekharappa, S., Athanassiadou, A., Papapetropoulos T, Johnson, W.G., Lazzarini, A.M., Duvoisin, R.C., Di Iorio, G., Golbe, L.I., Nussbaum, R.L. (1997). Mutation in the alpha-synuclein gene identified in families with Parkinson's disease. *Science* 276:2045-2047.

Samii, A., Nutt, J.G., Ransom, B.R. (2004). Parkinson's disease. *Lancet* 363:1783-1793.

Satake, W., Nakabayashi, Y., Mizuta, I., Hirota, Y., Ito, C., Kubo, M., Kawaguchi, T., Tsunoda, T., Watanabe, M., Takeda, A., Tomiyama, H., Nakashima, K., Hasegawa, K., Obata, F., Yoshikawa, T., Kawakami, H., Sakoda, S., Yamamoto, M., Hattori, N., Murata, M., Nakamura, Y., Toda, T. (2009) Genome-wide association study identifies common variants at four loci as genetic risk factors for Parkinson's disease. *Nat Genet* 41:1303-1307.

Schapira, A.H., Cooper, J.M., Dexter, D., Jenner, P., Clark, J.B., Marsden, C.D. (1989). Mitochondrial complex I deficiency in Parkinson's disease. *Lancet* 1:1269.

Schapira, A.H. (2008). Mitochondria in the aetiology and pathogenesis of Parkinson's disease. *Lancet Neurol* 7:97-109.

Schlossmacher, M.G., Mollenhauer, B. (2010). Biomarkers research in Parkinson's disease: objective measures needed for patient stratification in future cause-directed trials. *Biomarkers Med* 4:647-650.

Scholz, S.W., Houlden, H., Schulte, C., Sharma, M., Li, A., Berg, D., Melchers, A., Paudel, R., Gibbs, J.R., Simon-Sanchez, J., Paisan-Ruiz, C., Bras, J., Ding, J., Chen, H., Traynor, B.J., Arepalli, S., Zonozi, R.R., Revesz, T., Holton, J., Wood, N., Lees, A., Oertel, W., Wüllner, U., Goldwurm, S., Pellecchia, M.T., Illig, T., Riess, O., Fernandez, H.H.,

Rodriguez, R.L., Okun, M.S., Poewe, W., Wenning, G.K., Hardy, J.A., Singleton, A.B., Del Sorbo, F., Schneider, S., Bhatia, K.P., Gasser T. (2009). SNCA variants are associated with increased risk for multiple system atrophy. *Ann Neurol* 65:610-614.

Shi, M., Bradner, J., Hancock, A.M., Chung, K.A., Quinn, J.F., Peskind, E.R., Galasko, D., Jankovic, J., Zabetian, C.P., Kim, H.M., Leverenz, J.B., Montine, T.J., Ginghina, C., Kang, U.J., Cain, K.C., Wang, Y., Aasly, J., Goldstein, D., Zhang, J. (2011). Cerebrospinal fluid biomarkers for Parkinson disease diagnosis and progression. *Ann Neurol* 69:570-580.

Shin, Y., Klucken, J., Patterson, C., Hyman, B.T., McLean, P.J. (2005) The co-chaperone carboxyl terminus of hsp70-interacting protein (CHIP) mediates {alpha}-synuclein degradation decisions between proteasomal and lysosomal pathways. *J Biol Chem* 208:23727-23734.

Shults, C.W. (2006). Lewy bodies. *Proc Natl Acad Sci USA*103:1661-1668.

Shtilerman, M.D., Ding, T.T., Lansbury, P.T. Jr. (2002). Molecular crowding accelerates fibrillization of alpha-synuclein: could an increase in the cytoplasmic protein concentration induce Parkinson's disease? *Biochemistry* 41:3855–3860.

Siderowf, A., Xie, S.X., Hurtig, H., Weintraub, D., Duda, J., Chen-Plotkin, A., Shaw, L.M., Van Deerlin, V., Trojanowski, J.Q., Clark, C. (2010). CSF amyloid {beta} 1-42 predicts cognitive decline in Parkinson disease. *Neurology* 75:1055-1061.

Sidransky, E., Nalls, M.A., Aasly, J.O., Aharon-Peretz, J., Annesi, G., Barbosa, E.R., Bar-Shira, A., Berg, D., Bras, J., Brice, A., Chen, C.M., Clark, L.N., Condroyer, C., De Marco, E.V., Dürr, A., Eblan, M.J., Fahn, S., Farrer, M.J., Fung, H.C., Gan-Or, Z., Gasser, T., Gershoni-Baruch, R., Giladi, N., Griffith, A., Gurevich, T., Januario, C., Kropp, P., Lang, A.E., Lee-Chen, G.J., Lesage, S., Marder, K., Mata, I.F., Mirelman, A., Mitsui, J., Mizuta, I., Nicoletti, G., Oliveira, C., Ottman, R., Orr-Urtreger, A., Pereira, L.V., Quattrone, A., Rogaeva, E., Rolfs, A., Rosenbaum, H., Rozenberg, R., Samii, A., Samaddar, T., Schulte, C., Sharma, M., Singleton, A., Spitz, M., Tan, E.K., Tayebi, N., Toda, T., Troiano, A.R., Tsuji, S., Wittstock, M., Wolfsberg, T.G., Wu, Y.R., Zabetian, C.P., Zhao, Y., Ziegler, S.G. (2009). Multicenter analysis of glucocerebrosidase mutations in Parkinson's disease. *N Engl J Med* 361:1651-1661.

Simón-Sánchez, J., Schulte, C., Bras, J.M., Sharma, M., Gibbs, J.R., Berg, D., Paisan-Ruiz, C., Lichtner, P., Scholz, S.W., Hernandez, D.G., Krüger, R., Federoff, M., Klein, C., Goate, A., Perlmutter, J., Boninm M., Nalls, M.A., Illig, T., Gieger, C., Houlden, H., Steffens, M., Okun, M.S., Racette, B.A., Cookson, M.R., Foote, K.D., Fernandez, H.H., Traynor, B.J., Schreiber, S., Arepalli, S., Zonozi, R., Gwinn, K., van der Brug, M., Lopez, G., Chanock, S.J., Schatzkin, A., Park, Y., Hollenbeck, A., Gao, J., Huang, X., Wood, N.W., Lorenz, D., Deuschl, G., Chen, H., Riess, O., Hardy, J.A., Singleton, A.B., Gasser, T. (2009). Genome-wide association study reveals genetic risk underlying Parkinson's disease. *Nat Genet* 41:1308-1312.

Simonsen, A.H., McGuire, J., Hansson, O., Zetterberg, H., Podust, V.N., Davies, H.A., Waldemar, G., Minthon, L., Blennow, K. (2007). Novel panel of cerebrospinal fluid biomarkers for the prediction of progression to Alzheimer dementia in patients with mild cognitive impairment. *Arch Neurol* 64:366-370.

Singleton, A.B., Farrer, M., Johnson, J., Singleton, A., Hague, S., Kachergus, J., Hulihan, M., Peuralinna, T., Dutra, A., Nussbaum, R., Lincoln, S., Crawley, A., Hanson, M., Maraganore, D., Adler, C., Cookson, M.R., Muenter, M., Baptista, M., Miller, D.,

Blancato, J., Hardy, J., Gwinn-Hardy, K. (2003). Alpha-synuclein locus triplication causes Parkinson's disease. *Science* 302:841.

Sjögren, M., Davidsson, P., Wallin, A., Granérus, A.K., Grundström, E., Askmark, H., Vanmechelen, E., Blennow, K. (2002). Decreased CSF-beta-amyloid 42 in Alzheimer's disease and amyotrophic lateral sclerosis may reflect mismetabolism of beta-amyloid induced by disparate mechanisms. *Dement Geriatr Cogn Disord* 13:112-118.

Spies, P.E., Melis, R.J., Sjögren, M.J., Rikkert, M.G., Verbeek, M.M. (2009). Cerebrospinal fluid alpha-synuclein does not discriminate between dementia disorders. *J Alzheimers Dis* 16:363-369.

Spillantini, M.G., Goedert, M. (2000). The alpha-synucleinopathies: Parkinson's disease, dementia with Lewy bodies, and multiple system atrophy. *Ann N Y Acad Sci* 920:16-27.

Tayebi, N., Walker, J., Stubblefield, B., Orvisky, E., LaMarca, M.E., Wong, K., Rosenbaum, H., Schiffmann, R., Bembi, B., Sidransky, E. (2003). Gaucher disease with parkinsonian manifestations: does glucocerebrosidase deficiency contribute to a vulnerability to parkinsonism? *Mol Genet Metab* 79:104-109.

Tipton, K.F. & Singer, T.P. (1993). Advances in our understanding of the mechanisms of the neurotoxicity of MPTP and related compounds. *J Neurochem* 61:1191-1206.

Tokuda, T., Salem, S.A., Allsop, D., Mizuno, T., Nakagawa, M., Qureshi, M.M., Locascio, J.J., Schlossmacher, M.G., El-Agnaf, O.M. (2006). Decreased alpha-synuclein in cerebrospinal fluid of aged individuals and subjects with Parkinson's disease. *Biochem Biophys Res Commun* 349:162-166.

Tokuda, T., Qureshi, M.M., Ardah, M.T., Varghese, S., Shehab, S.A., Kasai, T., Ishigami, N., Tamaoka, A., Nakagawa, M., El-Agnaf, O.M. (2010). Detection of elevated levels of α-synuclein oligomers in CSF from patients with Parkinson disease. *Neurology* 75:1766-1772.

Uverski, V.N. (2007). Neuropathology, biochemistry, and biophysics of alpha-synuclein aggregation. *J Neurochem* 103:17-37.

Valente, E.M., Abou-Sleiman, P.M., Caputo, V., Muqit, M.M., Harvey, K., Gispert, S., Ali, Z., Del Turco, D., Bentivoglio, A.R., Healy, D.G., Albanese, A., Nussbaum, R., González-Maldonado, R., Deller, T., Salvi, S., Cortelli, P., Gilks, W.P., Latchman, D.S., Harvey, R.J., Dallapiccola, B., Auburger, G., Wood, N.W. (2004). Hereditary early-onset Parkinson's disease caused by mutations in PINK1. *Science* 304:1158-1160.

Van Dijk, K.D., Teunissen, C.E., Drukarch, B., Jimenez, C.R., Groenewegen, H.J., Berendse, H.W., van de Berg, W.D.J. (2010). Diagnostic cerebrospinal fluid biomarkers for Parkinson's disease: a pathogenetically based approach. *Neurobiol Dis* 39:229-241.

van Kamp, G.J., Mulder, K., Kuiper, M., Wolters, E.C. (1995). Changed transferrin sialylation in Parkinson's disease. *Clin Chim Acta* 235:159-167.

Velayati, A., Yu, W.H., Sidransky, E. (2010). The role of glucocerebrosidase mutations in Parkinson disease and Lewy body disorders. *Curr Neurol Neurosci Rep* 10:190-198.

Vermes, I., Steur, E.N., Reutelingsperger, C., Haanen, C. (1999). Decreased concentration of annexin V in parkinsonian cerebrospinal fluid: speculation on the underlying cause. *Mov Disord* 14:1008-1010.

Vermes, I., Steur, E.N., Jirikowski, G.F., Haanen, C. (2004). Elevated concentration of cerebrospinal fluid tissue transglutaminase in Parkinson's disease indicating apoptosis. *Mov Disord* 19:1252-1254.

Waragai, M., Wei, J., Fujita, M., Nakai, M., Ho, G.J., Masliah, E., Akatsu, H., Yamada, T., Hashimoto, M. (2006). Increased level of DJ-1 in the cerebrospinal fluids of sporadic Parkinson's disease. *Biochem Biophys Res Commun* 345:967-972.

Werner CJ, Heyny-von Haussen R, Mall G, Wolf S. (2008). Proteome analysis of human substantia nigra in Parkinson's disease. *Proteome Sci* 6:8.

Willingham, S., Outeiro, T.F., DeVit, M.J., Lindquist, S.L., Muchowski, P.J. (2003). Yeast genes that enhance the toxicity of a mutant huntingtin fragment or alpha-synuclein. *Science* 302:1769–1772.

Zarranz, J.J., Alegre, J., Gómez-Esteban, J.C., Lezcano, E., Ros, R., Ampuero, I., Vidal, L., Hoenicka, J., Rodriguez, O., Atarés, B., Llorens, V., Gomez Tortosa, E., del Ser, T., Muñoz, D.G., de Yebenes, J.G. (2004). The new mutation, E46K, of alpha-synuclein causes Parkinson and Lewy body dementia. *Ann Neurol* 55:164-173.

Zimprich, A., Biskup, S., Leitner, P., Lichtner, P., Farrer, M., Lincoln, S., Kachergus, J,. Hulihan, M., Uitti, R.J., Calne, D.B., Stoessl, A.J., Pfeiffer, R.F., Patenge, N., Carbajal, I.C., Vieregge, P., Asmus, F., Müller-Myhsok, B., Dickson, D.W., Meitinger, T., Strom, T.M., Wszolek, Z.K., Gasser, T. (2004) Mutations in LRRK2 cause autosomal-dominant parkinsonism with pleomorphic pathology. *Neuron* 44:601-607.

4

Neuropsychological Functions and SPECT Neuroimaging in Parkinson's Disease

Lambros Messinis[1], Athanasios Papathanasiou[1], Epameinondas Lyros[1], George Gatzounis[2] and Panagiotis Papathanasopoulos[1]
[1]*Department of Neurology, Neuropsychology Section, University of Patras Medical School,*
[2]*Department of Neurosurgery, University of Patras Medical School,*
Greece

1. Introduction

Parkinson's disease (PD) is a chronic progressive neurodegenerative disorder, characterized by motor and non-motor signs. It was Charcot, who first in 1875 pointed out that 'psychic faculties are definitely impaired' and that 'the mind becomes clouded and the memory is lost'. Most patients with PD experience some degree of cognitive impairment, ranging from mild selective deficits to Parkinson's disease dementia (Dubois & Pillon, 1997). PD patients may also spend several years in a transition state called Mild Cognitive Impairment (MCI), which is now recognized as one of the cardinal non-motor manifestations of PD. It is a major cause of disability, and has been shown to be an important predictor for quality of life (Karlsen et al., 1998). Recent studies have reported a 21% prevalence rate of MCI in a large PD population and consider MCI as a risk factor for developing Parkinson's disease Dementia (PDD) (Caviness et al., 2007; Janvin et al., 2006; Levin et al., 1992). The neuropathophysiological basis of cognitive deficits in PD is complicated and includes degeneration of dopaminergic neurons mainly of the nigrostriatal pathway and to a lesser degree the mesocortical and mesolimbic pathways. The striatum is closely interrelated to cortical areas mainly to the frontal lobes. The neuropathophysiological puzzle is further complicated by multiple neurotransmitter deficits including noradrenalin, serotonin and acetylcholine pathway as well as Lewy body- type degeneration in cortical and limbic structures (Mandir & Vaughan, 2000). The direct dopaminergic connections between the ventral tegmental area and the prefrontal cortex may also influence changes in cognition (Cools 2006; Mattay et al., 2002). The pattern of cognitive impairment seen even in early PD mainly resembles that produced by frontal lobe damage, as the basal ganglia and prefrontal cortex are closely interrelated through anatomofunctional circuits (Alexander et al., 1986; Bondi et al., 1993) and include deficits mainly in cognitive flexibility, planning, working memory and learning.

Perfusion brain single photon emission computed tomography (SPECT) provides a well-established means of studying regional cerebral blood flow (rCBF) which is known to reflect cortical function. On the other hand Dopamine Transporter (DAT) SPECT imaging can be used as a marker for the degree of loss of dopaminergic nerve endings. It is well known that SPECT Neuroimaging can assist in the differential diagnosis of parkinsonian and dementia syndromes and DAT SCAN can also be helpful in differentiating tremors resulting from damage to the nigrostriatal dopaminergic terminals from those due to essential tremor, drug-induced or psychogenic causes (Benamer et al., 2000). SPECT can also be useful in monitoring disease progression as well as providing information about the pathophysiological process.

Numerous studies during the last decade have attempted to investigate differences and associations between cortical perfusion, nigrostriatal dopamine pathway and neuropsychological functions in demented and non demented patients with PD. These studies show a tendency towards increased hypoperfusion in parietal and temporal lobes in PDD as compared to the non demented PD patients (Derejko et al., 2006; Liu et al., 1992; Matsui et al., 2005).There are also conflicting results in the literature regarding PD patients with MCI ranging from either no difference compared to controls (Sawada et al.,1992; Spampinato et al., 1991) to hypoperfusion in the parietal (Wallin et al., 2007) and frontal areas (Antonini et al., 2001; Firbank et al., 2005; Paschali et al., 2009). Regarding rCBF and neuropsychological functions in different stages of PD, as dopaminergic nerve endings degenerate in PD there is progressive cortical hypoperfusion affecting mainly the frontal lobes in the early stages, extending to the parietal and temporal lobes in the late stages of Parkinson's disease. In parallel, neuropsychological performance gradually deteriorates as the disease progresses (Paschali et al., 2010).

In the present chapter we will discuss neuropsychological deficits seen early in the course of Parkinson's disease as well as clinical characteristics of dementia seen later in the course of PD. We will also discuss the underlying neurochemistry of these cognitive impairments and address the concept of heterogeneous nature of the observed cognitive dysfunction in PD as revealed by neuropsychological and neuroimaging studies with a focus on SPECT neuroimaging.

2. Epidemiology of PDD

2.1 Prevalence rates

The prevalence of dementia in PD was reported to range from 2% in early onset cases (Hietanen &Teravainen, 1988) to 81% in an unselected patient population (Martin et al., 1973). In a review of 27 studies, an average prevalence of 40% was found (Cummings JL 1988). Other community based studies have estimated the point prevalence for dementia in PD to be between 28% and 44% (Mayeux et al., 1992).One longitudinal study observed a 52% prevalence rate of dementia with over 4 years follow-up and 60% prevalence rate of dementia with over 12 years follow up in 233 patients with PD (Buter et al., 2008). Another prospective study of 249 patients with PD observed a 65% risk rate of dementia by age 85 years (Mayeux et al., 1990). A further prospective study of 86 patients with PD and 102 age-matched controls estimated that the relative risk for dementia was equal to 5.1 in patients with PD (Hobson et al., 2004). In another study conducted in the general population, the prevalence of dementia among patients with PD was 41% and the association with age was striking, i.e. the prevalence rate was zero in patients below the age of 50 and 69% in patients above 80 years old (Mayeux et al., 1992). The variation noted between different studies is probably due to different methods of cognitive assessment, how dementia was defined, the study populations chosen and the data collection methods.

2.2 Incidence rates

Incidence studies may provide a more accurate estimate of risk of dementia in PD because of their prospective nature. Incidence of dementia was found to be consistently higher in patients with PD than in persons without PD. The number of demented patients was found to be four times higher than expected over a period of 3 years (Mindham et al., 1982). In another prospective study, the incidence of dementia was six times higher in patients with PD than in controls (Aarsland et al., 2001). In a survey of 83 patients and 50 controls, who were free of dementia at baseline, followed over 10 and 14 years, the cumulative incidence rate was 38% and 53% respectively (Hughes et al.,2000; Read et al.,2001).

3. Neuropsychology of Parkinson's disease

3.1 Neuropsychological deficits in PD

Cognitive deficits in PD are found early in the disease process even before initiation of anti-parkinsonian treatment and resemble those commonly attributed to frontal lobe dysfunction. PD patients have been reported to have reduced cognitive speed and increased distractibility, problems in set formation and impairment in set shifting and maintaining, visuoperceptual deficits, deficits in executive functions such as self-directed planning and problem solving and deficits in working memory. Characteristically, Parkinson's disease patients fail to solve a novel task when relying on internal rather than external cues. Memory impairments, mainly depicted in decreased performance in free recall tasks, while recognition memory appears to be intact, are thought to represent defective retrieval strategies, that is inability for active organization of the material to be remembered

Dopamine restoration offers relief from many of the motor symptoms of Parkinson's disease and has also been shown to exert beneficial effects on certain aspects of cognition that involve mainly executive functions, while memory and visuospatial deficits seem to be less dopamine dependent. Moreover, dopaminergic medication may have deleterious effects on certain cognitive functions such as reversal learning. This has led to the formation of the dopamine overdose hypothesis, according to which, dopamine dosing that ameliorates motor symptoms by restoring dopamine concentrations in severely depleted brain areas such as the putamen may impair some aspects of cognition by overdosing other areas, which are less dopaminergically depleted early in the disease such as the caudate nucleus and ventral striatum (Cools et al., 2001.) The pathological basis of cognitive impairments in PD has been attributed to disruption of the "complex loop" which connects the caudate nucleus with the frontal association regions, via the thalamus or to loss of dopaminergic neurons in the ventro-tegmental area affecting meso-cortico-limbic pathways. As cognitive impairment in PD however, is inadequately explained by dopamine loss alone, alternative hypotheses have been raised implicating the underlying frontal cholinergic denervation as outlined in a following section of this chapter.

3.2 Mild cognitive impairment in PD

Parkinson's disease is often associated with mild cognitive impairment (MCI) and dementia. The term mild cognitive impairment is used in Parkinson's disease to include diverse neuropsychological deficits within the executive, mnemonic and visuospatial domains. Cognitive impairment in a single or in multiple domain(s) is common in non-demented patients with PD (Foltynie et al., 2004; Janvin et al., 2003) and more than 50% of patients with PD will develop dementia and cognitive impairment which ultimately affects quality of life (Schrag et al., 2000). The original MCI definition requires presence of subjective cognitive complaints (preferably by third party), objective evidence of impaired test performance and lack of significant functional impairment (Petersen et al.,1999).The following subtypes of MCI in patients with PD have been described. Amnestic MCI-single domain, amnesticMCI-multiple domain, Non-amnestic MCI-Single domain and Non-amnestic MCI-multiple domain (Aarsland D. et al,. 2010). In a study by Caviness et al., (2007) the majority of their patients had single domain MCI (67%), with either executive dysfunction (39%) or amnestic deficits (22%). Another study showed that the most prevalent subtypes of MCI in PD were single, non-amnestic domain (mostly executive dysfunction) in 44,7%, followed by multiple impaired domains in 39, 5% and single amnestic domain MCI in 15,8% (Janvin et al., 2006). In a recently published multicenter pooled analysis study, one quarter of patients with Parkinson's disease without dementia, had impairments in at least one cognitive domain. The most common MCI subtype was nonamnestic single domain (11,3%), followed by amnestic single domain MCI (8,9%).These results showed that memory impairment also represents an important aspect of cognitive impairment in PD, and deficits in attention-executive functions may not always be the predominant deficits in PD-MCI (Aarsland et al., 2010). Findings from the above studies, underline the necessity that standardized diagnostic criteria for Mild Cognitive Impairment in Parkinson's disease need to be better defined. Based on existing data (Emre et al., 2004) that pharmacological treatment with acetylcholinesterase inhibitors can improve cognitive impairment in PDD, new studies must be performed in order to investigate whether these or other medications can delay the progression from MCI to PDD.

3.3 Risk factors associated with development of PDD

Several risk factors are reported to be associated with PDD. These include age at onset, age at the time of the study, duration of illness, akinetic-rigid syndrome, depression and atypical neurological features (e.g., early occurrence of autonomic nervous system failure, symmetrical disease presentation, and moderate response to dopaminergic treatment). More severe cognitive impairments and higher risk for developing dementia have also been associated with the clinical manifestations of postural instability and gait disorder (Alves et al., 2006). Further, poor performance in verbal fluency tasks was found to be significantly and independently associated with PDD (Jacobs et al., 1995). In summary, up to 40% of patients with Parkinson's disease will develop dementia and the incidence is up to six times higher than aged matched controls. Older age at onset and atypical features seem to be the main risk factors. With regard to neural correlates of cognitive decline in PD the hypothesis has been raised that this might be due to the simultaneous effect of age-related and disease associated neuropathology (Levy, 2007). Furthermore, it has been shown that cognitive status of PD patients correlates with neuropathological stage showing deterioration as the disease process in the brain progresses following an upward path from the brainstem to the neocortex (Braak et al., 2005). However, the extent of cortical alpha-synuclein pathology was not predictive of cognitive impairment in an autopsy series (Parkkinen et al., 2005).

4. Clinical characteristics of PDD

4.1 Executive function

The phenotype of dementia associated with Parkinson's Disease is a dysexecutive syndrome in which executive function (defined as the ability to plan, organize and regulate goal directed behavior) impairment is the main feature (Litvan et al., 1991; Pillon et al., 1986; Pillon et al., 1991).These deficits include impairment in concept formation and rule finding, problem solving, set elaboration and planning, set shifting and set maintenance. Difficulties are due to shifting attention to novel stimuli, whereas preservative errors are less common (Levin et al., 1991).Verbal fluency has been extensively studied in PDD, where impaired performance is typical (Aarsland et al., 2003; Cahn-Weiner et al., 2002; Paolo et al., 1995).The results of these studies reveal that executive functions are impaired in PDD patients, probably more than in patients with AD.

4.2 Attention

Attention was found to be impaired in demented patients with Parkinson's disease, as shown by measures of attention such as cognitive reaction and vigilance (Litvan et al.,1991).There were also fluctuations in attention similar to those found in patients with dementia with Lewy bodies (Ballard et al., 2002). In a test involving letter cancellation, it was found that PDD and DLB groups were slower and showed more errors than an AD group (Noe et al., 2004). Another study employing a composite index of attention noted greater deficits in PDD than AD patients (Beatty et al., 2003). Finally, when attention was measured in terms of variability in performance over time in a series of reaction time tasks, it showed that 29% of the PDD patients had attentional fluctuations compared to 42% of those with DLB (Ballard et al., 2002). From the above findings, it appears that attention is impaired in PDD and may fluctuate more than AD.

4.3 Memory

Memory, including working memory, long term memory, visuospatial memory and procedural learning is significantly impaired in Parkinson's disease demented patients, but the impairment differs from the amnesia seen in patients with Alzheimer's disease. Memory complaint was reported to be the presenting problem in 67% of PDD patients, compared to 94% with DLB and 100% in AD (Noe et al.,2004).Short term memory has received a little attention, although digit span performance which is more an attentional test, does not appear to distinguish PDD and AD patients (Starkstein et al.,1996). Learning of new information is also impaired, but to a lesser degree than in patients with Alzheimer disease (Helkala et al., 1989; Pillon et al., 1991; Stern et al., 1993). Several studies have shown that demented patients with Parkinson's disease have impaired free recall, similar to Alzheimer's disease, but their recognition is better than free recall, which shows that new information is stored but not accessed (Helkala et al., 1989; Pillon et al.,1993). A very important assumption is that memory in demented patients with Parkinson's disease was related to executive function test scores (Pillon et al., 1993).Therefore, amnesia is not of a temporal-limbic type, because patients are able to store information, but is caused by difficulty with the accessing of memory traces, which reflects a deficiency in strategy, due to a dysexecutive syndrome (Dubois et al., 1997). Both verbal and visual memory are impaired in PDD, and the degree of this impairment is probably less than that seen in AD, and recognition may be less affected than recall in mild to moderate PDD.

4.4 Visuospatial dysfunction

Visuospatial dysfunction was noted in demented patients with Parkinson's disease and this impairment was more severe in demented patients with Parkinson's disease than with

Alzheimer's disease (but similar to DLB) with approximately similar dementia severity (Huber et al.,1989; Stern et al.,1993). Boller et al., (1984) found impairments in visuoperceptual and visuomotor tasks, independent of intellectual impairment; however patients with larger loss in motor function tended to show the largest visuospatial impairment. Visuospatial impairment in PD is seen especially in more complicated tasks, that require planning and strategy, therefore impairments in perceptual motor tasks may be in part due to problems in organization of behavioral-executive problems (Stern et al.,1983).

4.5 Language

Language is also impaired in patients with PDD, but to a lesser degree than Alzheimer's disease (Cummings et al., 1988; Huber et al., 1989).The domain that is reported to be more severe than in patients with Alzheimer's disease is verbal fluency (Huber et al., 1989; Stern et al., 1993). Naming difficulties, decreased information content of spontaneous speech and impaired comprehension of complex sentences were described in demented and non demented patients with PD, but to a lesser degree than Alzheimer's disease (Grossman et al., 1991; Grossman et al., 1992).

4.6 Construction and praxis

Typically, drawing tests are used to assess construction ability and praxis, either copying designs or drawing common objects. The clock drawing test is markedly impaired in PDD (Emre et al., 2004). It should be noted however, that apraxia is not a common feature of PDD, although impaired ideomotor praxis was described (Goldenberg et al., 1986; Huber et al., 1989). Impaired verbal fluency and naming difficulties may not reflect an original involvement of language function but may be related to dysexecutive syndrome (Grossman et al., 1991).

5. Neuropsychiatric manifestations in PD

5.1 Depression and anxiety

Symptoms of depression and anxiety are common in Parkinson's disease. Approximately 30-40% of patients with PD have depressive symptoms, with lower prevalence rates in population based studies (Leentjens et al 2008; Reijnders et al., 2008). Anxiety also affects up to 40% of patients with PD (Leentjens et al., 2008; Menza et al., 1993; Richard 2005). Depression and anxiety can be off-period phenomena and respond to antiparkinsonian medication (Maricle et al., 1995; Nissenbaum et al., 1987; Siemers et al., 1993; Witjas et al., 2002).The pathophysiology of these symptoms is complex and probably includes dopaminergic, serotonergic and noradrenergic mechanisms. The raphe nuclei and locus coeruleus are structures which appear to be involved in depression, early in the course of Parkinson's disease (Braak et al., 2004). There is also clear evidence that dopaminergic dysfunction also plays a role. Dopaminergic projections from the ventral tegmentum of the midbrain to the medial temporal and orbitofrontal regions are affected in post mortem studies (Torack & Morris, 1988).There is also evidence that limbic noradrenergic/dopaminergic pathways are dysfunctional in PD patients with depression compared to those without (Remy et al.,2005). The main characteristics of depression are low mood and lack of interest or pleasure, one of which is required for a diagnosis of depression in most classifications. Other features are altered appetite or sleep, weight change, loss of libido, reduced memory, psychomotor retardation, loss of energy, feelings of guilt, and suicidal ideation which can overlap with the symptoms of PD, making diagnosis of depression in PD difficult (Gotham et al., 1986; Myslobodsky et al, 2001).The most common anxiety disorders in PD are panic attacks which are often noted during off-periods, generalized anxiety disorder, simple and social phobias. Outside off-periods, anxiety may be part of an underlying depressive disorder (Mondolo et al., 2007). The most commonly used diagnostic classification for depression and anxiety is the DSM IV-TR . For screening purposes the Hamilton depression scale, Beck depression inventory, Hospital anxiety and depression scale and Geriatric depression scale have been shown to be valid in depression of PD. However, it's very important to remember that diagnosis of depression should only be made using clinical criteria rather than scales. Several rating scales for anxiety have been used in patients with PD, but their validity needs to be assessed further (Leentjens et al., 2008). Regarding the management of these symptoms, the first important issue, is to determine whether the depression and/or anxiety symptoms occur during off-periods. If so, then the adjustment of antiparkinsonian medication is required. In most cases with mild depression, which are the majority, non-pharmacological intervention is the treatment of choice, ranging from counseling - patient education to cognitive-behavioral therapy (Cole & Vaughan, 2005).The most useful first step in treatment is the optimization of the existing dopaminergic medication. Other pharmacological agents used for depression of PD include tricyclic antidepressants, tricyclic-related drugs (trazodone), selective serotonin reuptake inhibitors (SSRI), the serotonin and noradrenaline re-uptake inhibitors (SNRI) venlafaxine, the selective noradrenaline re-uptake inhibitor reboxetine and the presynaptic alpha2 adrenoreceptor antagonist mirtazapine.

5.2 Apathy and fatigue

Apathy and fatigue are two common non motor manifestations in PD, which contribute to disability and are attributed to basal ganglia pathology and disturbances in frontal-subcortical connections (Dujardin et al., 2007). Reported prevalence for apathy ranges from 17% to 70% (Isella et al.,2002; Levy et al.,1998;Starkstein et al.,1992) and is influenced by the extend of cognitive impairment and depressive symptoms in the sample and the tools used (Pluck & Brown,2002; Shulman, 2000). Apathy in the absence of depression occurs in 4-30% of cases, whereas reported prevalence for depression in the absence of apathy is 6-28% and for combination of apathy-depression is 12-47% (Aarsland et al., 1999; Dujardin et al., 2007; Isella et al., 2002). Fatigue is reported in up to 1/3 of patients with PD (Friedmann et al., 2007), and has a prevalence rate of 32-58%. However, fatigue outcome is influenced by the definitions of fatigue and the assessment tool that was used (Alves et al., 2004). Fatigue is also associated with depression, cognitive deficits and daytime sleepiness (Rochester et al., 2004). Apathy refers to a set of behavioral, emotional and cognitive features with reduced interest and motivation in goal-directed behaviors (Marin, 1997). The impact of apathy is considerable, the patient is inactive and this leads to greater functional decline and disability (Aarsland et al., 1999).The role of depression and cognitive impairment in apathy is considerable. There are conflicting reports in the literature whether apathy and depression combined are more common than apathy without depression or depression without apathy (Isella et al., 2002). Fatigue can be classified as peripheral and central (Voon & Lang, 2004). Peripheral fatigue is a physiological phenomenon that involves lack of energy associated with muscular fatigue, and is measured objectively by decreased force generation or the inability to sustain repetitive movements (Lou et al., 2001). Central fatigue is generally described as an abnormal degree of persistent tiredness, weakness or exhaustion that can be mental, physical or both in the absence of motor and physical impairment (Lou et al., 2001). Physical fatigue represents the sense of physical exhaustion and lack of energy to perform physical tasks despite the ability to do so. Mental fatigue refers to the effects experienced during and after prolonged periods of demanding cognitive activities that require sustained mental efficiency. Fatigue exerts its main effects on quality of life, depression, and disability in PD and is the major determinant of work-related disability (Martinez-Martin et al., 2006; Zesiewicz et al., 2007). For apathy and fatigue, co-existence of depression and cognitive deficits and their overlap with motor signs of PD, contribute to diagnostic challenges. For apathy, Marin's criteria of reduced goal-directed behavior, cognition and emotional concomitants of goal-directed behavior are the most widely used (Marin, 1997). Distinguishing apathy from depression requires evidence for emotional features such as low mood, reduced levels of pleasure, guilt and anxiety in patients with a concurrent depressive disorder. A number of fatigue-rating scales have been developed for the general population and for specific conditions (Dittner et al.,2004).The Parkinson's fatigue scale was developed as a disease specific scale and is widely used (Brown et al.,2005).Treatments for both apathy and fatigue include illness education to families and patients about depression, fatigue, apathy and cognitive decline in PD, behavioral strategies to maximize executive functions and use of medication to treat mood disorders and cognitive impairment. It's very important to know that improvement of comorbid conditions may be sufficient to relieve apathy and fatigue. Non pharmacological strategies with an individualized daily schedule and structure with varied activities and group therapy help to maintain a satisfactory activity level. Possible medications include dopamine agonists, psychostimulants, modafinil and testosterone (Campbell & Duffy, 1997; Friedman et al., 2007).

5.3 Hallucinations and psychosis

The main psychotic symptoms noted in PD include, visuoperceptual symptoms such as visual hallucinations, illusions, and delusions. Auditory hallucinations may also occur but usually together with visual hallucinations. Psychotic symptoms may be mild or severe, occur either in combination or alone, may be accompanied by behavioral disturbances and require hospitalization. Psychotic features may affect up to 50% of patients with PD (Graham et al.,1997) and when present, tend to be persistent and progressive (Factor et al.,2003).The typical visual hallucinations consist of persons, familiar or not, and less often animals or objects. They are usually complex and stereotype and often occur in dim light, and at night. The neuropsychiatric symptoms in PD tend to cluster into distinct syndromes. It's very important, for the clinician to examine for these phenomena because these symptoms are not always reported voluntarily. Some patients may deny or refuse to report these symptoms, therefore the clinician should also ask relatives. There are several rating scales that can be utilized, although no one is generally accepted. Item 2 of UPDRS subscale 1 and the neuropsychiatric inventory are most often used. More detailed assessments can be made using specific scales such as the Parkinson psychosis rating scale. Psychotic symptoms develop from extrinsic and intrinsic factors. It was previously considered that visual hallucinations in patients with Parkinson's disease were caused by dopaminergic medications. However, it is now generally accepted that although dopaminergic drugs and especially dopamine agonists, can contribute to psychosis, other factors may be more important such as dementia, visuospatial impairment, old age and advanced disease stage. It is now well known that psychotic symptoms may occur during the night and are associated with sleep disturbances and vivid dreams that may lead to hallucinations. Non pharmacological approaches such as information about the nature of these phenomena may help. A cognitive approach is also very useful, such as distraction or re-directing attention. Improvement of light conditions and visual aids may also help (Diederich et al., 2003). It's crucial to search for general medical conditions such as infection, pain, metabolic disorders, dehydration, and recent changes in medication. Concerning the pharmacological approach for psychotic symptoms in patients with PD, the reduction of dose or number of drugs may reduce these symptoms without worsening the motor condition. For example anticholinergic drugs must be withdrawn first. It is better to withdraw selegiline first, amantadine and dopamine agonists before changing the L-dopa dose. The drug that is recommended is clozapine, which has been shown to reduce visual hallucinations without worsening motor features. Other agents such as risperidone and olanzapine are less effective and with a higher risk for worsening motor symptoms, cognitive decline and confusion (Miyasaki et al., 2006). Finally, initial open label reports on quetiapine were promising although two placebo controlled trials were negative.

5.4 Sleep disorders

Between 60-98% of patients with Parkinson's disease experience a sleep disorder (Stacy, 2002). These disorders include excessive daytime sleepiness, sleep attacks, advanced sleep phase syndrome, early morning awakenings and Rapid Eye Movement Sleep Behavior Disorder (RBD). Advanced stages of PD are associated with circadian rhythm disruption. Only few of these sleep disorders are treatable with dopaminergic therapy, and in fact, many are the side effects of treatment. The pathophysiological mechanism of circadian rhythm disruption in PD is not fully understood, and is complicated by the concomitant use of PD medications, as well as other medications such as antidepressants and stimulants, which are known to disrupt sleep architecture. RBD may respond to night-time clonazepam or melatonin (Gagnon et al., 2006). Modafinil 200-400mg per day is effective in treatment of excessive daytime sleepiness and the sedative effects of anti parkinsonian medications (Adler et al., 2003). Finally, nocturnal administration of sodium oxybate has been found to improve excessive daytime sleepiness and fatigue in patients with Parkinson's disease (Ondo et al., 2008).

6. SPECT neuroimaging

Perfusion brain single photon emission computed tomography (SPECT) provides a well-established means of studying regional cerebral blood flow (rCBF) which is known to reflect cortical function. On the other hand Dopamine Transporter (DAT) SPECT imaging can be used as a marker for the degree of loss of dopaminergic nerve endings. It is well known that SPECT Neuroimaging can assist in the differential diagnosis of parkinsonian and dementia syndromes and DAT SCAN can also be helpful in differentiating tremors resulting from damage to the nigrostriatal dopaminergic terminals from those due to essential tremor, drug-induced or psychogenic causes (Benamer et al., 2000). SPECT can also be useful in monitoring disease progression as well as providing information about the pathophysiological process in PD (Burn et al., 2003). Numerous studies during the last decade have attempted to investigate differences and associations between cortical perfusion, nigrostriatal dopamine pathway and neuropsychological functions in demented and non demented patients with PD. These studies show a tendency towards increased hypoperfusion in parietal and temporal lobes in PDD as compared to the non demented PD patients (Derejko et al., 2006; Liu et al., 1992; Matsui et al., 2005).There are also conflicting results in the literature regarding PD patients with MCI ranging from either no difference compared to controls (Sawada et al., 1992; Spampinato et al.,1991) or to hypoperfusion in the parietal (Wallin et al.,2007) and frontal areas (Antonini et al.,2001; Firbank et al.,2005; Paschali et al.,2009). Regarding rCBF and neuropsychological functions in different stages of PD, as dopaminergic nerve endings degenerate in PD there is progressive cortical hypoperfusion affecting mainly the frontal lobes in the early stages, extending to the parietal and temporal lobes in the late stages of Parkinson's disease. In parallel, neuropsychological performance gradually deteriorates as the disease progresses (Paschali et al., 2010).

7. Studies investigating correlations between cortical perfusion, nigrostriatal dopamine pathway and neuropsychological functions in PD patients

A study using 18F fluorodeoxyglucose positron emission tomography and neuropsychological tests identified a cognitive network associated with hypermetabolism of the medial and anterior temporal lobe, pons and cerebellum, concomitant to metabolic decreases in the parieto-occipital cortex that was related to mnemonic and visuospatial deficits in non-demented PD patients (Mentis, et al., 2002)

Another FDG-PET study in non-demented PD patients revealed a correlation of performance on tests of memory, visuospatial function and perceptual motor speed with a cognitive pattern characterized by metabolic reductions in frontal and parietal association areas and relative increases in the cerebellar vermis and dentate nuclei which was not altered by routine antiparkinsonian treatment (Huang, et al., 2007)

Marie et al. (1995) found verbal working memory performance to correlate positively with resting brain glucose metabolism in the dorsolateral prefrontal cortex. The same group in another study reported a correlation between working memory functions and striatal uptake of [^{11}C]-S-nomifensine, a radioligand for the presynaptic dopamine and noradrenaline transporters (Marie et al., 1999). Holthoff-Deto et al. (1997) found that deficits in paired associate learning in a subgroup of moderately to severe PD patients was shown to correlate with [^{18}F] dopa binding in the caudate nucleus. Further, Muller et al. (2000) found impaired prefrontal cognitive functions and preserved short-term memory, in a combined neuropsychological and neuroimaging study of twenty PD patients without dementia or depression. DAT density in the putamen as evaluated by [^{123}I]β-CIT SPECT was related to the severity of motor deficits and cognitive functions correlated with the integrity of both striatal compartments. The authors concluded that the striatum is part of a neuronal network mediating prefrontal cognitive tasks. Another study by Antonini et al (2001) found significant decrements in frontal lobe perfusion in PD patients without cognitive impairment. This data is consistent with the presence of reduced frontal lobe activity and may be related to reduced dopaminergic input from the basal ganglia to this region. Conversely, in the demented group, the study found more diffused cortical perfusion defects involving the temporal and parietal cortex. This finding is consistent with the neuropathological finding that neocortical cholinergic activity is depleted in patients with

PDD. In a longitudinal of 44 consecutive patients at an early stage of PD by Dujardin and colleagues (2004), 3 years after diagnosis, a proportion of patients showed reduced overall cognitive efficiency, a subcorticofrontal syndrome and more severe motor symptoms as measured by the motor UPDRS score. At the time of diagnosis, best predictors of this progression were specific cognitive scores, such as the interference index from the Stroop word-colour test and the number of animal nouns named on the semantic word fluency task, as well as more general variables such as the educational level and the MMSE score. Other indices that contributed to a lesser extent were specific cognitive scores, such as delayed recall in the Grober&Buschke test, the Mattis DRS score and SPECT measurements such as the left Temporal-Insular, Left Temporal-Parietal-Occipital, Right Temporal-Insular and Left lenticular nucleus regional cerebral blood flow.

In another study, Osaki et al (2005) identified regions with a reduced regional cerebral blood flow using the 3D-Stereotactic Surface Projection [^{123}I] IMP-SPECT in cases for which the original diagnosis was PD. Multiple hypoperfusion areas were also observed in this analysis. There were significant correlations between clinical manifestations and regional hypoperfusion, namely between the presence of dementia and the bilateral posterior cingulated areas, and between fluctuating cognition and the bilateral parietal association areas, medial parietal lobes and dorsal occipital lobes. Derejko and colleagues (2006) observed significantly greater bilateral temporal and left parietal decrease of regional cerebral blood flow in PDD patients as compared to a group without cognitive impairment. This pattern of perfusion deficits described as 'a posterior' type of hypoperfusion resembles the one mostly described in Alzheimer's disease, except that defects were often unilateral, whereas predominantly bilateral defects are seen in AD. Hypoperfusion within the left temporal cortex with additional hyperperfusion in the ipsilateral thalamus were the most significant factors associated with cognitive decline and dementia.

In a study by Firbank et al (2005) the aim was to monitor perfusion changes over a one-year period in subjects with PDD compared to a group with DLB, and also healthy controls, and to relate any perfusion changes to cognitive impairment or motor functioning. The authors hypothesized that cortical (parieto-occipital) changes would be associated with worsening of cognitive function, and basal ganglia changes with progression of motor features. The main finding of this study was a bilateral increase in perfusion in the putamen of DLB patients over a year, and a correlation between increased striatal perfusion and worsening motor symptoms in both PDD and DLB. The authors postulate, that this is associated with continued dopaminergic degeneration, a process which may appear more pronounced in DLB because of the relatively more intact nigrostriatal dopaminergic system at the baseline scan compared to PDD, perhaps due to the shorter duration of Parkinsonism. In another study by Colloby et al (2005), the authors investigated the progression of dopaminergic degeneration in patients with DLB, PD and PDD and healthy controls using serial SPECT imaging with ^{123}I-FP-CIT, a marker for dopamine transport, using a semi-automated region of interest approach. This study found that serial FP-CIT over 1 year demonstrated progressive dopaminergic loss compared with controls in DLB, PD and PDD, and showed that serial dopaminergic SPECT may be useful in monitoring disease progression in DLB, PD as well as PDD. Dementia severity and motor impairment were predictors of percentage decline, suggesting that dopaminergic loss may play an important role in the development of cognitive as well as motor features.

In another study comparing SPECT findings between patients with PD and DLB by Chang et al (2008), significant perfusion differences in bilateral temporal areas were noted between the DLB and PD groups, with a lower perfusion index in the DLB group. On the other hand, Rossi and colleagues (2009) concluded that neither FP-CIT nor ECD-SPECT investigations were able to discriminate between DLB and PDD in vivo. These findings might support the theory that PDD and DLB share clinical and neurobiological characteristics within a Parkinson-Dementia spectrum. Moreover, the perfusional cortical pattern of both PDD and DLB is unrelated to dopaminergic impairment evaluated either clinically or by means of ^{123}I-FP-CIT SPECT and it may be due to different neurochemical systems impairment. Wallin et al (2007) note in their study that reductions of cortical blood flow in PD patients with cognitive impairment indicate cortical brain dysfunction. In the PDD group, the regional cerebral blood flow reductions were extensive and bilaterally symmetric, involving both anterior and posterior brain regions. In the PD-MCI group, individual variations were seen, but a nonsignificant reduction in the posterior brain regions was the most prominent finding. These findings suggest once more that there is an associatiom between the degree of cognitive impairment and the magnitude of cortical brain dysfunction in PD patients. In addition, hypoperfusion in the left inferior parietal lobule and supramarginal gyrus has been reported in a small group of PD-MCI patients with low performance in the frontal assessment battery (Matsui et al., 2006).

In another study by Nobili et al (2009), that investigated cortical dysfunction in PD-MCI patients, the authors found a posterior parietal-occipital hypoperfusion pattern in PD-MCI, maximally expressed in the comparison with both healthy subjects and common amnestic MCI patients, and more slightly in comparison with cognitively unimpaired PD patients. These findings are consistent with the hypothesis that PD patients with MCI of the amnestic type may be at high risk of developing PDD, by sharing a similar posterior pattern of cortical dysfunction. Finally, a recent study by Nobili and colleagues (2010) showed that the associations between nigrostriatal and cognitive functions are different for the nigro-caudate and for the nigro-putaminal endings in PD, whereas in the control group nigrostriatal and cognitive functions are not correlated. In de novo PD patients, the nigro-caudate dysfunction is significantly correlated to executive functions. This result is in keeping with other studies, highlighting the relationships between nigro-caudate impairment and executive dysfunction in PD. In this study, the motor severity of the disease was not correlated to executive functions and just marginally to caudate uptake.

A PET study using an alpha4beta2*-nAChR-specific radioligand provided in vivo evidence that there is a broad reduction of alpha4beta2*-nAChR availability in patients with PD without clinically manifest dementia or depression compared with healthy volunteers. Reduced alpha4beta2*-nAChR binding in patients with PD within the subcortical and cortical regions was associated with the severity of mild cognitive or depressive symptoms (Meyer et al., 2009)

8. Studies contributing to the neuropsychological and SPECT neuroimaging literature in PD conducted at the University of Patras Medical School

In our first study (Paschali et al., 2009) we examined relationships between neuropsychological functions and brain single photon emission computed tomography (SPECT) regional cerebral blood flow observed at presurgical evaluation for deep brain stimulation (DBS) of the subthalamic nucleus (STN) in advanced PD patients. Twenty advanced non-demented PD patients, candidates for DBS surgery, underwent perfusion brain SPECT study and neuropsychological assessment prior to surgery (range 30-50 days). Patients were further assessed using the Unified Parkinson's Disease Rating Scale (UPDRS) and Hoehn and Yahr (H&Y) scale. During all assessments patients were on standard medication. Neurogam Software, which permits voxel by voxel analysis, was used to compare the brain perfusion of PD patients with a normal database adjusted for sex and age. Neuropsychological scores were compared to age, education and sex- adjusted normative databases. Our results indicated that the distribution of rCBF showed significant differences when compared to an age and sex-adjusted normative database. We found impaired blood flow in 17 (85%) of our patients in the left prefrontal lobe, in 14 (70%) in the right prefrontal lobe and in 11 (55%) in the left frontal and right parietal lobes. Neuropsychological testing revealed that 18 (90%) of our patients had significant impairments in measures of executive functions (set-shifting) and 15 (75%) in response inhibition. Furthermore we found significant correlations between measures of visual attention, executive functions and the right frontal lobe region. The presence of widespread blood flow reduction was observed mainly in the frontal lobes of non-demented patients with advanced PD. Furthermore, performance on specific cognitive measures was highly related to perfusion brain SPECT findings. Frontal lobe dysfunctions in PD have also been reported from other studies as mentioned above. In a recent review by Zgaljardic et al., (2003), frontostriatal circuit impairments in PD were described and it was suggested that the anterior cingulated cortex was related to conflict monitoring, motivation, response initiation and apathy. Moreover, they showed that the dorsolateral prefrontal cortex was related to working memory, set shifting, conditioned associate learning, set maintenance and memory retrieval, while the orbitofrontal cortex was related to stimulus-driven behavior, disinhibition, and impulse control.

In our second study (Paschali et al., 2010), we investigated differences and associations between cortical perfusion, nigrostriatal dopamine pathway and neuropsychological functions in different stages of PD. We recruited 53 non-demented PD patients divided into four groups according to the Hoehn and Yahr staging system and 20 healthy controls who were used in the comparison of the neuropsychological findings. Each patient underwent two separate brain single photon emission computed tomography (SPECT) studies (perfusion and dopamine transporter binding) as well as neuropsychological evaluation. Perfusion images of each patient were quantified and compared with a normative database provided by the Neurogam software manufacturers. Mean values obtained from the cortical areas and neuropsychological measures in the different groups were also compared by analysis of covariance (ANCOVA) controlling for disease duration and educational level. We found cognitive deficits especially in the late PD stages (HY 3, 4, 5) compared to the early stages (HY 1, 2) and associations between cognitive decrements and cortical perfusion deterioration mainly in the frontal and posterior cortical areas. Compared with controls, PD patients showed impairments of cognition and cerebral perfusion that increased with clinical severity. Furthermore, we found a significant correlation between the performance on the phonemic fluency task and regional cerebral blood flow in the left frontal lobe. Dopamine transporter binding in the left caudate nucleus significantly correlated with blood flow in the left dorsolateral prefrontal cortex, but not with measures of executive functions. We reached the conclusion that there are significant cognitive and perfusion deficits associated with PD progression, implying a multifactorial neurodegeneration process apart from dopamine depletion in the substantia nigra pars compacta. As dopaminergic nerve endings degenerate in PD, there is a progressive cortical hypoperfusion affecting mainly the frontal lobes in the early stages, extending to the parietal and temporal lobes in the late stages of the disease. In parallel, neuropsychological performance gradually deteriorates as the disease progresses. The findings of this study support the multifactorial degeneration process in PD, as the degeneration of the nigrosrtiatal pathway of dopamine alone, cannot explain the perfusion and cognitive deficits in PD progression

9. Conclusions

DAT reduction correlates with dopamine neuron loss in the substantia nigra and striatum which is characteristic for PD. Neuropsychological deficits in the disease cannot be explained by dopamine loss alone as indicated by neuroimaging studies using DAT radiotracers. Thus further evidence is provided through these studies that additional changes occur in the brains of PD patients. Studies of regional cerebral blood flow in PD as an indicator of cognitive impairment show a more diffuse reduction in cortical metabolism as a result of disease progression and transition to dementia. On the other hand the identification of certain metabolic brain networks associated with cognitive functions in non-demented PD patients may provide a tool in clinical trials targeting the progression of non-motor manifestations of the disease and the possible efficacy of new drugs to be tested in PD. The differential diagnosis between PDD and other parkinsonian syndromes with dementia may be assisted but is not yet clearly established by PET and SPECT. The recent development of novel radioligands for use in PET studies point to the role of other neurotransmitter deficits such as the cholinergic deficit in cognitive impairment in PD. SPECT neuroimaging may therefore be useful not only in understanding the pathophysiology of the disease and cognitive impairment but also for clinical monitoring in research studies in PD.

10. References

Aarsland, D. et al. (1999). Range of neuropsychiatric disturbances in patients with Parkinson's disease. *J Neurol Neurosurg Psychiatry*, 67, 492-496.

Aarsland, D. et al. (2001). Risk of dementia in Parkinson's disease: a community -based, prospective study. *Neurology*, 56, 730-36.

Aarsland, D., Cummings, J. & Larsen, J. (2001). Neuropsychiatric differences between Parkinson's disease with dementia and Alzheimer's disease. *Intern Journ of Geriatric Psychiatry*, 16, 184-191.

Aarsland, D. et al. (2003). Performance on the dementia rating scale in Parkinson's disease with dementia and dementia with Lewy bodies: comparison with progressive supranuclear palsy and Alzheimer's disease. *J Neurol Neurosurg Psychiatry*, 74, 1215-1220.

Aarsland, D. et al. (2010). Mild cognitive impairment in Parkinson disease, A multicenter pooled analysis. *Neurology*, 75, 12, 1062-1069.

Adler, CH. et al. (2003). Randomized trial of modafinil for treating subjective daytime sleepiness in patients with Parkinson's disease. *Mov Disord*, 18, 287-293.

Alexander, GE.; Delong, MR & Strick, PL. (1986). Parallel organization of functionally segregated circuits linking basal ganglia and cortex. *Annu Rev Neurosci*, 9, 357-81.

Alves, G. et al. (2004). Is fatigue an independent and persistent symptom in patients with Parkinson's disease? *Neurology*, 63, 1908-1911.

Alves, G. et al. (2006). Changes in motor subtype and risk for incident dementia in Parkinson's disease. *Mov Disord*, 21(8), 1123-30.

Antonini, A. et al. (2001). Perfusion ECD/SPECT in the characterization of cognitive deficits in Parkinson's disease. *Neurol Sci*, 22, 45-46.

Ballard, CG. et al. (2002). Fluctuations in attention: PD dementia vs DLB with parkinsonism. *Neurology*, 59, 1714-1720.

Beatty, WW. et al. (2003). Analyzing the subcortical dementia syndrome of Parkinson's disease using the RBANS. *Arch Clin Neuropsychol*, 18, 509-520. Benamer, HTS. et al. (2000). Accurate differentiation of Parkinsonism and essential tremor using visual assessment of ^{123}I-FP-CIT SPECT imaging : the ^{123}I-FP-CIT study group. *Mov Disord*, 15, 503-510.

Boller, F. et al. (1984). Visuospatial impairment in Parkinson's disease : role of perceptual and motor factors. *Arch Neurol*, 41, 485-90.

Bondi, MW.; Kaszniak, AW.; Bayles, KA. &Vance, KT. (1993). Contribution of frontal system dysfunction to memory and perceptual abilities in Parkinson's disease. *Neuropsychology*, 7, 89-102.

Braak, H. et al. (2004). Stages in the development of Parkinson's disease-related pathology. *Cell Tissue Res*, 318, 121-134.

Braak, H. et al. (2005). Cognitive status correlates with neuropathological stage in Parkinson disease. Neurology, 64, 1404-1410.

Brown, RG. et al. (2005). The Parkinson fatigue scale. *Parkinsonism Relat Disord*, 11, 49-55.

Burn, D. & O'Brien, J. (2003). Use of Functional Imaging an Parkinsonism and Dementia. *Movement Disorders*, 18, Suppl.6, S88-S95.

Buter, TC. et al. (2008). Dementia and survival in Parkinson's disease: a 12-year population study. *Neurology*, 70 (13), 1017-22.

Cahn-Weiner, DA. et al. (2002). Cognitive and behavioral features discriminate between Alzheimer's and Parkinson's disease. *Neuropsychiatry Neuropsychol Behav Neurol* , 15, 79-87.

Campbell, JJ. & Duffy, DJ. (1997). Treatment strategies in amotivated patients. *Psychiatr Ann*, 27, 44-49.

Caviness, J. et al. (2007). Defining Mild Cognitive Impairment in Parkinson's disease. *Movement Disorders*, 22, 9, 1272-1277.

Chang, C.-C. et al. (2008). ^{99m}Tc-ethyl cysteinate dimer brain SPECT findings in early stage of dementia with Lewy bodies and Parkinson's disease patients: a correlation with neuropsychological tests. *European Journal of Neurology*, 15, 61-65.

Cole, K. & Vaughan, FL. (2005). The feasibility of using cognitive behavior therapy for depression associated with Parkinson's disease: a literature review. *Parkinsonism Relat Disord*, 11, 269-276.

Colloby, SJ. et al. (2005). Progression of dopaminergic degeneration in dementia with Lewy bodies and Parkinson's disease with and without dementia assessed using ^{123}I-FP-CIT SPECT. *European Journal of Nuclear Medicine and Molecular Imaging*, 32, 10, 1176-1185.

Cools, R.; Barker, RA.; Sahakian, BJ. & Robbins, TW. (2001). Enhanced or impaired cognitive function in Parkinson's disease as a function of dopaminergic medication and task demands. *Cereb Cortex*, 11, (12), 1136-43.

Cools, R. (2006). Dopaminergic modulation of cognitive function –implications for L-DOPA treatment in Parkinson's disease. *Neurosci Biobehav Rev,* 30, 1-23.

Cummings, JL.; Darkins, A.; Mendez, M.; Hill, MA. & Benson, DF. (1988). Alzheimer's disease and Parkinson's disease: comparison of speech and language alterations. *Neurology*, 38, 680–84.

Cummings, JL. (1988). Intellectual impairment in Parkinson's disease : clinical, pathologic, and biochemical correlates. *J Geriatr Psychiatry Neurol,* 1, 24-36.

Derejko, M. et al. (2006). Regional cerebral blood flow in Parkinson's disease as an indicator of cognitive impairment. *Nuclear Medicine Communications*, 27, 945-951.

Diederich, NJ.; Pieri, V. & Goetz, CG. (2003). Coping strategies for visual hallucinations in Parkinson's disease. *Mov Disord, 18, 831-832.*

Dittner, AJ. et al. (2004). The assessment of fatigue : a practical guide for clinicians and researchers. *J Psychosom Res,* 56, 157-170.

Dubois, B. & Pillon, B. (1997). Cognitive deficits in Parkinson's disease. *Neurol*, 244, 2-8.

Dujardin, K. et al. (2004). Cognitive and Spect characteristics predict progression of Parkinson's disease in newly diagnosed patients. *J Neurol,* 251, 1383-1392.

Dujardin, K. et al. (2007). Characteristics of apathy in Parkinson's disease. *Mov Disord*, 22, 778-784.

Emre, M. et al. (2004). Rivastigmine for dementia associated with Parkinson's disease. *N Engl J Med*, 351, 2509-2518.

Emre, M. (2004). Dementia in Parkinson's disease : cause and treatment
Curr Opin Neurol, 17 (4), 399-404.

Factor, SA. et al. (2003). Longitudinal outcome of Parkinson's disease patients with psychosis. *Neurology*, 60, 1756-1761.

Firbank, M.; Burn, D.; McKeith, I. & O'Brien, J. (2005). Longitudinal study of cerebral blood flow SPECT in Parkinson's disease with dementia, and dementia with Lewy bodies. *International Journal of Geriatric Psychiatry*, 20, 776-782.

Foltynie, T. et al. (2004). The cognitive ability of an incidence cohort of Parkinson's patients in the UK. The CamPaIGN study. *Brain*,127 (Pt3), 550-560.

Friedman, JH. et al. (2007). Fatigue in Parkinson's disease : a review. *Mov Disord*, 22, 297-308.

Gagnon, JF.; Postuma, RB. & Montplaisir, J. (2006). Update on the pharmacology of REM sleep behavior disorder. *Neurology*, 67, 742-747.

Goldenberg, G.; Wimmer, A.; Auff, E. & Schnaberth, G. (1986). Impairment of motor planning in patients with Parkinson's disease: evidence from ideomotor apraxia testing. *J Neurol Neurosurg Psychiatry*, 49, 1266–72.

Gotham, AM. et al. (1986). Depression in Parkinson's disease : a quantitative and qualitative analysis. *J Neurol Neurosurg Psychiatry*, 49, 381-389.

Graham, JM.; Grunewald, RA. & Sagar, HJ.(1997). Hallucinosis in idiopathic Parkinson's disease. *J Neurol Neurosurg Psychiatry*, 63, 434-440.

Grossman, M. et al. (1991). Sentence comprehension and praxis deficits in Parkinson's disease. *Neurology*, 41, 1620-26.

Grossman, M. et al. (1992). Sentence comprehension in Parkinson's disease: the role of attention and memory. *Brain Lang*, 42, 347-84.

Helkala, EL.; Laulumaa, V.; Soininen, H. & Riekkinen, PJ. (1989) Different error pattern of episodic and semantic memory in Alzheimer's disease and Parkinson's disease with dementia. *Neuropsychologia*, 27, 1241–48.

Hietanen, M. & Teravainen, H. (1988). The effect of age of disease onset on neuropsychological performance in Parkinson's disease. *J Neurol Neurosurg Psychiatry*, 51, 244-49.

Hobson, P. & Meara, J. (2004). Risk and incidence of dementia in a cohort of older subjects with Parkinson's disease in the United Kingdom. *Mov Disord*, 19 (9), 1043-9.

Holthoff-Detto, VA. et al. (1997). Functional effects of stiatal dysfunction in Parkinson disease. *Arch Neurol*, 54 (2), 145-50.

Huang, C. et al. (2007). Metabolic brain networks associated with cognitive function in Parkinson's disease. *Neuroimage*, 34 (2), 714-23.

Huber, SJ.; Shuttleworth, EC. & Freidenberg, DL. (1989). Neuropsychological differences between the dementias of Alzheimer's and Parkinson's diseases. *Arch Neurol*, 46, 1287–91.

Hughes, TA. et al. (2000). A 10-year study of the incidence and factors predicting dementia in Parkinson's disease. *Neurology*, 54, 1596-602.

Isella, V. et al. (2002). Clinical, Neuropsychological and morphometric correlates of apathy in Parkinson's disease. *Mov Disord*, 17, 366-371.

Jacobs, DM. et al. (1995). Neuropsychological characteristics of preclinical dementia in Parkinson's disease. *Neurology*, 45, 1691-96.

Janvin, C. et al. (2003). Neuropsychological profile of patients with Parkinson's disease without dementia. *Dement Geriatr Cogn Disord*, 15, 126-131.

Janvin, C. et al. (2006). Subtypes of Mild Cognitive Impairment in Parkinson's Disease: Progression to Dementia. *Movement Disorders*, 21, 9, 1343-1349.

Karlsen, KH. et al. (1998). Quality of life measurements in patients with Parkinson's disease: a community based study. *Eur. J Neurol*, 5, 443-450.

Leentjens, et al. (2008). Anxiety rating scales in Parkinson's disease: critique and recommendations. *Mov Disord*, 23, 2015-2025.

Levin, et al. (1991). Visuospatial impairment in Parkinson's disease. *Neurology*, 41, 365–69.

Levin, BE.; Tomer, R. & Rey, GJ. (1992). Cognitive impairments in Parkinson's disease. *Neurol. Clin*, 10, 471-8.

Levy, G. (2007). The relationship of Parkinson disease with aging. *Arch Neurol*, 64 (9), 1242-6.

Levy, ML. et al. (1998). Apathy is not Depression. *J Neuropsychiatry Clin Neurosci*, 10, 314-319.

Liu, RS. et al. (1992). Cognition and 99Tcm-HMPAO SPECT in Parkinson's disease. *Nucl Med Commun*, 13, 744-8.

Litvan, I.; Mohr, E.; Williams, J.; Gomez, C. & Chase, TN. (1991). Differential memory and executive functions in demented patients with Parkinson's and Alzheimer's disease. *J Neurol Neurosurg Psychiatry*, 54, 25–29.

Lou, JS. et al. (2001). Exacerbated physical fatigue and mental fatigue in Parkinson's disease. *Mov Disord*, 16, 190-196.

Mandir, AS. & Vaughan, C. (2000). Pathophysiology of Parkinson's disease. *Int Rev Psychiatry*, 12, 270-80.

Maricle, RA. et al. (1995). Dose-response relationship of levodopa with mood and anxiety in fluctuating Parkinson's disease: a double-blind, placebo-controlled study. *Neurology*, 45, 1757-1760.

Marie, RM. et al. (1995). PET imaging of neocortical monoaminergic terminals in Parkinson's disease. *J Neyral Transm Park Dis Dement Sect*, 9 (1), 55-71.

Marie, RM. et al. (1999). Relationships between striatal dopamine denervation and frontal executive tests in Parkinson's disease. *Neurosci Lett*, 260, 77-80.

Marin, RS. (1997). Differential diagnosis of apathy and related disorders of diminished motivation. *Psychiatr Ann*, 27, 30-33.

Martin, WE.; Loewenson, RB.; Resch, JA.& Baker, AB. (1973). Parkinson's disease: clinical analysis of 100 patients. *Neurology*, 23, 783-790.

Martinez-Martin, P. et al. (2006). Impact of fatigue in Parkinson's disease : the fatigue impact scale for daily use. *Qual Life Res*, 15, 597-606.

Matsui, H. et al. (2005). N-isopropyl-p-123I iodoamphetamine single photon emission computed tomography study of Parkinson's disease with dementia. *Intern Med*, 44, 1046-50.

Matsui, H. et al. (2006). Frontal assessment battery and brain perfusion image in Parkinson's disease. *J Geriatr Psychiatry Neurol*, 19, 41-45.

Mattay, VS. et al. (2002). Dopaminergic modulation of cortical function in patients with Parkinson's disease. *Ann. Neurol*, 51, 156-64.

Mayeux, R. et al. (1990). An estimate of the incidence of dementia in idiopathic Parkinson's disease. *Neurology*, 40, 1513-17.

Mayeux, R. et al. (1992). A population-based investigation of Parkinson's disease with and without dementia: relationship to age and gender. *Arch Neurol*, 49, 492-97.

Mentis, MJ. et al. (2002). Relationships among the metabolic patterns that correlate with mnemonic, visuospatial, and mood symptoms in Parkinson's disease. *Am J Psychiatry*, 159 (5), 746-54.

Menza, et al. (1993). Parkinson's disease and anxiety: comorbidity with depression. *Biol Psychiatry*, 34, 465-470.

Meyer, PM. et al. (2009). Reduced alpha4beta2*-nicotinic acetylcholine receptor binding and its relationship to mild cognitive and depressive symptoms in Parkinson disease. *Arch Gen Psychiatry*. 66 (8), 866-77.

Mindham, RH.; Ahmed, SW.; & Clough, CG. (1982). A controlled study of dementia in Parkinson's disease. *J Neurol Neurosurg Psychiatry*, 45, 969-74.

Miyasaki, JM. et al. (2006). Practice parameter: evaluation and treatment of depression,psychosis, and dementia in Parkinson's disease (an evidence-based review):report of the Quality Standards Subcomittee of the American Academy of Neurology. *Neurology*, 66, 996-1002.

Mondolo, F. et al. (2007). Evaluation of anxiety in Parkinson's disease with some commonly used rating scales. *Neurol Sci*, 28, 270-275.

Muller, U. et al. (2000). Striatal $[^{123}I]\beta$-CIT SPECT and prefrontal cognitive functions in Parkinson's disease. *J Neural Transm*, 107, 303-319.

Myslobodsky, M.,et al. (2001). Are patients with Parkinson's disease suicidal? *J Geriatr Psychiatry Neurol*, 14, 120-124.

Nissenbaum, H.. et al. (1987). Mood swings associated with the on-off phenomenon in Parkinson's disease. *Psychol Med*, 17, 899-904.

Nobili, F. et al. (2009). Amnestic Mild Cognitive Impairment in Parkinson's Disease: A Brain Perfusion SPECT Study. *Movement Disorders*, 24, 3, 414-421.

Nobili, F. et al. (2010). Cognitive-Nigrostriatal Relationships in De Novo, Drug-Naïve Parkinson's Disease Patients : A [I-123]FP-CIT SPECT Study. *Movement Disorders*, 25, 1, 35-43.

Noe, .E et al. (2004). Comparison of dementia with Lewy bodies to Alzheimer's disease and Parkinson's disease with dementia. *Mov Disord*, 19, 60-67.

Ondo, WG. et al. (2008). Sodium oxybate for excessive daytime sleepiness in Parkinson disease : an open-label polysomnographic study. *Arch Neurol*, 65, 1337-1340.

Osaki, Y. et al. (2005). Three-Dimensional Stereotactic Surface Projection SPECT Analysis in Parkinson's Disease With and Without Dementia, *Movement Disorders*, 20, 8, 999-1005.

Paolo, AM. et al. (1995). Differentiation of the dementias of Alzheimer's and Parkinson's disease with the dementia rating scale. *J Geriatr Psychiatry Neurol*, 8, 184-188.

Parkkinen, L. et al. (2005). Alpha-synuclein pathology does not predict extrapyramidal symptoms or dementia. *,Ann Neurol*, 57 (1), 82-91.

Paschali, A. et al. (2009). Neuropsychological functions and rCBF-SPECT in Parkinson's disease patients considered candidates for deep brain stimulation. *Eur J Nucl Med Mol Imaging*, 36, 1851-1858.

Paschali, A. et al. (2010). SPECT neuroimaging and neuropsychological functions in different stages of Parkinson's disease. Eur J Nucl Mol Imaging, 37 (6), 1128-40.

Petersen, RC. et al. (1999). Mild cognitive impairment : clinical characterization and outcome. *Arch Neurol*, 56, 303-308.

Pillon, B.; Dubois, B.; Lhermitte, F. & Agid, Y. (1986). Heterogeneity ofcognitive impairment in progressivesupranuclear palsy, Parkinson's disease, and Alzheimer's disease. *Neurology*, 36, 1179–85.

Pillon, B.; Dubois, B.; Ploska, A. & Agid, Y. (1991). Severity and specificity of cognitive impairment in Alzheimer's,Huntington's, and Parkinson's diseases and progressive supranuclear palsy. *Neurology*, 41, 634–43.

Pillon, B. et al. (1993). Explicit memory in Alzheimer's disease, Huntington's disease, and Parkinson's disease. *Arch Neurol*, 50, 374-379.

Pluck, GC. & Brown, RG. (2002). Apathy in Parkinson's disease. *J Neurol* Neurosurg *Psychiatry*, 73, 636-642.

Read, N. et al. (2001). Dementia in Parkinson's disease: incidence and associated factors at 14-years of follow up. *Parkinsonism Relat Disord* ,7 (suppl), S109.

Reijnders, JS. et al. (2008). A systematic review of prevalence studies of depression in Parkinson's disease. *Mov Disord*, 23, 183-189.

Remy, P. et al. (2005). Depression in Parkinson's disease : loss of dopamine and noradrenaline innervations in the limbic system. *Brain*, 128, 1314-1322. Richard, IH. (2005). Anxiety disorders in Parkinson's disease. *Adv Neurol*, 96, 42-55.

Rochester, L. et al. (2004). Attending to the task: interference effects of functional tasks on walking in Parkinson's disease and the roles of cognition, depression, fatigue and balance. *Arch Phys Med Rehabil*, 85, 1578-1585.

Rossi, C. et al.(2009). "Parkinson-dementia" diseases : A comparison by double tracer SPECT studies. *Parkinsonism and Related Disorders*, 15, 762-766.

Sawada, H. et al. (1992). SPECT findings in Parkinson's disease associated with dementia. *J Neurol Neurosurg Psychiatry*, 55, 960-3.

Schrag, A.; Jahanshahi, M. & Quinn, N. (2000). What contributes to quality of life in patients with Parkinson's disease? *J Neurol Neurosurg Psychiatry*, 69, 308-312.

Shulman, LM. (2000). Apathy in patients with Parkinson's disease. *Int Rev Psychiatry*, 12, 298-306.

Siemers, ER. et al. (1993). Anxiety and motor performance in Parkinson's disease. *Mov Disord*, 8, 501-506.

Spampinato, U. et al. (1991). 99mTc-HMPAO SPECT and cognitive impairment in Parkinson's disease: a comparison with dementia of the Alzheimer type. *J Neurol Neurosurg Psychiatry*, 54, 787-92.

Stacy, M. (2002). Sleep disorders in Parkinson's disease : epidemiology and management. *Drugs Aging*, 19, 733-739.

Starkstein, SE. et al. (1992). Reliability, validity and clinical correlates of apathy in Parkinson's disease. *J Neuropsychiatry Clin Neurosci*, 4, 134-139.

Starkstein, SE. et al. (1996). Neuropsychological and psychiatric differences between Alzheimer's disease and Parkinson's disease with dementia. *J Neurol Neurosurg Psychiatry*, 61, 381-387.

Stern, Y. et al. (1983). Perceptual motor dysfunction in Parkinson's disease: a deficit in sequential and predictive voluntary movement. *J Neurol Neurosurg Psychiatry*, 46, 145-51.

Stern, Y.; Richards, M.; Sano, M. & Mayeux, R. (1993). Comparison of cognitive changes in patients with Alzheimer's and Parkinson's disease. *Arch Neurol*, 50, 1040–45.

Torack, RM. & Morris, JC. (1988). The association of ventral tegmental area histopathology with adult dementia. *Arch Neurol*, 45, 497-501.

Voon, V. & Lang, E. (2004). Antidepressants in the treatment of psychosis with comorbid depression in Parkinson disease. *Clinical Neuropharmacol*, 27, 90-92.

Wallin, A. et al. (2007). Posterior cortical brain dysfunction in cognitively impaired patients with Parkinson's disease - a rCBF-Scintigraphy study. *Acta Neurol Scand*, 116, 347-354.

Witjas, T. et al. (2002). Nonmotor fluctuations in Parkinson's disease: frequent and disabling. *Neurology*, 59, 408-413.

Zesiewicz, TA. et al. (2007). Social security disability insurance in Parkinson's disease. *Disabil Rehabil*, 29, 1934-1936.

Zgaljardic, DJ. et al. (2003). A review of the cognitive and behavioral sequale of Parkinson's disease: relationship to frontostriatal circuitry. *Cogn Behav Neurol*, 16, 193-210.

5

Imaging Dyskinesias in Parkinson's Disease

Marios Politis and Clare Loane
Centre for Neuroscience, Hammersmith Hospital, Imperial College London, United Kingdom

1. Introduction

Parkinson's disease (PD) is a neurodegenerative movement disorder characterised by the motor features of tremor, rigidity and bradykinesia. These features are associated with the loss of dopaminergic (DA) neurons in the substantia nigra pars compacta and a subsequent deficiency in striatal DA, which is required for the effective control of movements. However, there is evidence of a more diffuse pathology in PD (Braak et al., 2004) with other, non-DA neutotransmitter systems possibly playing a role (Kish et al., 2003, 2008; Remy et al., 2005; Albin et al., 2008; Politis et al., 2010a).

To date, regular administration of the direct metabolic precursor for DA, L-3, 4-dihydroxyphenylalanine (L-DOPA) remains the most effective treatment of PD symptomatology. L-DOPA therapy is most optimally effective in the early stages of the disease and long term use leads to the appearance of motor complications such as involuntary movements, so-called L-DOPA-induced dyskinesia (LID). LID represents a debilitating complication of L-DOPA therapy in PD and is experienced by the vast majority of patients (estimates range between 40-90% between 4 and 10 years after initiation of L-DOPA therapy) (Racol et al, 2000; Ahlskog and Muenter, 2001). The mechanisms underlying LID remain obscure. It is known that LID is observed following DA therapy and that there is a time-lag between the initiation of DA therapy and the emergence of LID. Risk factors commonly associated with the development of LID include PD severity, L-DOPA dose and duration of L-DOPA therapy.

Positron emission tomography (PET) neuroimaging provides a useful tool for assessing *in vivo* functionality of basal ganglia in the PD brain. As such, the use of specific radiotracers permits insight into the integrity of both pre- and postsynaptic DA function, which could help elucidate some of the pathophysiological mechanisms underlying LID. Furthermore, over the last decade or so, PET studies have provided evidence that non-DA neurotransmitter systems may be involved in the development of LID. For example, PET has been used to investigate the role of different neuropeptides in LID, such as opioids and NK1, preliminary findings implicating the role of adenosine A_{2A} receptors and more recently promising results have emerged suggesting that the serotonergic system may possess a valuable role in the emergence of LID in PD.

Taken together, the *in vivo* findings to date have provided valuable information regarding the function of various neurotransmitter systems in the occurrence of LID and support the use of PET brain imaging to further explore these investigations. Considering the promising evidence suggesting that non-DA neurotransmitter systems may have a role in the pathogenesis of LID, further manipulation of these systems may offer an alternative

therapeutic approach in abating LID and preventing their initial development. Such investigations are vital as consequences of LID are pertinent to both the patients' quality of life and healthcare services and costs.
This chapter will review the use of PET imaging in the attempt to delineate the possible mechanisms underlying LID in PD. The imaging data available to date will be discussed supporting these mechanisms in relation to both DA and non-DA neurotransmitter systems including opioid, adenosinergic, glutamatergic and serotonergic systems.

2. LID in PD: incidence and phenomenology

LID is a common complication of L-DOPA treatment. It has been estimated to occur in approximately 40-50% of PD patients 4-6 years post-initiation of L-DOPA treatment (Ahlskog and Muenter, 2001) rising to approximately 90% after 10 years of treatment with an estimated incidence of approximately 10% per year of treatment (Rascol et al., 2000). Studies suggest that LID often initiates in the foot, ipsilateral to the side most affected by PD (Marconi et al., 1994). Somatotopically, the foot area corresponds to the dorsolateral striatum, an area which has been shown to be affected by DA denervation in the early stages of PD and is innervated by the ventrolateral portion of the substantia nigra (Fearnley et al., 1991).
The phenomenology of LID is diverse, encompassing: chorea, athetosis, dystonia, stereotypy and ballism. However, there are three many types of LID observed in PD patients in relation to their L-DOPA treatment. The most common is called 'peak-dose' LID which is characterised by both choreic and dystonic movements occurring during L-DOPA peak plasma concentration (60-90 minutes following L-DOPA administration) (Contin et al., 2000), i.e. when the L-DOPA is optimally abating PD motor symptoms. This type of LID is characterised by a sequence of Improvement-Dyskinesia-Improvement (IDI) and can often be improved by reducing the L-DOPA dose (for review see, Fahn, 2000). A less common form of LID is termed 'biphasic' dyskinesia. This form of LID follows a sequence opposite to the peak-dose form, of Dyskinesia-Improvement-Dyskinesia (DID). A further, form of LID termed 'yo-yo' dyskinesia does not follow an Improvement-Dyskinesia sequence with the involuntary movements appearing and abating at various points throughout the L-DOPA-dose cycle, therefore, it does not seem to be related to L-DOPA dosing (Nutt and Wooton, 1995). Finally, an unusual form of LID occurring when the patient is in an 'off' state, i.e. they are not taking any L-DOPA medication and is termed 'off-phase' dyskinesia. This form of LID has been observed in patients following surgical interventions, such as deep brain stimulation (DBS) and neural transplantation with fetal tissue (Freed et al., 2001; Hagell et al., 2002; Olanow et al., 2003). The off-phase dyskinesia observed following neural transplantation are named, 'graft-induced' dyskinesia (GID) and currently is not known whether they share the same pathogenic mechanisms as LID.
The initial presentation of LID is often mild with the majority of patients preferring to continue the L-DOPA therapy reaping the therapeutic benefits while experiencing some form of LID, rather than terminate L-DOPA therapy with its associated decrease in mobility (Hung et al, 2010). Fatigue and exhaustion levels increase as LIDs develop and there is increased risk of injury for the patient. LID usually appear at the point where the disease is advancing and larger L-DOPA doses are required (Thanvi et al., 2007).
Despite the increased frequency and the clinical significance, the underlying mechanisms of LID in PD are not clear. It has been suggested that the development of LID may be

dependent on several clinical risk factors including, disease severity, extent of DA denervation, and dose and duration of L-DOPA treatment. However, considerable efforts have been devoted to developing neuroimaging techniques to study the basal ganglia (the set of structures most affected by DA denervation leading to PD motor symptoms) (Eidelberg and Edwards, 2000; Feigin et al., 2001; Eidelberg, 2009). PET imaging in particular has provided a useful *in vivo* tool to assess the DA as well as other neurotransmitter systems in relation to LID in PD.

3. Animal models of LID

Two animals models commonly used to investiagte LID pathogenesis are the 1-methyl 4-phenyl 1,2,3,6-tetrahydropyridine [MPTP]-lesioned primate model and 6-hydroxydopamine [6-OHDA]- lesioned rat model. MPTP is a lipophillic substance which can efficiently cross the blood-brain-barrier and subsequently inhibit complex 1 of the mitrochondrial respiratory chain (Heikkila et al., 1985) thus inducing parkinsonian, behavioural, neurochemical and pathological effects (Jenner et al., 1984). The 6-OHDA rat model utilises the 6-OHDA, a nonspecific catecholaminergic toxin. Following administration of the toxin *via* sterotaxial surgery, induction of unilateral lesions along the nigrostrial pathway allow permenant DA depletion and observation of Parkinsonian deficits can be achieved. In both models, L-DOPA is administered to reproduce human LID (dyskinetic group) and compared to at least one control group (non-dyskinetic group) which may or may not be lesioned, but will not have LID induced.

To date, findings from these studies appear to corroborate what is observed clinically; that is, the degree of DA denervation is associated with LID development. However, interesting findings from MPTP-treated models, revealed that primates which did not develop parkinsonian motor symptoms, did go on to develop LID, indicating that the threshold of DA denervation required to induce LID is lower than that of PD sympotmatology (Sassin et al., 1975). Furthermore, LID has been effectively induced in normal, unlesioned primates (Mones et al., 1973). Indeed, L-DOPA dosage in animal studies are invariably much higher than in patients studies or administered in clinic and as such may explain the swift development of LID (Di Monte et al., 2000). Nonetheless, 6-OHDA-lesioned rats has demonstrated that daily administration of L-DOPA induces LID, emerging 20-30 minutes after administration (Lundblad et al., 2002). This observation is comparable to the peak-dose dyskinesia observed in PD patients. Again in 6-OHDA-lesioned rats, L-DOPA dose was shown to modulate dyskinesia development, i.e. a therapeutic dose of L-DOPA (6-10 mg/kg L-DOPA/day) produced LID in nearly all rats within 2-3 weeks compared to a larger L-DOPA dose (50 mg/kg L-DOPA/day) which shortened latency, and increased the severity and incidence of LID induced (Lundblad et al., 2010).

Furthermore, L-DOPA leading to a priming effect has been demonstrated in both 6-OHDA-lesioned rats and MPTP-lesioned primates, with recurrence of LID appearing more readily compared to primates who did not receive any L-DOPA or were only partially lesioned (Cenci et al., 1998; Pearce et al., 1998; Andersson et al., 1999; Johansson et al., 2001; Maratos et al., 2001; Delfino et al., 2004). Moreover, primates who were lesioned, exhibited LID after a single dose of L-DOPA compared to partially lesioned primates where several doses were require before any LID developed (Di Monte et al., 2000). However, it has also been shown that the paradigm of lesion induction or pulsatility of L-DOPA treatment may play a role in LID induction (Jenner, 2003; Schneider et al., 2003). The extent of nigrostrital DA neuronal

loss required before LID is exhibited in 6-OHDA-lesioned rats has been proposed as 80% denervation, indicating that DA denervation is no soley responsible for the induction of LID in rats, and likely not the sole contributory factor in PD patients either (Winkler et al., 2002).
It is generally thought that both presynaptic (production, storage, release and reuptake of DA by dopaminergic neurons in the nigrostriatal pathway) and postsynaptic (receptor and second messenger signaling pathway status in striatal neurons) DA components are critical for the development of LID. A presynaptic mechanism proposed as a contributary factor of LID development relates to the administration of L-DOPA resulting in a dramatic increase in synaptic DA levels subsequently leading to an alteration in the degree of DA receptor stimulation (Carta et al., 2006). Clinically this pathologic mechanism corresponds to peak-dose dyskinesias (de la Feunte-Fernandez et al., 2001, 2004). It has been suggested that a decrease in the pre-synaptic 'buffering' is not dependent upon the degree of pre-synaptic denervation (Sassin et al., 1975).
Postsynaptically, LID may result from dysplastic changes occuring following the destruction of DA input to the striatum and subsequent L-DOPA administration (Hirsch et al., 2000). Alterations at the synpase level may cause a 'denervation sensitivity' and as such modifying the downstream cascade including the second messenger and signalling pathways ultimately leading to the developemnt of dyskinesia (Cenci and Lundblad, 2006; Ulusoy et al., 2010). However, dissociating changes induced by each compartment independently is complicated by the fact that following destruction of the presynaptic DA neurons, plastic changes of the postsynaptic neurons occur simultaneously (Nadjar et al., 2009; Ulusoy et al., 2010).

4. Positron emission tomography

PET is a nuclear imaging technique which allows *in vivo* estimations of important physiological parameters, such as, glucose metabolism and neuroreceptor binding (Table 1.). In PET, radioisotopes bound to specific tracers are administered to an individual *via* an intravenous (IV) injection. After administration, the radiotracer will decay by positron emission, whereby a positron will be emitted (a particle with the opposite electrical charge but same mass as an electron) and then collide and annihilate with an electron, producing a pair of photons. These photons are subsequently detected by the scintillator in the scanner. These measurements allow the final outcome of estimation of the distribution of the radiotracer over time in the brain. The development of various radiotracers for PET has allowed the *in vivo* assessment of various physiological processes in PD which can be applied for the investigation of pathophysiologic mechanisms underlying both motor and non-motor symptomatology. For example, 18-FDG PET has been implemented to assess glucose brain metabolism in PD patients with dementia (Peppard et al., 1992; Goto et al., 1993) and ^{11}C-PK11195 for microglial activation estimation for monitoring disease progression (Ouchi et al., 2005; Teune et al., 2010)
PET has high sensitivity and specificity for detecting striatal DA deficiency, the core pathological feature of PD, and as such provides an excellent tool for gaining greater understanding of the underlying pathological mechanisms leading to the development of LID in PD. The function of the presynaptic DA system in LID pathogenesis has utilised the tracers; ^{11}C-methylphenidate (MP) which targets the DA transpoter (DAT) (Sossi et al., 2007; Troiano et al., 2009), ^{11}C-dihydrotetrabenaine (DHTBZ) which targets the vesicular

monoamine transporter 2 (VMAT2) (Troiano et al., 2009) and Fluorine-18-6-fluoro-L-DOPA (18F-dopa) targeting aminoacid decarboxylase (AADC) PET (de la Feunte-Fernandez et al., 2000). The postsynaptic DA system has been assessed using ^{11}C-raclorpide (RAC) trageting D2/D3 receptors (Kishore et al., 1997; Tortonsen et al., 1997; de la Fuente-Fernandez et al., 2001; Pavese et al., 2006; Turjanski et al., 2007) and ^{11}C-SCH23390 which targets D1 receptors (Kishore et al., 1997; Turjanksi et al., 2007). Due to emerging evedence that non-DA neurotransmitter systems may play a role in the pathogeneisis of dyskinesia tracers such as ^{11}C-diprenorphine (Piccini et al., 1997) and ^{18}F-L829165 (Whone et al., 2002) have permitted *in vivo* investgation of the neuropeptides, μ, κ, δ opioid sites and NK1 receptors respectively. The adenosinergic system has been investiagted with ^{11}C-SCH442416 as a measure of A_{2A} receptors (Ramlackhansingh et al., 2010), the serotonergic system using ^{11}C-DASB as a measure of 5-HT1A binding (Politis et al., 2010b) and the glutamatergic system with ^{11}C-CNS5161 as a marker of activated N-methyl-D-aspartate receptor (NMDA) receptor channels (Ahmed et al., 2010). Knowledge regarding the underlying mechanisms of LID in PD has been greatly advanced by the use of PET imaging tools.

PET tracer	Target	Assessment	Reference
^{11}C-methylphenidate (MP)	DAT	Presynaptic DA system	Sossi et al., (2007); Troiano et al., (2009)
^{11}C-dihydrotetrabenazine (DHTBZ)	VMAT2	Presynaptic DA system	Troiano et al., (2009)
Fluorine-18-6-fluoro-L-DOPA (^{18}F-dopa)	AADC	Monaminergic systems: -Presynaptic DA system - Noradrenergic system - Serotonergic system	de la Feunte-Fernandez et al., (2000)
^{11}C-raclopride (RAC)	D2/D3 receptors	Postsynaptic DA system	Turjanski et al., (2007); Kishore et al., (1997); Tortonsen et al., (1997); de la Fuente-Fernandez et al., (2001); Pavese et al., (2006)
^{11}C-SCH23390	D1 receptors	Postsynaptic DA system	Turjanski et al., (2007); Kishore et al., (1997)
^{11}C-DASB	5-HT1A receptors	Serotonergic system	Politis et al., (2010a)
^{11}C-diprenorphine	μ, κ, δ, opioid sites	Opioid system	Piccini et al., (1997)
^{11}C-SCH442416	Adenosine A_{2A} receptors	Adenosinergic system	Ramlackhansingh et al., (2010)
^{18}F-L829165	NK1 receptors	Substance P	Whone et al., (2002)
11C-CNS 5161	NMDA receptors	Glutamatergic system	Ahmed et al., (2010)

Table 1. PET tracers used to image dyskinesias in PD

5. PET imaging and LID

5.1 Dopaminergic system

The role of DA denervation in the pathogenesis of PD has resulted in the DA neurotransmitter system to have received the most attention in PET studies to date. As both pre- and postsynaptic DA mechanisms are though to be involved in dyskinesia pathogenesis and pathophysiology, the opportunity to choose specific tracers targeting each system independently with PET is an important asset of the technique. A study utilising ^{18}F-dopa PET, a measure of the presynaptic DA system by targeting L-aromatic-amino-acid-decarboxylase (AADC) has reported a 28% decrease in presynaptic terminal function in the putamen in PD subjects who had a fluctuating motor response to L-DOPA ('wearing-off' effect) compared to patients who had a stable response to L-DOPA (de la Feunte-Fernandex et al., 2000). The results of this study suggest two things, i) the observed differences between the groups provides support for the 'storage hypothesis'. This hypothesis states that loss of DA terminals, i.e unable to store and subsequently release DA for use, in the nigrostriatal pathway is responsible for the motor complications observed in PD patients ii) The reported results may reflect an altered 'buffering' capacity of the DA terminals in response to differences in the degree of nigrostriatal damage between groups. However, one limitation of the study relates to the considerable overlap between the two groups studied. This may be indicative of other factors playing a role, such as, postsynaptic mechanisms and increased turnover of DA in the synapse. Another study of presynaptic mechanisms in relation to LID which utilized ^{11}C-methylphenidate (DA transporter [DAT] marker) demonstrated that higher DAT levels were directly related to lower DA turnover and lower changes in the synaptic DA concentration (Sossi et al., 2007). DAT is crucially involved in maintaining consistent levels of DA in the synapse and terminals. Therefore, a decrease in DAT may lead to an increase in DA turnover and higher oscillations in synaptic DA concentration, thus potentially predisposing a PD patient to the occurrence of LID as the disease processes. A more recent study assessing PD patients with motor fluctuations (27/36 patients presenting LID) using ^{11}C-methylphenidate (MP) and DHTBZ PET in combination, demonstrated that putaminal MP/DTBZ was decreased in the motor fluctuating group compared to PD patients with a stable response to L-DOPA (Troiano et al., 2009). These findings add further support for presynaptic alterations playing a role in the appearance of LID due to continued DAT downregulation leading to increased levels of extracellular DA.

In order to assess the postsynaptic DA mechanisms ^{11}C-SCH23390 and RAC have been used in combination to investigate the avaliability of the D1 receptor and D2 receptor subtypes respectively, in two groups of PD patients, one with LID and without LID (Kishore et al., 1997; Turjanski et al., 1997). Findings from these studies suggest that postsynaptic DA D1 and D2 mechanisms are possibly not involved in the pathophysiology of LID in PD. The results demonstrate that the mean D1 receptor availability is within normal range in the caudate nucleus and putamen and mean D2 receptor availability in the putamen during the baseline condition in both groups of PD patients. However, mean D2 receptor availability is reduced in both groups in the caudate nucleus by around 15% in each. It may be that the reductions observed in the caudate are a result of disease progression and not due to the development of LID.

However, utilisation of RAC PET in conjunction with L-DOPA challenge can be used in order to assess *in vivo* increases in synaptic DA by measuring decreases of D2 receptor availability (Tedroff et al., 1996; Endres et al., 1997; de al Fuente-Fernandez et al., 2001, 2004). One of the early RAC PET studies revealed a decrease of RAC binding in the putamen by 23% following a single dose of L-DOPA administered IV compared to 10%

decrease in PD patients with a stable response to L-DOPA (Tortenson et al., 1997), which is suggestive of exogenous L-DOPA provoking greater DA release in the putamen of dyskinetic patients than stable responders. Moreover, Unified Parkinson's Disease Rating Scale (UPDRS) scores in the 'off' medication state were inversely correlated with the reduction of putaminal RAC binding. From these data, it appears that as the disease progresses (as evidenced by the decline in motor function measured by the UPDRS), the regulation of DA release following exogenous administration of L-DOPA is impaired. The cause for this is suggested as the impaired regulation of DA back into the synapse after L-DOPA administration is due to the remaining terminals increased DA synthesis and as such, DAT is unable to compensate by reuptaking the excess DA. Another RAC PET study reported that synaptic levels of DA in PD patients with motor fluctuations were three times higher than in those with a stable response to L-DOPA one hour following administration of an L-DOPA challange (de al Fuente-Fernandez et al., 2001). This result may explain the rapid response to the medication in the motor fluctuating group. Furthermore, stable responders maintained increased DA levels for four hours after L-DOPA administration compared to patients with motor fluctuations, whose synaptic DA levels dropped to baseline ('off') state. More recently, another RAC PET study reported a positive correlation between the presence of LID with increased levels of DA in the synapse (Pavese et al., 2006). More specifically, dyskinetics cases showed significantly decreased levels of putaminal RAC binding reflecting greater levels of synaptic DA, following L-DOPA administration compared to non-dyskinetics. Moreover, the authors correlated L-DOPA induced increases in synaptic DA with corresponding motor scores. It was found that rigidity and bradykinesia but not tremor correlated with DA release in the putamen.

5.2 Opioid system

Opioid neuropeptides are abundant in the basal ganglia as well as the thalamus and association cortex (Haber et al., 1985). Opioid involvement in the pathophysiology of PD has been previously hypothesised from post-mortem studies, however many of these studies are inconsistent with inconclusive and conflicting findings (Rinne et al., 1983; Delay-Goyet et al., 1987; Fernandez et al., 1994). Enkephalin and dynorphin are transmitted by the functionally distinct y-aminobutyric acid (GABA)ergic pathway transmits these neuropeptides to the globus pallidus (both external [GPe] and internal [GPi]) and have been suggested to play a neuromodulatory role in the control of movements (Austin and Kalavis, 1990). It has been suggested that LID may result due to a reduction in the inhibitory output from the thalamus to the GPi (Crossman, 1990). 6-OHDA-lesioned rats have demonstrated an increase of enkephalin in the GPe and striatum following L-DOPA administration (Engberg et al., 1991; Taylor et al., 1992) and MPTP-treated primates have demonstrated high levels of enkephalin gene expression in the putamen of primates exhibiting LID (Jolkkon et al., 1995). Altered opiod transmission in the development of LID has been investigated using ^{11}C-Diprenorphine PET (Piccini et al., 1997). This study demonstrated that dyskinetic PD patients had reduced binding in both striatal (caudate nucleus and putamen) and extra-striatal (thalamus and anterior cingulate) regions compared to PD patients who had a stable response to L-DOPA and no LID. Little is known regarding impact of a dysfunctional opioid system on LID development, however, these results are suggestive that an involvement is possible, considering it is established that the opiod system is involved in the pathophysiology of PD.

5.3 NK1 receptors

^{18}F-L829165 is a selective marker of Neurokinin-1 (NK1) receptor availability. NK1 receptors belong to the family of neuropeptides called Tachykinins and can be found in both the central and peripheral nervous system. A more recent, although, preliminary study has been reported a reduction in thalamic NK1 availability in dyskinetic PD patients while remaining within the normal range in PD with a stable response to L-DOPA (Whone et al., 2002). Overall, these *in vivo* findings are suggestive that the presence of elevated levels of endogenous neuropeptides in the basal ganglia of dyskinetic PD patients may be, in part, responsible for the development of LID.

5.4 Adenosinergic system

There is neurochemical evidence that A_{2A} receptors functionally appose the action of D2 receptors on GABAnergic striatopallidal neurons (Ferre and Fuxe, 1992; Ferre et al., 1993; Fuxe et al., 1993) raising the possibility that A_{2A} antagonists may be able to contribute to the anti-parkinsonian therapeutic benefit observed in DA replacement therapy. Indeed, animal studies have shown that lesioning one side of the DA nigrostriatal pathway by 6-OHDA revealed that blockade of A_{2A} receptors markedly increased the number of contralateral rotations induced buy a threshold dose of L-DOPA or by stimulation of DA receptor stimulation (Pinna et al., 1996; Pollack and Fink, 1996; Fenu et al., 1997; Le Moine et al., 1997). Thus blockade of A_{2A} receptors and as such potentiating DA transmission may contribute to the restoration of motor impairment observed in animal models of PD.

Early clinical data suggests that A_{2A} agonists do not suppress LID in PD patients once LID is established (Hauser et al., 2003), however, preclinical data suggests that a possible role of A_{2A} blockade in the reduction of initial LID emergence when combined with L-DOPA (Pinna et al., 2001). However, the potential therapeutic benefit of A_{2A} agonists are yet to be fully delineated as conflicting evidence has been reported (Lundblad et al., 2003).

To date only one preliminary imaging study has been undertaken to assess the potential role of A_{2A} receptors in LID pathogenesis. The recent study utilised ^{11}C-SCH442416 PET as a marker of A_{2A} receptor function in six PD patients with LID, six PD patients without LID and three healthy controls (Ramlackhansingh et al., 2010). Both PD groups withdrew from medication prior to the scan. Spectral analysis was used to calculate regional volumes of A_{2A} receptor binding distribution in the striatum and thalamus. Results showed a significant increase of striatal A_{2A} binding in the PD patients with LID compared to the PD group without LID and healthy controls which demonstrated a similar degree of striatal A_{2A} binding. Thalamic A_{2A} binding was similar across all three groups. The authors concluded that their results provide a rationale for the use of A_{2A} receptor agonists in the clinical management of LID.

5.5 Glutamatergic system

Glutamate is an excitatory neurotransmitter in the basal ganglia which acts through ionotropic, amino acid derivative, N-Methyl-D-aspartate (NMDA) and the non-NMDA trasnmembrane receptors for glutamate, -amino-3-hydroxy-5-methyl-4-isoxazolepropionic acid (AMPA) and kainite and G-protein coupled metabotropic receptor sybtypes. Within the striatum, NMDA receptors mostly contain the subtypes, NR1, NR2A and NR2B subtypes (Küppenbender et al., 2000). Animal models of PD, including the 6-OHDA-lesioned rat model and MPTP-treated primates, have demonstrated an increase of glutamate neurotransmittion in association with hyperphosphorylation of these receptor subtypes and the development and maintenance of LID.

To date, only one study has attempted to investigate abnormal glutamate function *in vivo* in PD patients in relation to LID (Ahmed et al., 2010). ^{11}C-CNS 5161 PET binds to the MK801 site in the activated voltage-gated ion channels with high affinity (Biegon et al., 2007), and as such, striatal and cortical NMDA glutamate ion channel activity can be assessed in relation to LID. A recent study of 18 PD patients divided into those with LID and those with a stable response to L-DOPA underwent two ^{11}C-CNS 5161 PET scans, one while 'ON' following administration of L-DOPA and another while functionally 'OFF' any DA medication. Results showed reduced binding in the caudate, putamen and motor cortex of the stable responders following administration of L-DOPA. This is in contrast to the LID PD group suggesting that there is a relatively enhanced glutamate receptor activity in the motor areas of this group. The authors suggest that their results justify a rationalization of glutamate antagonist use in the attempt to improve LID in PD patients. However, the authors accept the study is limited by the fact that ^{11}C-CNS 5161 is a selective agonist for MNDA receptors therefore does not provide any information regarding other glutamate receptor subtypes. Although they do suggest that it is likely that other receptor subtypes also become sensitive to L-DOPA.

5.6 Serotonergic system

L-DOPA acts in the early stages of the disease by being taken up into the spared DA terminals, whereby it is converted to DA, stored in synaptic vesicles and then released in an activity-dependent manner. As the disease progresses, there are less DA terminals avaliable for this conversion and as such, it has been suggested that other cell types may become involved in the decarboxylation of L-DOPA in the advanced disease. Serotonergic neurons express AADC and vesicular monamine transporter 2 (VMAT-2), which are involved in the conversion of L-DOPA and which is involved in the storage of DA respectively (Arai et al., 1994, 1995, 1996). Moreover, serotonin neurons in the dorsal and median raphe nuclei innervate the striatum (Lavoie and Parent, 1990; Nicholson et al., 2002). The presence of AADC and VMAT-2 in serotonin neurons provides the possible opportunity for L-DOPA derived DA to be formed, stored and released, thus acting as a 'false neurotransmitter' in serotonergic terminals. However, serotonergic neurons are unable to handle DA release in a regulated manner. Auroreceptor-mediated feedback control and reuptake *via* DAT maintain extracellular DA levels within a narrow physiological range in the DA synapes. The process of DA reuptake allows effective elimination of excess DA from the synaptic cleft, with the D2 autoreceptor maintaining the release from DA terminals in response to changes in the extracellular DA levels (Venton et al., 2003; Cragg et al., 2004) within the desired range. As serotonin neurons do not possess this autoregulatory mechanism, any DA released from serotonergic terminals is likely to generate excessive swings in extracellular levels of DA in response to L-DOPA administration (Carta et al., 2007). To date, the possible role of serotonin in LID has been studied primarily in animal models of PD (Ng et al., 1970, 1971;

Hollister et al., 1979; Lavoie and Parent, 1990; ; Arai et al., 1994, 1995, 1996; Tanaka et al., 1990; Brotchie et al., 2000; Luginer et al., 2000; Obeso et al., 2000; Nicholson et al., 2002; Maeda et al., 2005; Carta et al., 2007) with only one *in vivo* preliminary results being reported thus far (Politis et al., 2010b).

Animal studies utilising 6-OHDA- lesioned rat (Carta et al., 2007; Munoz et al., 2009) and MPTP-trated primates (Munoz et al., 2008) has reported an almost-complete abolition of the dyskinetic movements induced by chronic L-DOPA treatment when DA release is blocked from the serotonin neurons using 5-HT1A and 5-HT1B autoreceptor agonists without compromisnig the therapeutic benefit of L-DOPA on motor symptoms. Furthermore, the authors demonstrated that the combination of 5-HT1A and 5-HT1B agnosits prevented the developemnt of LID in MPTP-tratemed primates (Munoz et al., 2008). Therefore, the authors suggets that combining 5-HT1A and 5-HT1B agonists may be a favourable treated strategy for PD patients.

Clinical trials have been undertaken testing the 5-HT1A agonist, Sarizotan in more than 1000 PD patients (PADDY-1 and PADDY-2). Unfortunately these trials were unable to meet their primary endpoint which may have been a result of the low dose (1mg) administered in the phase III study compared to the dose (2 – 5mg) administered and proven effective in the phase II study (Bara-Jimenez et al., 2005).

Overall, it appears that there may be a competition for storage at the serotonergic synapse, between L-DOPA derived DA and serotonin. It is suggested that this competetion may lead to a depletion in serotonin content thus an over-activation of serotonin terminals which are attempting to compensate for the reduced binding to the presynaptic serotonin autoreceptors. Subsequently there is an excessive release of DA from these neurons, triggering the LID.

To date only preliminary data has been reported relating the serotonergic system to the pathophysiology of LID in PD patients with PET (Politis et al., 2010b). The authors conducted a RAC PET study and medication challenges with suprathreshold doses of L-DOPA and Buspirone (5-HT1A agonist) in 16 PD patients with LID and 12 PD patients with a stable response to L-DOPA therapy. The authors aimed to investiagte the possibility that relatively preserved striatal 5-HT terminals may cause or aggravate LID by mishandling exogenous L-DOPA and releasing DA as a false neurotransmitter.

Dyskinetic patients demonstrated an 18% decrease in putaminal RAC binding compared to an 8% reduction in the stable PD responder group. This result reflects an increase of DA synaptic turnover in the dyskinetic group as also shown in previous studies (de la Fuente-Fernandez et al., 2001; Pavese et al., 2006). However, administration of 5-HT1A agonist, buspirone preceding the administration of L-DOPA in the dyskinetic PD group revealed a normalization of putaminal synaptic DA at comparable levels to those of the stable PD responders as this was judged by the 12% decrease of their putaminal RAC binding. The authors also demonstrated that clinically, the administration of L-DOPA and Buspirone in combination significantly attenuated LID. Therefore, the authors suggest that the use of 5-HT agonists, which dampen the transmitter release from 5-HT neurons, alleviating excessive synaptic DA levels and thus attenuating LID, is justified.

6. Dyskinesias following neural transplantation

The progressive declination of the clinical course of PD and the resulting motor complications of LID has resulted in more sophisticated therapeutic approaches in tackling PD symptomatology and medication side-effects. One such approach has been implemented in the way of DA-rich fetal ventral mesencephalic (VM) tissue transplantation in the striatum of PD patients. The rationale for such a procedure is based on the hypothesis that PD is the result of DA denervation in the nigostriatal pathway and striatum and that transplanation of DA neurons could restore DA levels and reverse motor disability. Clinical trials on VM transplantation have been undertaken in the past two decades. Unfortunately results regarding motor symptom relief have been inconsistent with many patients developing motor complications termed GIDs, whereby these patients appear to develop these involuntary movements whilst 'OFF' their DA medication. It is not currently understood if GIDs share the same pathophysiology and pathogenesis as LID induced by L-DOPA therapy. It has been suggested that GIDs develop as a result of graft fiber outgrowth causing an increase in DA release (Freed et al., 2001) or due to an underadequate degree of DA release as DA reinnervation has failed (Ma et al., 2002).

Animal studies may have provided an insight in to the pathogenesis of GIDs in PD patients following VM tissue transplantaion. DA rich grafts have been shown to improve LID in animals (Lee et al., 2000). However, transplantation of fetal serotonergic neurons into the striatum of 6-OHDA-lesioned rats has been shown to exacerbate LID by up to 70% compared to pre-transplantation scores (Carlsson et al., 2007, 2009). Considering the evidence that other cells may be involved in the conversion, storage and release of DA, it is possible that this effect occurs as a consequence of abnormal handling of DA. Recent work has shown that serotonin neurons are involved in the development of GIDs despite the successful recovery of motor function. Utilising ^{11}C-DASB PET, a selective marker for serotonin tranporter (SERT) binding, in two patients who developed GID following neural transplantation, it has been demonstrated that PD patients developing GIDs following VM tissue transplantation, exhibited excessive serotonergic innervation in the grafted striatum (Politis et al., 2010c). Furthermore, following the administration of the 5-HT1A buspirone, the GIDs were markedly reduced indicating that the motor complication arose from serotonergic hyperinnervation. It is not known, however, if the mechanisms underlying GID are the same for LID, but nonetheless, this study provides the first *in vivo* evidence for the serotonergic hypothesis in the development of motor complications in PD.

7. Conclusion

Risk factors of LID development appear to be relatively established including degree of DA denervation, L-DOPA dose and duration of L-DOPA therapy. The advent of PET imaging has enabled much progress in understanding the mechanisms underlying LID. LID likely results from a combination of factors including, alteration of various neurotransmitter systems, abnormal synaptic plasticity and an altered firing pattern within the basal ganglia.
LID is a troublesome side effect of DA therapy and currently there is no treatment. As such, it results in decreased quality of life for PD patients and in increased health care costs. Although the DA system appears to be primarily implicated in the PD pathological process, results from animal and *in vivo* studies provide evidence that non-DA neurotransmitter systems may have a role in the pathogenesis of LID. Manipulation of these systems may offer an alternative therapeutic approach in abating LID and preventing their initial

development. Furthermore, as more sophisticated therapeutic approaches for alleviating the symptoms of PD are considered, it is imperative that these potential motor complications are fully understood in order to avoid their development. The use of PET imaging, although expensive and not widely available, provides an excellent tool for predictive validity of *in vivo* patient studies which will ultimately minimise the risk of failure in future clinical and cell therapy trials.

8. References

Ahlskog, JE., Muenter, MD. Frequency of levodopa-related dyskinesias and motor fluctuations as estimated from the cumulative literature. *Mov Disord.* Vol. 16 no.3, (May 2001) pp. 448-58, ISSN 1531-8257.

Ahmed, I., Bose, SK., Pavese, N., Ramlackhansingh, A., Turkheimer, F., Hotton, G., Hammers, A., Brooks, DJ. Glutamate NMDA receptor dysregulation in Parkinson's disease with dyskinesias. *Brain.* (March 2011)

Albin, RL., Koeppe, RA., Bohnen, NI., Wernette, K., Kilbourn, MA., Frey, KA. Spared caudal brainstem SERT binding in early Parkinson's disease. *J Cereb Blood Flow Metab.* Vol.28, No.3, (March 2008) pp. 441-4

Andersson, M., Hilbertson, A., Cenci, M.A. Striatal fosB expression is causallylinked with L-dopa-induced abnormal involuntary movements and the associated upregulation of striatal prodynorphin mRNA in a rat model of Parkinson's disease. *Neurobiol. Dis.* Vol.6 No.6, (December 1999) pp. 461–474

Austin, MC., Kalivas, PW. Enkephalinergic and GABAergic modulation of motor activity in the ventral pallidum. *J Pharmacol Exp Ther.* Vol.252 No. 3 (March 1990) pp. 1370-1377

Arai, R., Karasawa, N., Nagatsu, I. Dopamine produced from L-DOPA is degraded by endogenous monoamine oxidase in neurons of the dorsal raphe nucleus of the rat: an immunohistochemical study. *Brain Res.* Vol. 722 No,1-2 (May 1996) pp. 181-4

Biegon, A., Gibbs, A., Alvarado, M., Ono, M., Taylor, S. In vitro and in vivo characterization of [3H]CNS-5161–a use-dependent ligand for the N-methyl-D-aspartate receptor in rat brain. *Synapse.* Vol.61 No. 8 (August 2007) pp. 577–86

Braak, H., Ghebremedhin, E., Rub, U., Bratzke, H., Del Tredici, K.. Stages in the development of Parkinson's diseaserelated pathology, *Cell Tissue Res.* Vol.318 No.1 (Oct 2004) pp. 121-134

Brotchie, JM. The neural mechanisms underlying levodopa-induced dyskinesia in Parkinson's disease. *Ann Neurol.* Vol.47(No.4 Suppl. 1) (April 2000) pp. S105e12. discussion S12e4.

Calon, F., Rajput, AH., Hornykiewicz, O., Bedard, PJ., Di Paolo, T. Levodopa-induced motor complications are associated with alterations of glutamate receptors in Parkinson's disease. *Neurobiol Dis.* Vol.14 No.3 (December 2003) pp. 404–16

Carlsson, T., Carta, M., Winkler, C., Björklund, A., Kirik, D.. Serotonin neuron transplants exacerbate L-DOPA-induced dyskinesias in a rat model of Parkinson's disease. *J Neurosci.*Vol.27 No.30 (July 2007) pp. 8011-22

Carlsson, T., Carta, M., Muñoz, A., Mattsson, B., Winkler, C., Kirik, D., Björklund, A. Impact of grafted serotonin and dopamine neurons on development of L-DOPA-induced dyskinesias in parkinsonian rats is determined by the extent of dopamine neuron degeneration. *Brain*. Vol.132 No.2 (February 2009) pp. 19-35

Carta M, Lindgren HS, Lundblad M, Stancampiano R, Fadda F, Cenci MA. Role of striatal L-DOPA in the production of dyskinesia in 6-hydroxydopamine lesioned rats. *J Neurochem*. Vol.96 No.6 (March 2006) pp. 1718-27

Carta, M., Carlsson, T., Kirik, D., Björklund A. Dopamine released from 5-HT terminals is the cause of L-DOPA-induced dyskinesia in parkinsonian rats. *Brain*. Vol. 130 No.7 (July 2007)pp. 1819-33.

Cenci, M.A., Lee, C.S., Bjorklund, A. L-Dopa-induced dyskinesia in the rat is associated with striatal overexpression of prodynorphin- and glutamic acid decarboxylase mRNA. *Eur. J. Neurosci.* Vol.10 No.8 (August 1998) pp. 2694–2706.

Cenci, MA., Lundblad, M. Post- versus presynaptic plasticity in L-DOPA-induced dyskinesia. *J Neurochem*. Vol.99 No.2 (October 2006) pp. 381-92.

Contin, M., Riva, R., Martinelli, P., Cortelli, P., Albani, F., Baruzzi, A.. Pharmacodynamic modeling of oral levodopa: clinical application in Parkinson's disease. *Neurology*. Vol.43 No.2 (Febuary 1993) pp. 367-71.

Cragg, SJ., Baufreton, J., Xue, Y., Bolam, JP., Bevan, MD. Synaptic release of dopamine in the subthalamic nucleus. *Eur J Neurosci.* Vol.20 No.7 (October 2004) pp. 1788-802.

Crossman, AR. A hypothesis on the pathophysiological mechanisms that underlie levodopa- or dopamine agonist-induced dyskinesias in Parkinson's disease: implication for future strategies in treatment. *Mov Disord.* Vol.5 No.2 (1990) pp. 100-108

Delay-Goyet, P., Zajac, JM., Javoy-Agid, F., Agid, Y., Roques, BP. Regional distribution of mu, delta and kappa opioid receptors in human brains from controls and parkinsonian subjects. *Brain Res.* Vol.414 No.1 (June 1987) pp. 8-14

de la Fuente-Fernández, R., Lu, JQ, Sossi, V., Jivan, S., Schulzer, M., Holden, JE., Lee, CS., Ruth,TJ., Calne. DB., Stoessl, AJ.. Biochemical variations in the synaptic level of dopamine precede motor fluctuations in Parkinson's disease: PET evidence of increased dopamine turnover. *Ann Neurol*. Vol.49 No.3 (March 2001) pp.298-303.

de la Fuente-Fernández R, Sossi V, Huang Z, Furtado, S., Lu, JQ., Calne, DB., Ruth, TJ., Stoess,l AJ. Levodopa-induced changes in synaptic dopamine levels increase with progression of Parkinson's disease: implications for dyskinesias. *Brain*. Vol.127 Pt.12 (December 2004)pp. 2747-54.

Delfino, M.A., Stefano, A.V., Ferrario, J.E., Taravini, I.R., Murer, M.G., Gershanik, O.S. Behavioral sensitization to different dopamine agonists in a parkinsonian rodent model of drug-induced dyskinesias. *Behav. Brain Res.* Vol.152 No. 2(July 2004) pp.297–306.

Di Monte, DA., McCormack, A., Petzinger, G., Janson, AM., Quik, M., Langston, WJ. Relationship among nigrostriatal denervation, parkinsonism, and dyskinesias in the MPTP primate model. *Mov Disord.* Vol.15 No.3 (May 2000) pp. 459-66.

Eidelberg, D. Metabolic brain networks in neurodegenerative disorders: a functional imaging approach.*Trends Neurosci*. Vol.32 No.10 (October 2009) pp. 548-57.

Endres, CJ., Kolachana, BS., Saunders, RC., Su, T., Weinberger, D., Breier, A., Eckelman, WC., Carson, RE.. Kinetic modeling of [11C]raclopride: combined PET-microdialysis studies. *J Cereb Blood Flow Metab*. Vol.17 No.9 (September 1997) pp. 932-42.

Engberg, TM., Susel, Z., Kuo, S., Gerfen CR, Chase TN. Levodopa replacement therapy alters enzyme activities in striatum and neuropeptide content in striatal output regions of 6-hydroxydopamine lesioned rats. Vol.552 No.1 *Brain Res* (June 1991) pp. 113-118

Eskow, KL., Gupta, V., Alam, S., Park JY, Bishop C. The partial 5-HT(1A) agonist buspirone reduces the expression and development of l-DOPA-induced dyskinesia in rats and improves l-DOPA efficacy. *Pharmacol Biochem Behav*. Vol. 87 No, 3 (Aug-Sep 2007) pp. 306-14.

Fahn, S. The spectrum of levodopa-induced dyskinesias. Vol.47(No. 4 Suppl 1) *Ann Neurol*. (April 2000) pp. S2-9.

Fearnley, JM., Lees, AJ. Striatonigral degeneration. A clinicopathological study. *Brain*. Vol.113 (Pt 6) (December 1990) pp.1823-42.

Fenu, S. Pinna A, Ongini E, Morelli M. Adenosine A2A receptor antagonism potentiates Ldopa- induced turning behaviour and c-fos expression in 6- hydroxydopamine-lesioned rats. *Eur. J. Pharmacol*. Vol.321 No.2 (February 1997) pp. 143–147

Fernandez, A., De Ceballos, ML., Jenner, P., Marsden, CD. Neurotensin, substance P, delta and mu opioid receptors are decreased in basal ganglia of Parkinson's disease patients. *Neuroscience*. Vol.61 No.1 (July 1994)pp. 73-79

Ferre´, S. and Fuxe, K. Dopamine denervation leads to an increase in the intramembrane interaction between adenosine A2 and dopamine D2 receptors in the neostriatum. *Brain Res*. Vol.594 No.2 (November 1992) pp.124–130

Ferre´, S. O'Connor, WT., Fuxe, K., Ungerstedt, U. The striopallidal neuron: a main locus for adenosine–dopamine interactions in the brain. *J. Neurosci*. Vol.13 No.12 (December 1993) pp. 5402–5406

Freed, CR., Greene, PE., Breeze, RE., Tsai, WY., DuMouchel, W., Kao, R., Dillon, S., Winfield, H., Culver, S., Trojanowski, JQ., Eidelberg, D., Fahn, S. Transplantation of embryonic dopamine neurons for severe Parkinson's disease. *N Engl J Med* Vol.344 No. 10 (March 2001) pp. 710-719.

Fuxe, K. Ferré, S., Snaprud, P., von Euler, G., Johansson, B, Ferdholm, B. Antagonistic A2A/D2 receptor interactions in the striatum as a basis for adenosine/dopamine interactions in the central nervous system. *Drug Dev. Res*. Vol. 28 No.3 (March 1993) pp. 374–380

Goto, I., Taniwaki, T., Hosokawa, S., Otsuka, M., Ichiya, Y., Ichimiya, A. Positron emission tomographic (PET) studies in dementia. *J Neurol Sci*. Vol.114 No.1 (January 1993) pp. 1-6.

Haber, SN., Watson, SJ. The comparative distribution of enkephalin, dynorphin and substance P in the human globus pallidus and basal forebrain. *Neuroscience* Vol.14 No.4 (1985) pp. 1001-1024.

Hagell, P., Piccini, P., Björklund, A., Brundin, P., Rehncrona, S., Widner, H., Crabb, L., Pavese, N., Oertel, WH., Quinn, N., Brooks, DJ., Lindvall, O. Dyskinesias following neural transplantation in Parkinson's disease. *Nat Neurosci.* Vol.5 No.7 (July 2002) pp. 627-8.

Hauser, RA. Hubble, JP., Truong, DD.,and the Istradefylline US-001 Study Group. Randomized trial of the adenosine A2A receptor antagonist istradefylline in advanced PD. *Neurology* Vol.61 No.3 (August 2003) pp. 297–303.

Heikkila, RE., Nicklas, WJ., Vyas, I., Duvoisin, RC. Dopaminergic toxicity of rotenone and the 1-methyl-4-phenylpyridinium ion after their stereotaxic administration to rats: implication for the mechanism of 1-methyl-4-phenyl-1,2,3,6-tetrahydropyridine toxicity. *Neurosci Lett.* Vol.62 No.3 (December 1985) pp. 389-94.

Hirsch, EC. Nigrostriatal system plasticity in Parkinson's disease: effect of dopaminergic denervation and treatment. *Ann Neurol.* Vol.47 (No.4 Suppl 1) (April 2000) S115-20; discussion S120-1

Hollister, AS., Breese, GR., Mueller, RA. Role of monoamine neural systems in L-dihydroxyphenylalanine-stimulated activity. *J Pharmacol Exp Ther* Vol.208 No.1 (January 1979) pp. 37-43.

Iravani, MM., Tayarani-Binazir, K., Chu, WB.,Jackson, MJ., Jenner, P. In 1-methyl-4-phenyl-1,2,3,6-tetrahydropyridine-treated primates, the selective 5-hydroxytryptamine 1a agonist (R)-(+)-8-OHDPAT inhibits levodopa-induced dyskinesia but only with\ increased motor disability. *J Pharmacol Exp Ther.* Vol.319 No.3 (December 2006) pp. 1225-34.

Jenner, P., Rupniak, NM., Rose, S., Kelly, E., Kilpatrick, G., Lees, A., Marsden, CD. 1-Methyl-4-phenyl-1,2,3,6-tetrahydropyridine-induced parkinsonism in the common marmoset. *Neurosci Lett.* Vol.50 No.1-3 (September 1984) pp. 85-90.

Jenner, P. The MPTP-treated primate as a model of motor complications in PD: primate model of motor complications. *Neurology* Vol.61 No.6 (September 2003) S4–11.

Johansson, P.A., Andersson, M., Andersson, K.E., Cenci, M.A., 2001. Alterations in cortical and basal ganglia levels of opioid receptor binding in a rat model of Ldopa-induced dyskinesia. *Neurobiol. Dis.* Vol.8 No.2 (April 2001) pp. 220–239.

Jolkkonen, J., Jenner, P., Marsden, CD. L-Dopa reverses altered gene expression of substance P but not enkephalin in the caudate-putamen of common marmosets treated with MPTP. *Brain Res.* Vol.32 No.2 (September 1995) pp. 297-307

Kish, SJ. Biochemistry of Parkinson's disease: is a brain serotonergic deficiency a characteristic of idiopathic Parkinson's disease? *Adv Neurol.* Vol.91 (2003) pp. 39-49.

Kish, SJ., Tong, J., Hornykiewicz, O., Rajput, A., Chang, LJ., Guttman, M., Furukawa, Y. Preferential loss of serotonin markers in caudate versus putamen in Parkinson's disease. *Brain.* Vol.131 Pt.1 (January 2008) pp. 120-31.

Kishore, A., De la Fuente-Fernandez R, Snow BJ, et al. Levodopa-induced dyskinesias in idiopathic Parkinsonism (IP): a simultaneous PET study of dopamine D1 and D2 receptors. *Neurology.* Vol. 47 (1997) A327.

Küppenbender, KD., Standaert, DG., Feuerstein, TJ., Penney, JB Jr., Young, AB., Landwehrmeyer, GB. Expression of NMDA receptor subunit mRNAs in neurochemically identified projection and interneurons in the human striatum. *J Comp Neurol* Vol.419 No.4 (April 2000) pp. 407–21.

Lavoie B, Parent A. Immunohistochemical study of the serotoninergic innervation of the basal ganglia in the squirrel monkey. *J Comp Neurol.* Vol.299 No.1 (September 1990) pp. 1-16.

Lee, CS., Cenci, MA., Schulzer, M., Björklund, A. Embryonic ventral mesencephalic grafts improve levodopa-induced dyskinesia in a rat model of Parkinson's disease. *Brain.* Vol.123 Pt.7 (July 2000) pp. 1365-79.

Le Moine, C. Svenningsson, P., Fredholm, BB., Bloch, B. Dopamine-adenosine interactions in the striatum and the globus pallidus: inhibition of striatopallidal neurons through either D2 or A2A receptors enhances D1 receptormediated effects on c-fos expression. *J. Neurosci.* Vol.17 No.20 (October 1997) pp. 8038–8048

Lindgren, HS., Andersson, DR., Lagerkvist, S, Nissbrandt, H., Cenci, MA.. L-DOPA-induced dopamine efflux in the striatum and the substantia nigra in a rat model of Parkinson's disease: temporal and quantitative relationship to the expression of dyskinesia. *J Neurochem.* Vol.112 No.6 1465-76.

Luginger, E., Wenning, GK., Bosch, S., Poewe, W. Beneficial effects of amantadine on L-dopa-induced dyskinesias in Parkinson's disease. *Mov Disord.* Vol.15 No.5 (September 2000) pp. 873-88.

Lundblad, M., Andersson, M., Winkler, C., Kirik, D., Wierup, N., Cenci, MA. Pharmacological validation of behavioural measures of akinesia and dyskinesia in a rat model of Parkinson's disease. *Eur J Neurosci.* Vol.15 No.1 (January 2002) pp.120-32.

Lundblad, M. Vaudano, E., Cenci, MA. Cellular and behavioural effects of the adenosine A2a receptor antagonist KW-6002 in a rat model of LDOPA- induced dyskinesia. *J. Neurochem.* Vol.84 No.6 (March 2003) pp. 1398–1410

Ma, Y., Feigin, A., Dhawan, V., Fukuda, M., Shi, Q., Greene, P., Breeze, R., Fahn, S., Freed, C., Eidelberg, D. Dyskinesia after fetal cell transplantation for parkinsonism: a PET study. *Ann Neurol.* Vol.52 No.5 (November 2002) pp. 628-634.

Maeda, T., Nagata, K., Yoshida, Y., Kannari., K . Serotonergic hyperinnervationinto the dopaminergic denervated striatum compensates for dopamine conversion from exogenously administered L-DOPA. *Brain Res.* Vol. 1046 No.1-2 (June 2005) pp.230-3.

Marconi, R., Lefebvre-Caparros, D., Bonnet, AM., Vidailhet, M., Dubois, B., Agid, Y.. Levodopa-induced dyskinesias in Parkinson's disease phenomenology and pathophysiology. *Mov Disord.* Vol.9 No.1

Maratos, E.C., Jackson, M.J., Pearce, R.K., Jenner, P. Antiparkinsonian activity and dyskinesia risk of ropinirole and L-dopa combination therapy in drug naive MPTP-lesioned common marmosets (Callithrix jacchus). *Mov. Disord.* Vol.16 No.4 (July 2001) pp. 631–641.

Mones, RJ. Experimental dyskinesias in normal rhesus monkeys. In: Barbeau A, Chase TN, Paulson GW, eds. Advances in Neurology, vol 1. New York, NY: Raven Press, 1973 pp.665–669.

Nadjar, A., Gerfen, CR., Bezard, E. Priming for l-dopa-induced dyskinesia in Parkinson's disease: a feature inherent to the treatment or the disease? *Prog Neurobiol.* Vol.87 No.1 (January 2009) pp. 1-9.

Nash, JE., Brotchie, JM. Characterisation of striatal NMDA receptors involved in the generation of parkinsonian symptoms: intrastriatal microinjection studies in the 6-OHDA-lesioned rat. *Mov Disord.* Vol.17 No.3 (May 2002) pp. 455–66.

Nicholson, SL., Brotchie, JM. 5-hydroxytryptamine (5-HT, serotonin) and Parkinson's disease - opportunities for novel therapeutics to reduce the problems of levodopa therapy. *Eur J Neurol.* Vol.9 Suppl 3 (November 2002) pp.1-6.

Ng, KY., Chase, TN., Colburn, RW., et al. L-Dopa-induced release of cerebral monoamines. *Science.* Vol.170 No.953 (October 1970) pp. 76-7.

Ng, KY., Colburn, RW., Kopin, IJ. Effects of L-dopa on efflux of cerebral monoamines from synaptosomes.*Nature.* Vol.230 No.5292 (April 1971) pp. 331-2

Nutt, JG., Woodward, WR., Carter, JH., Gancher, ST.. Effect of long-term therapy on the pharmacodynamics of levodopa. Relation to on-off phenomenon. *Arch Neurol.*Vol.49-No.11 (November 1992) pp.1123-30.

Oh, JD., Russell, DS., Vaughan, CL., Chase, TN., Russell, D. Enhanced tyrosine phosphorylation of striatal NMDA receptor subunits: effect of dopaminergic denervation and L-DOPA administration. *Brain Res.* Vol.813 No.1 (November 1998) pp. 150–9.

Olanow, CW., Goetz, CG., Kordower, JH., Stoessl, AJ., Sossi, V., Brin, MF., Shannon, KM., Nauert, GM., Perl, DP., Godbold, J., Freeman, TB. A double-blind controlled trial of bilateral fetal nigral transplantation in Parkinson's disease. *Ann Neurol.* Vol.54 No.3 (Septmber 2003) pp. 403-414.

Ouchi, Y., Yoshikawa, E., Sekine, Y., Futatsubashi, M., Kanno, T., Ogusu, T., Torizuka, T. Microglial activation and dopamine terminal loss in early Parkinson's disease. *Ann Neurol.* Vol57. No.2 (February 2005) pp.168-75.

Pavese, N., Evans, AH., Tai, YF., Hotton, G., Brooks, DJ., Lees, AJ., Piccini, P. Clinical correlates of levodopa-induced dopamine release in Parkinson disease: a PET study. *Neurology.* Vol.67 No.9 (November 2006) pp.1612-7.

Pearce, R.K., Jackson, M., Smith, L., Jenner, P., Marsden, C.D., 1995. Chronic L-dopa administration induces dyskinesias in the MPTP-treated common marmoset (Callithrix jacchus). Mov. Disord. 10, 731–740.

Pearce, R.K., Banerji, T., Jenner, P., Marsden, C.D., 1998. De novo administration of ropinirole and bromocriptine induces less dyskinesia than L-dopa in the MPTPtreated marmoset. Mov. Disord. 13, 234–241.

Peppard, RF., Martin, WR., Carr, GD., Grochowski, E., Schulzer, M., Guttman, M., McGeer, PL., Phillips, AG., Tsui, JK., Calne, DB. Cerebral glucose metabolism in Parkinson's disease with and without dementia. *Arch Neurol.* Vol.49 No. 12 (December 1992) pp. 1262-8.

Piccini, P., Weeks, RA., Brooks, DJ. Alterations in opioid receptor binding in Parkinson's disease patients with levodopa-induced dyskinesias. *Ann Neurol.* Vol.42 No.5 (November 1997) pp. 720-6.

Pinna, A. di Chiara, G., Wardas, J., Morelli, M. Blockade of A2A adenosine receptors positively modulates turning behaviour and c-Fos expression induced by D1 agonists in dopamine-denervated rats. *Eur. J. Neurosci.* Vol.8 No.6 (June 1996) pp.1176- 1181

Pinna, A. Fenu, S., Morelli, M. Motor stimulant effects of the adenosine A2A receptor antagonist SCH 58261 do not develop tolerance after repeated treatment in 6-hydroxydopamine-lesioned rats. *Synapse* Vol.39 No.3 (March 2001) pp. 233–238

Politis M, Wu K, Loane C, Kiferle, L., Molloy, S., Brooks, DJ., Piccini, P. Staging of serotonergic dysfunction in Parkinson's Disease: An in vivo 11C-DASB PET study. *Neurobiol Dis.* Vol.40 No. 1

Politis, M., Wu, K., Loane, C., Kiferle, L., Molloy, S., Bain, P., Brooks, DJ., Piccini ,P. Serotonergic involvement in L-DOPA-induced dyskinesia [abstract]. *Mov Disord.* Vol.25(Suppl 3) (2010) S658.

Politis, M., Wu, K., Loane, C., Quinn, NP., Brooks, DJ., Rehncrona, S., Bjorklund, A., Lindvall, O., Piccini, P. Serotonergic Neurons Mediate Dyskinesia Side Effects in Parkinson's Patients with Neural Transplants. *Sci Transl Med.* Vol.2 No.38 (June 2010c) pp. 38-46.

Pollack, AE. and Fink, JS. Synergistic interaction between an adenosine antagonist and a D1 dopamine agonist on rotational behavior and striatal c-Fos induction in 6-hydroxydopamine-lesioned rats. *Brain Res.* Vol.743 No.1-2 (December 1996) pp. 124–130

Ramlackhansingh, AF., Bose, SK., Ahmed, I., Turkheimer, FE., Pavese, N., Brooks, DJ. Adenosine A(2A) Receptor Availability in Parkinson's Disease Patients with and without Levodopa Induced Dyskinesias Studied with [C-11]SCH442416 PET. *62nd Annual Meeting of the American-Academy-of-Neurology,* 10 Apr 2010 - 17 Apr 2010. 74:A588-A588.

Rascol, O., Brooks, DJ., Korczyn, AD., De Deyn, PP., Clarke, CE., Lang, AE. A five-year study of the incidence of dyskinesia in patients with early Parkinson's disease who were treated with ropinirole or levodopa. 056 Study Group. *N Engl J Med.* Vol.342 No. 20 (May 2000) pp. 1484–91.

Remy, P., Doder, M., Lees, A., Turjanski, N., Brooks, D. Depression in Parkinson's disease: loss of dopamine and noradrenaline innervation in the limbic system. *Brain.* Vol.128 Pt.6 (June 2005) pp. 1314-22.

Rinne, UK., Rinne, JK., Rinne, JO., Laakso, K., Tenovuo, O., Lönnberg, P., Koskinen, V. Brain enkephalin receptors in Parkinson's disease. *J Neural Transm.* (suppl 19) (1983) pp. 163-17 1

Sassin, JF. Drug-induced dyskinesias in monkeys. In: Meldrum BS, Marsden CD, eds. *Advances in Neurology,* vol 10. New York, NY: Raven Press, 1975:47–54.

Schneider, J.S., Gonczi, H., Decamp, E. Development of levodopa-induced dyskinesias in parkinsonian monkeys may depend upon rate of symptom onset and/or duration of symptoms. *Brain Res.* Vol.990 No. 1-2 (November 2003) pp. 38–44.

Sivam, SP.Dopamine dependent decrease in enkephalin and substance P levels in basal ganglia regions of postmortem parkinsonian brains. *Neuropeptides.* Vol.18 No.4(April 1991) pp.201-7.

Sossi, V., de la Fuente-Fernández, R., Schulzer, M.,. Dopamine transporter relation to dopamine turnover in Parkinson's disease: a positron emission tomography study. *Ann Neurol.* Vol.62 No.5 (2007) pp.468-74.

Tanaka, H., Kannari, K., Maeda, T.Tomiyama, M., Suda, T., Matsunaga, M. Role of serotonergic neurons in L-DOPA-derived extracellular dopamine in the striatum of 6-OHDA-lesioned rats. *Neuroreport* Vol.10 No.3 (February 1999) pp. 631-4.

Taylor, MD., De Ceballos, ML., Rose, S.,Jenner, P., Marsden, CD. . Effects of unilateral 6-hydroxydopamine lesion and prolonged ~-3,4 dihydroxyphenylalanine treatment on peptidergic systems in rat basal ganglia. *Eur J Pharmacol.* Vol.219 No. 2(August 1992) pp.183-192

Tedroff J, Pedersen M, Aquilonius SM, Hartvig, P., Jacobsson, G., Långström, B. Levodopa-induced changes in synaptic dopamine in patients with Parkinson's disease as measured by [11C]raclopride displacement and PET. *Neurology.* Vol.45 No.6 (May 1996) pp. 1430-6.

Teune, LK., Bartels, AL., de Jong, BM., Willemsen, AT., Eshuis, SA., de Vries, JJ., van Oostrom, JC., Leenders, KL. Typical cerebral metabolic patterns in neurodegenerative brain diseases. *Mov Disord.* Vol.25 No.14 (October 2010) pp. 2395-404.

Thanvi B, Lo N, Robinson T. Levodopa-induced dyskinesia in Parkinson's disease: clinical features, pathogenesis, prevention and treatment. *Postgrad Med J.* Vol.83 No.980 (June 2007) pp. 384-8.

Tomiyama, M., Kimura, T., Maeda, T., Kannari, K, Matsunaga., M, Baba,. M.. A serotonin 5-HT1A receptor agonist prevents behavioral sensitization to L-DOPA in a rodent model of Parkinson's disease. *Neurosci Res.* Vol.52 No.2 (June 2005)pp. 185-94.

Troiano, AR., de la Fuente-Fernandez, R., Sossi, V., Schulzer, M., Mak, E., Ruth, TJ., Stoessl, AJ. PET demonstrates reduced dopamine transporter expression in PD with dyskinesias. *Neurology.* Vol.72 No. 14 (April 2009) pp. 1211-6.

Turjanski, N., Lees, AJ., Brooks, DJ. In vivo studies on striatal dopamine D1 and D2 site binding in L-dopa-treated Parkinson's disease patients with and without dyskinesias. *Neurology.* Vol.49 No.3 (September 1997) pp. 717-23.

Torstenson, R., Hartvig, P., Långström, B., Westerberg, G., Tedroff, J.. Differential effects of levodopa on dopaminergic function in early and advanced Parkinson's disease. *Ann Neurol.* Vol.41 No.3 (April 1997) pp. 334-40.

Ulusoy, A., Sahin, G., Kirik, D. Presynaptic dopaminergic compartment determines the susceptibility to L-DOPA-induced dyskinesia in rats. *Proc Natl Acad Sci U S A.* Vol.107 No.29 (July 2010) pp.13159-64.

Venton, BJ., Michael, DJ., Wightman, RM. Correlation of local changes in extracellular oxygen and pH that accompany dopaminergic terminal activity in the rat caudate-putamen. *J Neurochem*. Vol.84 No.2 (January 2003) pp. 373-81.

Whone, AL., Rabiner, EA., Arahata, Y., Luthra, SK., Hargreaves, R., Brooks, DJ. Reduced substance P binding in Parkinson's disease complicated by dyskinesias: an F-18-L829165 PET study. *Neurology*. Vol.58 No. (2002) A488-49.

Winkler, C., Kirik, D., Björklund ,A., Cenci, MA. L-DOPA-induced dyskinesia in the intrastriatal 6-hydroxydopamine model of parkinson's disease: relation to motor and cellular parameters of nigrostriatal function. *Neurobiol Dis*. Vol.10 No.2 (July 2002) pp.165-86.

6

Combinations of Markers Provide Clues to the Underlying Neurodegenerative Disorder in REM Sleep Behavior Disorder

Tomoyuki Miyamoto[1] and Masayuki Miyamoto[2]

[1]*Department of Neurology, Dokkyo Medical University, Koshigaya Hospital,*

[2]*Department of Neurology, Center of Sleep Medicine, Dokkyo Medical University, Japan*

1. Introduction

REM sleep behavior disorder (RBD) is characterized by dream-enacting behaviors and unpleasant dreams, and presents a risk for self-injury and harm to others due to abnormal REM sleep during which control of muscle tonus is lacking (REM sleep without atonia) (Schenck et al., 1986; Schenck et al., 2002; American Academy of Sleep Medicine 2005). RBD is a heterogeneous disease entity consisting of a variety of manifestations (Schenck et al., 2002; Gagnon et al. 2006; Postuma et al., 2006, 2009; Maetzler et al., 2009). Idiopathic RBD (iRBD), which develops in middle age or later and progresses chronically, in particular is a common clinical manifestation of Lewy body-related syndrome and is regarded as a clinical entity from pathological aspects. For example (Table 1), it has been elucidated that iRBD is often accompanied by soft motor signs, olfactory and color identification deficits, decreased cardiovascular and respiratory changes between REM and Non-REM sleep, reduced cardiac ^{123}I-metaiodobenzylguanidine (123I-MIBG) uptake, impairment of visual memory and visuo-spatial construction revealed by neuropsychological testing, EEG slowing during wakefulness or sleep, and decreased strial dopaminergic innervation and reduced pre-synaptic strial dopamine transporter binding on SPECT or positron emission topography (PET) scans, which are considered as non-motor symptoms of Parkinson's disease (PD) (Becker et al., 2002; Gagnon et al., 2006; Miyamoto et al., 2006; Miyamoto et al., 2008). Furthermore, despite the limited number of pathological reports on iRBD, the characteristics of iRBD have been supported to have a close relationship with Lewy body pathology (Boeve et al., 2007). Therefore, additional clinical features that could distinguish iRBD with Lewy body-related alpha-synucleinopathies from iRBD due to other causes would be helpful in clinical practice.

Transcranial ultrasound imaging of the substantia nigra
Olfactory dysfunction
Impairment of visual functions
Visualization of postganglionic sympathetic cardiac neurons by 123I-metaiodobenzylguanidine (MIBG) scintigraphy
MRI
Cognitive decline
Affective symptoms
Motor testing
Sleep disturbance
REM sleep behavior disorder
Daytime sleepiness
Fatigue
Insomnia

Table 1. Early diagnosis of Parkinson's disease

2. Polysomonography

Loss of REM sleep atonia is the essential hallmark of RBD. Abnormal activity of phasic REM sleep components is essential for the induction of dream-enacting behaviors during REM sleep in iRBD. Motor-behavioral episodes in RBD are significantly more likely to occur in association with phasic than with tonic periods of REM sleep (Figure 1). Excessive tonic and phasic EMG activity during REM sleep has been shown to increase over time in subjects with iRBD (Iranzo et al. 2009). This finding suggests that, in subjects with iRBD, there is an underlying progressive pathologic process damaging the brainstem structures that modulate REM sleep. Out of a group of potential predictive markers, higher % tonic EMG activity was the most predictive of development of PD (Postuma et al. 2009).

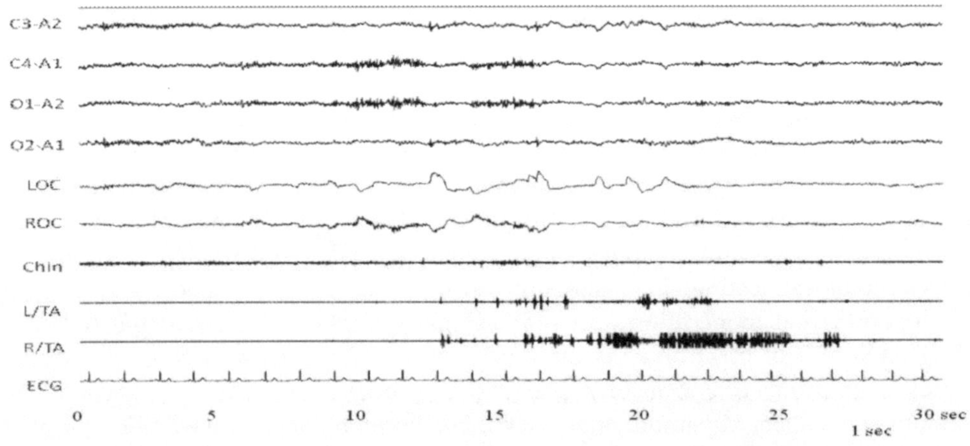

Fig. 1. Stage of RWA in a patient idiopathic REM sleep behavior disorder. The recording shows sustained elevation of submental and tibialis anterior (TA) EMG concomitant with phasic EMG elevation. EEG bears the characteristic feature of REM sleep, low voltage activity with mixed frequency, and EOG demonstrates clusters of rapid eye movements. RWA, REM sleep without atonia; EOG, electrooculogram.

3. Olfactory dysfunction

Olfactory disturbance is present in most PD or pure autonomic failure (PAF) cases (Doty et al., 1995; Goldstein et al., 2009; Silverira-Moriyama et al., 2009). The deficit in olfaction in PD contrasts with previous reports of preserved or only mildly reduced olfaction in patients with atypical parkinsonism such as a tauopathy or multiple system atrophy (MSA) (Doty et al., 1993; Wenning et al., 1995). In dementia patients, neuropathologic studies reported neuronal alterations in several subcortical structures such as the olfactory tract/bulb, anterior olfactory nucleus, orbito-frontal cortex, hippocampus, and amygdala in the olfactory system (Hubbard et al., 2007). Olfactory abnormalities have been reported in Alzheimer's disease (AD), but anosmia appears to be common in dementia with Lewy bodies (DLB) but not in pure AD (McShane et al., 2001). A Lewy body variant of AD had an increased frequency of anosmia compared with "pure" AD (Olichney et al., 2005). Furthermore, olfactory impairment is more marked in patients with mild dementia with Lewy bodies than in those with mild AD (Williams et al., 2009). In addition to reduced odor identification prior to the onset of PD, olfactory dysfunction has been frequently recognized in patients with incidental Lewy body disease (ILBD) (Ross et al. 2006). Also, neuropathological olfactory bulb alpha-synuclein has high specificity and sensitivity for Lewy body formation in confirmed cases of PD and DLB (Beach et al., 2009). On the basis of pathological studies of a large number of autopsy cases, Braak et al. proposed a hypothesis as to the onset and advancement pattern of PD in that the disease developed from the medulla and olfactory bulb and extended to the pons and substantia nigra (SN) (Braak et al., 2003). In the Honolulu-Asia Aging Study of Japanese Americans, 2,267 males without PD and dementia at the time of olfaction testing were followed-up, and more subjects who developed olfactory dysfunction in the first 4-year follow-up period developed PD than those who did not develop olfactory dysfunction (Ross et al., 2008). Another study clinically followed patients with idiopathic hyposmia to determine the percentage of patients who developed idiopathic PD after a 4-year interval. 7% of the individuals with idiopathic hyposmia had developed clinical PD, and 13% presented with abnormalities of the motor system. (Haehner et al., 2007). In a prospective study involving first-degree relatives of PD patients, a low score on three olfactory processing tasks was associated with an increased risk of developing PD within 5 years (Ponsen et al., 2009). The point of view that reduced odor identification is manifested at the very beginning of the development of PD has been supported. These reports indicate that the rhinencephalon may be an area of selective vulnerability for alpha-synuclein accumulation (Sengoku et al., 2008) and iRBD that develops in middle age or after progresses mostly to Lewy body diseases among synucleinopathies such as PD and DLB, which have some pathological features in common. In Fantini's and Postuma's cohorts (Fantini et al., 2006; Postuma et al., 2006), the olfactory deficit as revealed by the University of Pennsylvania Smell Identification Test found in most iRBD patients shares similarities with that described in PD. We also found that reduced odor identification as revealed by the Odor Stick Identification Test for Japanese were similar in patients with iRBD and PD and distinct from a control group (Miyamoto et al., 2009).

4. Color discrimination

Color vision abnormalities are among the non-motor clinical characteristics of PD (Prise et al., 1992; Büttner et al., 1995), and impairments in color discrimination and contrast sensitivity in PD are progressive over time (Diederich et al., 2002). The severity of the axial motor symptoms has been shown to be more closely related to visual dysfunction than mental function. Most patients with PD showed more marked impairment along the red-green axis than the blue-yellow axis (Oh et al., 2011), and this pattern contrasts with that typically seen in aging-predominant blue-yellow axis deficiency (Archibald et al., 2009). Color discrimination deficits also have been reported in iRBD, a potential forerunner of PD (Postuma et al., 2008). In their prospective study, they found that two potential preclinical markers of neurodegeneration, olfaction and color vision, indeed identify early-stage synucleinopathy-mediated neurodegenerative diseases (Figure 2). Compared to those remaining diseases free, patients destined to develop disease had poorer baseline olfaction and color vision. In most cases, abnormalities are measurable up to at least 5 years before disease onset , and progress slowly in the preclinical stages (Postuma et al., 2011).

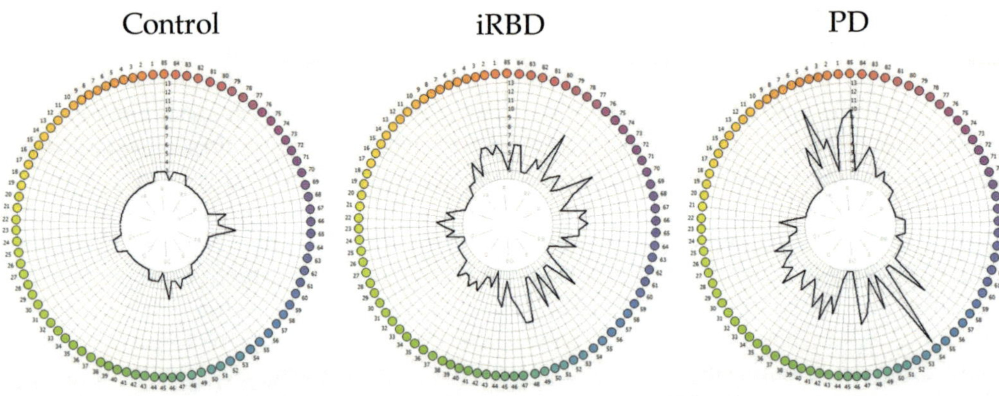

Fig. 2. Farnsworth-Munsell 100 Hue test (FMT).

The total error score for a patient with iRBD or PD was higher than that of a control subject. iRBD, idiopathic REM sleep behavior disorder. PD, Parkinson's disease.

5. Magnetic resonance imaging studies

We detected an increase (compared with reference values from another institution) in the choline/creatine ratio on protein magnetic resonance spectroscopy (1H-MRS) in the pons of a 69-year-old man with iRBD. Since other ratios were normal, the investigators interpreted these findings as demonstrating functional impairment at the cell membrane level (Miyamoto et al., 2000). Iranzo and coworkers performed 1H-MRS in a larger sample of patients with iRBD (n = 15) to determine if midbrain or pontine tegmentum abnormalities could be detected compared with matched controls (n = 15) (Iranzo et al., 2002). No significant differences in N-acetylaspartate/creatine, choline/creatine, and myoinosito/creatine ratios were found between patients and controls, which they interpreted as suggesting that marked mesopontine neuronal loss or 1H-MRS-detectable metabolic disturbances do not occur in iRBD. Recently, Unger and coworkers described diffusion tensor imaging changes in patients with iRBD (Unger et al., 2010). They found important microstructural abnormalities in the white matter of the brain stem, as well as in the right SN, olfactory region, left temporal lobe, fornix, and the right visual stream of patients with iRBD (n =12), which are known to be involved in REM sleep regulation and/or to indicate neurodegenerative pathology in early PD. In another recent study (Scherfler et al., 2010), Statistical Parametric Mapping localized significant decreases in fractional anisotropy in the tegmentum of the midbrain and rostral pons and increases in mean diffusivity within the pontine reticular formation overlapping with a cluster of decreased fractional anisotropy in the midbrain. Voxel-based morphometry revealed increases in gray matter densities in both hippocampi of iRBD patients. A concomitant fractional anisotropy decrease and mean diffusivity increase are thought to be correlates of neuronal and myelin damage leading to depletion of barriers restricting water molecular motion. As a result, anisotropy, which is a measure of the degree of alignment of cellular structures within fiber tracts, decreases and the magnitude of diffusion, a measure of extracellular fluid volume, increases. Cortical gray matter volume increases are likely to be related to sprouting of new connections, dendritic spine growth, and modification in the strength of existing connections. Their findings are in line with a ^{99m}Tc-ethylene cysteinate dimer SPECT study (Mazza et al., 2006) reporting increased cerebral blood flow in the hippocampus of patients with iRBD suggesting hypermetabolism, which would fit the concept of increased gray matter volume in the hippocampus. Further functional imaging studies are warranted to investigate the pathogenesis beyond the structural gray matter density changes and cerebral blood flow increases in the hippocampus in iRBD.

6. Transcranial ultrasound sonography

Enlarged SN hyperechogenicity (SN+) assessed by transcranial ultrasound sonography (TCS) is present in about 90% of PD patients, independent of age and disease stage. SN+ may ultimately be considered an imaging marker for disease progression in PD. It also may be useful as a screening tool to detect individuals at risk for developing PD.

Using age-corrected data, motor signs of PD were shown to begin when the decrease in the percentage of [^{123}I] FP-CIT binding ratios in the putamen was 46-64% (Booij et al., 2001). There was a significant correlation between the extension of the echogenic SN area and striatal β-CIT binding(Weise et al., 2009). They discussed the possibility that extension of SN echogenicity may be a consequence of degeneration of dopaminergic neurons in the SN rather than an independent and mechanistically unrelated phenomenon. ^{18}Fluoro-DOPA uptake was lowest in patients with PD followed by individuals with SN+ and finally healthy controls without SN+ (Behnke et al., 2009). On the other hand, a lack of correlation between SN echogenicity and striatal FP-CIT uptake was found (Spiegel et al., 2006; Doepp et al., 2008). They hypothesized that the pathogenic substrate of SN+ is different from that associated with degeneration of dopaminergic SN projection neurons. Furthermore, in asymptomatic and symptomatic *parkin* mutation carriers, echogenic SN areas were found to be enlarged(Walter et al., 2004). Brain parenchyma sonography demonstrated SN+ in concordance with abnormal nigrostriatal ^{18}F-dopa PET in all symptomatic and 3 asymptomatic *Parkin* mutation carriers. Thus, they suggested SN+ as an early marker for detection of preclinical parkinsonism. Moreover, SN+ is a stable marker because the area of echogenicity is not related to the disease stage and was found not to change during the course of disease progression over a 5-year follow-up period (Berg et al., 2005). Thus, SN+ may reflect a pathogenic process that initiates the degeneration of dopaminergic neurons but does not reflect its morphological substrate.

The clinical interest and utility of the findings of our study (Figure 3) are that hyperechogenic alterations in the area of the SN may be suggestive of the existence of preclinical dopaminergic dysfunction and of an underlying neurodegenerative disorder associated with nigrostriatal dysfunction in those with iRBD. Approximately 9% of the healthy population exhibits the same ultrasound signal, which is found in those with subclinical impairment of the nigrostriatal system as detected by 18F-labeled dopa PET examinations (Berg et al., 1999; Berg et al., 2002; Behnke et al., 2009). SN+ subjects have an approximately twofold probability for the combined occurrence of the risk markers for impaired motor performance and hyposmia versus those with SN− and SN+ is more regularly observed in subjects with higher Unified Parkinson's Disease Rating Scale (UPDRS) motor scores, in particular in subjects with UPDRS scores above 3 (Berg et al., 2010). This observation indicates that the ultrasound feature may serve as a marker for nigrostriatal vulnerability in affected healthy persons or in those in the premotor phase of PD. The frequency of iRBD patients with SN+ was 37.3% (Stockner et al., 2009) or 41.2% (Iwanami et al., 2010). The finding of an increased frequency of SN+ in a subgroup of individuals with an a priori increased risk for PD supports the potential role of SN+ as a risk marker for PD. Our recent study compared FMT-PET findings between patients with iRBD grouped according to the presence or absence of SN+ (Miyamoto et al., in press). 6-[^{18}F]-FMT is also a good substrate for aromatic L-amino acid decarboxylase (AADC) but is not metabolized by catechol-O-methyl-transferase . Thus, 6-[^{18}F]-FMT uptake has approximately twice the sensitivity of 6-[18F]fluoro-L-dopa uptake and more fully represents the extent of AADC activity (Asari et al., 2011). We found that enlarged SN+ in patients with iRBD may be suggestive of nigrostriatal dopaminergic dysfunction as determined by FMT-PET. However, as there was no significant correlation between the area of SN+ and the degree of 6-[^{18}F]-FMT uptake, it may be that two parameters have different characteristics from each other. In other words, the area of SN echogenicity is thought to be a stable marker, whereas dopaminergic tracer uptake changes with time. In a recent study (Iranzo et al., 2010), 19% of 43 patients developed a neurodegenerative syndrome such as PD, DLB or MSA 2.5 years after TCS and ^{123}I-FP-CIT SPECT and they noted that combined use of ^{123}I-FP-CIT SPECT and TCS is a potential strategy for early identification of iRBD patients who are at risk for development of a synucleinopathy. They also reported that one case of iRBD who developed MSA had decreased striatal ^{123}I-FP-CIT uptake and normal echogenic SN, and that this discrepancy might be explained by the fact SN+ is less frequent in MSA than in PD and DLB. Even those individuals with iRBD with a normal echogenic SN may be at risk of developing MSA. Therefore we need to follow up iRBD patients with regard to the risk for developing to not only PD or DLB but also MSA.

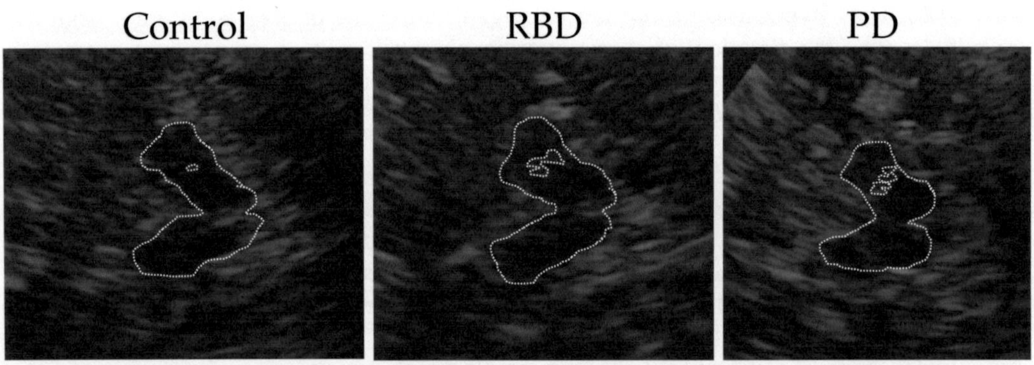

Fig. 3. Typical examples of transcranial ultrasound images of the midbrain encircled by dotted lines in control, iRBD and PD patients. The area of enlarged hyperechogenic substantia nigra signal was encircled on the ipsilateral side for planimetric measurement.

iRBD, idiopathic REM sleep behavior disorder. PD, Parkinson's disease.

7. PET and SPECT

Cognitively normal persons with dream-enactment behavior have a reduced cerebral metabolic rate of glucose (CMRgl) in brain regions known to be metabolically affected by DLB and AD (parietal, temporal, and posterior cingulate cortexes) and in several other regions, including the anterior cingulate cortex. The authors interpreted these findings as supporting further study of dream-enactment behavior as a possible risk factor for the development of DLB (Caselli et al., 2006). In another recent study, four patients were found to have diffuse areas of reduced CMRglc, predominantly in the occipital lobe, which is the preferentially affected region in DLB patients. In contrast, in five patients no such occipital hypometabolism was shown; instead, in those five patients hypometabolism was evident in the left anterior cingulate gyrus (Broadmann area (BA) 24), right frontal lobe (BA 32) and right anterior temporal lobe (BA 38), which are the preferentially affected regions in PD rather than DLB (Fujishiro H et al., 2010). The variability in the [^{18}F]-FDG PET scans of the present subjects raised the possibility that some iRBD patients with particular patterns may go on to develop PD or DLB. In terms of early intervention, it is important to determine which patterns on the [^{18}F]-FDG PET scans of iRBD patients are suggestive of underlying prodromal DLB or PD.

A single photon emission computed tomography imaging study showed that PD patients with visual hallucinations had perfusion reductions in the bilateral inferior parietal lobule, inferior temporal gyrus, precuneus gyrus and occipital cortex (Matsui et al., 2006). In a cerebral SPECT study (Shirakawa et al., 2002) that compared iRBD patients with a control group, a statistically significant decrease in blood flow was observed in the upper portion of the frontal lobe on the left and right sides and the pons in the iRBD group. According to another study (Mazza et al., 2006), there was increased perfusion in the pons and putamen bilaterally and in the right hippocampus, and decreased perfusion in frontal and temporoparietal cortices. They concluded that the similarity between the distribution of perfusional impairments found in iRBD and those observed in patients with early PD argues for a common pathophysiologic mechanism for these syndromes in at least the initial stages of these conditions. Our recent study (Hanyu et al., 2010), found decreased regional cerebral blood flow in the parietooccipital lobe (precuneus), limbic lobe, and cerebellar hemispheres in patients with iRBD. Such perfusion abnormalities are also common in patients with confirmed alpha-synucleinopathies (PD, DLB, or MSA).

Thus, based on these findings, as with [^{18}F]-FDG PET or SPECT findings in iRBD, a close relationship is indicated between PD and DLB, although the phenomenon is not observed constently with regard to the pathology of iRBD. The results of [^{18}F]-FDG PET or SPECT studies suggest that iRBD can be a presymptomatic stage of alpha-synucleinopathies.

Striatal binding of DTBZ-PET (Albin et al., 2000) was reduced in iRBD subjects compared with control subjects, suggesting reduced dopaminergic SN neuron numbers. 123I-IPT SPECT (Eisensehr et al., 2000) demonstrated a reduction of striatal dopamine transporter binding in iRBD which is indicative of a presynaptic dopaminergic deficit such as in PD patients. In a recent study (Kim et al., 2010), the dopamine transporter density of the subregions in the majority of RBD patients remained above the lower normal limit, although there was a significant group difference in CIT binding in the putamen between RBD and control subjects. In contrast, CIT binding in each region in most of the PD patients was below the normal range. In our study (Figure 4), a 6-[18F]-fluoro-meta-tyrosine PET (FMT/PET) template was superimposed onto each individual brain MRI for PD, iRBD, and control subjects. Regions of interest (ROIs) for the striatum and cerebellum were placed over each brain template. ROIs were manually drawn on the FMT/PET after overlapping with each brain MRI, and the striatal ROI was divided into the putamen and caudate. We proposed that FMT-PET imaging could assess the level of the presynaptic dopaminergic nerve for iRBD, PD, and control subjects. IRBD patients had no signs of parkinsonism and had neuroimaging evidence of an almost intact striatal dopaminergic innervation such as in controls. In contrast, PD patients have parkinsonism by definition and have loss of striatal dopaminergic innervation, as evidenced by decreased striatal uptake. We followed the present case by PET immediately after development of iRBD and at 2.5 years after the first scan (Miyamoto et al., 2010) . Nigrostriatal presynaptic dopaminergic function was normal 1 year after the diagnosis of iRBD and decreased by 4 ~ 6% per year, which is similar to that in PD (Nurmi et al., 2003). Nigrostriatal dopaminergic degeneration could be a part of the pathogenesis of RBD, but is not essential for the development of RBD.

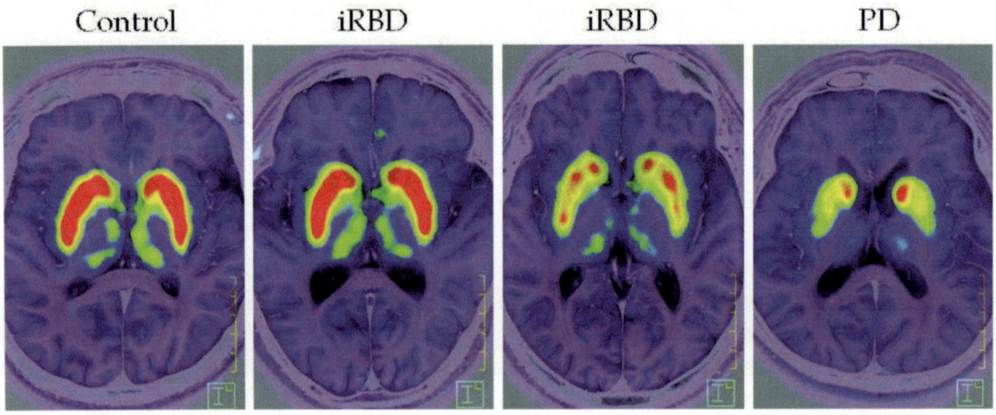

Fig. 4. 6-[18F]-fluoro-meta-tyrosine PET (FMT/PET) template superimposed onto each individual brain MRI for PD, iRBD, or control subjects. IRBD patients have no signs of parkinsonism and have neuroimaging evidence of almost intact striatal dopaminergic innervation such as in controls. Nor do they have reduced uptake such as in PD.

8. Cardiac ^{123}I-MIBG scintigraphy

There is evidence that 123I-MIBG cardiac uptake is markedly reduced in patients with Lewy body diseases such as PD, DLB, and PAF (Courbon et al., 2003; Kashihara et al., 2006; Yoshita et al., 2006). It was reported that cardiac 123I-MIBG imaging could distinguish between clinically diagnosed DLB and AD with high levels of sensitivity and specificity (Yoshita et al., 2006) . Interestingly, pathological findings occur even in patients with DLB who have no parkinsonism. Since PAF patients do not have parkinsonism or decreased striatal dopaminergic innervation, and since cardiac noradrenergic denervation occurs in both diseases, the pathogenetic mechanisms of cardiac noradrenergic denervation in Lewy body diseases differ from those producing parkinsonism and nigrostriatal dopaminergic denervation (Goldstein et al., 2009). A reduction in 123I-MIBG uptake in sympathetic terminals was observed in cases with early-phase PD and ILBD irrespective of the presence or absence of remarkable autonomic nerve injury (Courbon et al., 2003). As pathological evidence (Orimo et al., 2007; Orimo et al., 2008; Fujishiro et al., 2008), it has been proven that the Lewy body is present in cardiac sympathetic nerve postganglionic fibers, and it has been suggested that Lewy body-related pathology potentially causes severe denervation and reduced 123I-MIBG uptake in the cardiac postganglionic sympathetic nerves. The 123I-MIBG studies showed markedly decreased cardiac uptake in PD, DLB and PAF, which is a common feature of Lewy body diseases(Courbon et al., 2003; Kashihara et al., 2006; Yoshita et al., 2006).

We reported markedly reduced cardiac 123I-MIBG uptake in iRBD as well as in PD or DLB (Miyamoto et al., 2006; Miyamoto et al., 2008)(Figure 5). In our recent case report (Miyamoto et al., 2009), we described a small subset of iRBD patients who have relatively preserved uptake at RBD onset, but which then becomes lost over the follow-up period. If RBD precedes MSA, 123I-MIBG uptake is preserved over years; on the other hand, in iRBD patients, progression in the reduction in 123I-MIBG uptake occurs over years.

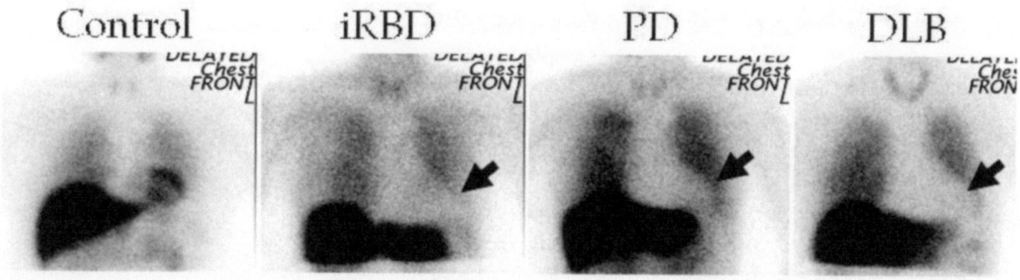

Fig. 5. Idiopathic RBD subject displayed reductions in cardiac ^{123}I-MIBG uptake (arrows) in contrast to a control subject. Uptake was also markedly reduced in a PD or DLB subject (arrows).

9. iRBD and relevance to Lewy body pathology

Men over the age of 50 years who have iRBD are at very high risk for future PD, DLB or MSA several years after the onset of RBD (Schenck et al., 1996; Iranzo et al., 2006; Postuma et al., 2009). Neuropathologic studies at autopsy of cases that had been diagnosed with RBD while alive showed that every case had Lewy bodies (Boeve et al., 2007). For example, cognitive abnormalities appeared 15 years after the onset of RBD and probable DLB was diagnosed, and eventually the presence of Lewy bodies was confirmed pathologically (Turner et al. 2000). Patients with ILBD were shown to have nigrostriatal pathological features that are intermediate between those in pathologically normal persons and those with PD (DelleDonne et al., 2008). Among the study participants with ILBD, decreased striatal dopaminergic immunoreactivity was documented for both tyrosine hydroxylase (TH) and vesicular monoamine transporter 2 (VMAT 2) in comparison with the pathologically normal subjects; the reductions were even greater in those with PD. Also, SN neuronal loss correlated with both striatal VMAT2 and TH. Thus, ILBD probably represents presymptomatic PD rather than nonspecific, age-related alpha-synuclein pathological changes.

In PD, approximately 60% of the nigrostrial neurons of the SN are degenerated before patients fulfill the clinical criteria of PD (Fearnkey et al., 1991). In some cases of PD, the patient appears to develop cortical disease before the motor signs of "stage 3" disease, whereas iRBD patients with ILBD could be diagnosed after longstanding disease with no evidence of motor or cognitive abnormalities (Uchiyama et al., 1995; Boeve et al., 2007). If progression of syncleinopathies is not universal, it is essential to understand why. Since a variety of symptoms of PD and disorders resembling PD have been elucidated, Langston (Langston et al., 2006) proposed a "Parkinson's complex" because parkinsonism would represent only the tip of the iceberg as typically viewed by both clinicians and researchers. However, when the disease process is measured by neuronal degeneration, the presence of Lewy bodies and neuritic pathology are widespread in the central and peripheral nervous systems. From this point of view, iRBD can be positioned as an earlier preclinical stage of PD or DLB or a variant of Lewy body-related alpha-synucleinopathies. To gain such an understanding, it is necessary to extract a group of patients with abnormalities in a combination of markers from among iRBD patients and provide follow-up, considering the possibility that some patients in that group may develop neurodegenerative disease (Figure 6). These steps may help elucidate the possibility that iRBD is part of the spectrum of conditions under the heading of alpha-synucleinopathies, such as PD, DLB, or MSA, or is a subtype of Lewy body-related alpha-synucleinopathy.

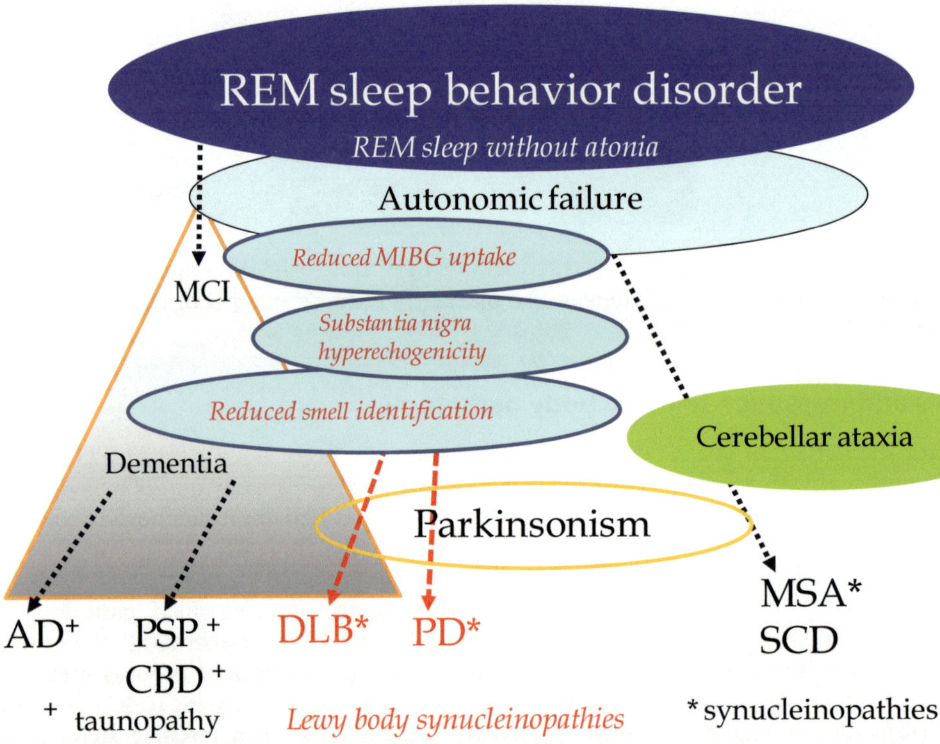

Fig. 6. Combinations of markers for neurodegenerative disease in patients idiopathic REM sleep behavior disorder. A longitudinal study of a large cohort of patients with RBD should identify which marker or combination of makers can predict progression toward a neurodegenerative disorder. The question is, does iRBD progress insidiously to PD, DLB or MSA, or does it remain static?

MCI, mild cognitive impairment, AD, Alzheimer disease, PSP, progressive supranuclear palsy, CBD, corticobasal degeneration, DLB, dementia with Lewy bodies, PD, Parkinson's disease, MSA, multiple system atrophy, SCD, spinocerebellar degeneration, iRBD, idiopathic REM sleep behaviour disorder.

10. Conclusion

Combinations of markers in iRBD were considered for the purpose of diagnosing neurodegenerative diseases such as PD, DLB or MSA at an early stage. Important advances have been made in the diagnosis of PD using imaging methods such as PET/SPECT or cardiac 123I-MIBG scintigraphy. However, while these methods are important in clinical research, they are complex, expensive, not widely available and inappropriate for the routine screening of large populations. Recent advances in the identification of biomarkers in iRBD offer diagnostic opportunities and point the way to new therapeutic strategies.

11. References

Albin, R.L., Koeppe, R.A., Chervin, R.D., Consens, F.B., Wernette, K., Frey, K.A. & Aldrich, M.S.(2000). Decreased striatal dopaminergic innervation in REM sleep beehavior disorder. Neurology 55, 1410-1420.

American Academy of Sleep Medicine. (2005). *International classification of sleep disorders, 2nd ed.: Diagnosis and cording manual,* American Academy of Sleep Medicine, Westchester Illinois, pp. 148-152.

Archibald, N.K., Clarke, M.P., Mosimann, U.P. & Burn, D.J. (2009). The retina in Parkinson's disease. Brain 132, 1128-1145.

Asari, S., Fujimoto, K., Miyauchi, A., Satou, T., Nakano, I. & Muramastu, S. (2011). Subregional 6-[18F]fluoro-L-m-tyrosine uptake in the striatum in Parkinson's disease. BMC Neurology 11:35.

Becker, G., Müller, A., Braune, S., Büttner, T., Benecke, R., Greulich, W., Klein, W., Mark, G.,Rieke J. & Thümler, R. (2002). Early diagnosis of Parkinson's disease. J Neurol 249 Suppl 3:III/40-48.

Beach, T.G., White, C.L. 3rd, Hladik, C.L., Sabbagh, M.N., Connor, D.J., Shill, H.A., Sue, L.I., Sasse, J., Bachalakuri, J., Henry-Watson, J., Akiyama, H. & Adler, C.H.; Arizona Parkinson's Disease Consortium. (2009). Olfactory bulb alpha-synucleinopathy has high specificity and sensitivity for Lewy body disorders. Acta Neuropathol 117, 169-174.

Boeve, B.F., Dickson, D.W., Olson, E.J., Shepard, J.W., Silber, M.H., Ferman, T.J., Ahlskog, J.E. & Benarroch, E.E. (2007). Insights into REM sleep behavior disorder pathophysiology in brainstem-predominant Lewy body disease._Sleep Med 8, 60-64.

Boeve, B.F., Silber, M.H., Saper, C.B., Ferman, T.J., Dickson, D.W., Parisi, J.E., Benarroch, E.E, Ahlskog, J.E., Smith, G.E., Caselli, R.C., Tippman-Peikert, M., Olsen, E.J., Lin, S.-C., Young, T., Wszolek, Z., Schenck, C.H., Mahowald, M. W., Castillo, P.R., Del Tredicci, K.D. & Braak, H. (2007). Pathophysiology of REM sleep behaviour disorder and relevance to neurodegenerative disease. Brain 130, 2770-2788.

Büttner, T., Kuhn, W., Müller, T., Patzold, T., Heidbrink, K., Przuntek, H. (1995). Distorted color discrimination in 'de novo' parkinsonian patients. Neurology 45, 386-387.

Braak, H., Del Tredici, K., Rüb, U., de Vos, R.A.I., Jansen Steur, E.N. & Braak, E. (2003).Staging of pathology related to sporadic Parkinson's disease. Neurobiol Aging 24, 197–211.

Caselli RJ, Chen K, Bandy D, Smilovici O, Boeve BF, Osborne D, Alexander GE, Parish JM, Krahn LE, Reiman EM. A preliminary fluorodeoxyglucose positron emission tomography study in healthy adults reporting dream-enactment behavior. Sleep. 2006 Jul 1;29(7):927-33.

Courbon, F., Brefel-Courbon, C., Thalamas, C., Alibelli, M.J., Berry, I., Montastruc, J.L.,Rascol, O. & Senard, J.M. (2003). Cardiac MIBG scintigraphy is a sensitive tool for detecting cardiac sympathetic denervation in Parkinson's disease. Mov Disord 18,890-897.

Diederich, N.J., Raman, R., Leurgans, S., Goetz, C.G. (2002). Progressive worsening of spatialand chromatic processing deficits in Parkinson disease. Arch Neurol 59, 1249-1252.

Diederich NJ, Mayer G, Möller JC, Oertel WH, Knake S. (2010). Diffusion tensor imaging in idiopathic REM sleep behavior disorder reveals microstructural changes in the brainstem, substantia nigra, olfactory region, and other brain regions. Sleep 33, 767-773.

Doty, R.L., Bromley, S.M. & Stern, M.B. (1995). Olfactory testing as an aid in the diagnosis of Parkinson's disease: development of optimal discrimination criteria. Neurodegeneration 4,93-97.

Doty, R.L., Golbe, L.I., McKeown, D.A., Stern, M.S., Lehrach, C.M. & Crawford, D. (1993). Olfactory testing differentiates between progressive supranuclear palsy and idiopathic Parkinson's disease. Neurology 43, 962-965.

Eisensehr, I., Linke, R., Tatsch, K., Kharraz, B., Gildehaus, J.F., Wetter, C.T., Trenkwalder, C., Schwarz, J. & Noachtar, S. (2003). Increased muscle activity during rapid eye movement sleep correlates with decrease of striatal presynaptic dopamine transporters. IPT and IBZM SPECT imaging in subclinical and clinically manifest idiopathic REM sleep behavior disorder, Parkinson's disease, and controls. Sleep 26, 507-512.

Fantini, M.L., Postuma, R.B., Montplaisir, J., et al. (2006). Olfactory deficit in idiopathic rapid eye movements sleep behavior disorder. Brain Research Bulletin 70:386-390.

Fearnley, J.M. & Lees, A.J. (1991). Aging and Parkinson's disease: substantia nigra regional selectivity.Brain 114, 2283-2301.

Fujishiro, H., Frigerio, R., Burnett, M., Klos, K.J., Josephs, K.A., Delledonne, A., Parisi, J.E., Ahlskog, J.E. & Dickson D.W. (2008). Cardiac sympathetic denervation correlates with clinical and pathologic stages of Parkinson's disease. Mov Disord 23, 1085-1092.

Fujishiro H, Psychogeriatrics 2010 Gagnon, J.F., Postuma, R., Mazza, S., Doyon, J. & Montplaisir, J. (2006). Rapid-eye-movement Sleep behaviour disorder and neurodegeneration diseases. Lancet Neurol 5, 424-432.

Haehner, A., Hummel, T., Hummel, C., Sommer, U., Junghanns, S. & Reichmann, H. (2007). Olfactory loss may be a first sign of idiopathic Parkinson's disease. Mov Disord 22, 839-842.

Hanyu, H, Inoue, Y, Sakurai, H, Kanetaka, H, Nakamura, M, Miyamoto, T, Sasai, T & Iwamoto, T. (2011). Regional cerebral blood flow changes in patients with idiopathic REM sleep behavior disorder. Eur J Neurol 18, 784-788.

Hubbard, P.S., Esiri, M.M., Reading, M., McShane, R. & Nagy, Z. (2007). Alpha-synucleinpathology in the olfactory pathways of dementia patients. J Anat 211,117-124.

Iranzo A, Santamaria J, Pujol J, Moreno A, Deus J, Tolosa E. (2002). Brainstem protonmagnetic resonance spectroscopy in idopathic REM sleep behavior disorder. Sleep 25, 867-870.

Iranzo, A., Molinuevo, J.L., Santamaría, J., Serradell, M., Martí, M.J., Valldeoriola, F. & Tolosa, E. (2006). Rapid-eye-movement sleep behaviour disorder as an early marker for a neurodegenerative disorder: a descriptive study. Lancet Neurol 5, 572-577.

Iranzo, A., Ratti, P.L., Casanova-Molla, J., Serradell, M., Vilaseca, I. & Santamaria, J. (2009). Excessive muscle activity increases over time in idiopathic REM sleep behavior disorder. Sleep 32, 1149-1153.

Kashihara, K., Ohno, M., Kawada, S. & Okumura, Y. (2006). Reduced cardiac uptake and enhanced washout of 123I-MIBG in pure autonomic failure occurs conjointly with Parkinson's disease and dementia with Lewy bodies. J Nucl Med 47, 1099-1101.

Kim, Y.K., Yoon, I-Y., Kim, J-M., Jeong, S-H., Kim, K.W., Shin, Y-K., Kim, B.S. & Kim, S.E. (2010). The implication nigrostriatal dopaminergic degeneration in the pathogenesis of REM sleep behaviour disorder. Eur J Neurol 17, 487-492.

Langston, J.W. (2006). The Parkinson's complex: parkinsonism is just the tip of the iceberg. Ann Neurol 59, 591-596.

Maetzler, W., Liepelt, I. & Berg, D. (2009). Progression of Parkinson's disease in the clinical phase: potential markers. Lancet Neurol 8, 1158-1171.

Matsui, H., Nishinaka, K., Oda, M., Hara, N., Komatsu, K., Kubori, T. & Udaka, F. (2006). Hypoperfusion of the visual pathway in parkinsonian patients with visual hallucinations. Mov Disord 21, 2140-2144.

McShane, R.H., Nagy, Z., Esiri, M.M., King, E., Joachim, C., Sullivan, N. & Smith, A.D. (2001). Anosmia in dementia is associated with Lewy bodies rather than Alzheimer's pathology. J Neurol Neurosurg Psychiatry 70, 739-743.

Miyamoto, T., Miyamoto, M., Inoue, Y., Usui, Y., Suzuki, K. & Hirata, K. (2006). Reduced cardiac 123I-MIBG scintigraphy in idiopathic REM sleep behavior disorder. Neurology 67, 2236-2238.

Miyamoto, T., Miyamoto, M., Suzuki, K., Nishibayashi, M., Iwanami, M. & Hirata, K. (2008). 123I-MIBG cardiac scintigraphy provides clues to the underlying neurodegenerative disorder in idiopathic REM sleep behavior disorder. Sleep 31, 717-723.

Miyamoto, T., Miyamoto, M., Iwanami, M., Suzuki, K., Inoue, Y. & Hirata, K. (2009). Odor identification as an indicator of idiopathic REM sleep behavior disorder. Mov Disord 24:268-273.

Miyamoto, T., Miyamoto, M., Iwanami, M. & Hirata, K. (2009). Three-year follow-up on the accumulation of cardiac (123) I-MIBG scintigraphy in idiopathic REM sleep behavior disorder. Sleep Med 10, 1066-1067.

Miyamoto, T., Orimo, S., Miyamoto, M., Hirata, K., Adachi, T., Hattori, R., Suzuki, M. & Ishii, K. (2010). Follow-up PET studies in case of idiopathic REM sleep behavior disorder. Sleep Med 11, 100-101.

Miyamoto, M., Miyamoto, T., Kubo, J., Yokota, N., Hirata, K. & Sato, T. (2000). Brainstem function in rapid eye movement sleep behavior disorder: the evaluation of brainstem function by proton MR spectroscopy (1H-MRS). Psychiatry Clin Neurosci 54, 350-351.

Miyamoto, M., Miyamoto, T., Iwanami M., Muramatsu, S., Asari, S., Nakano, I. & Hirata, K. (2011). Preclinical substantia nigra dysfunction in rapid eye movement sleep behavior disorder. Sleep Med (in press).

Nurmi, E., Bergman, J., Eskola, O., Vahlberg, T., Sonninen, P. & Rinne, J.O. (2003). Progression of dopaminergic hypofunction in striatal subregions in Parkinson's disease using [18F]CFT PET. Synapse 48, 109–115.

Oh, Y.S., Kim, J.S., Chung, S.W., Song, I.U., Kim, Y.D., Kim, Y.I. & Lee, K.S. (2011). Color vision in Parkinson's disease and essential tremor. Eur J Neurol 18, 577-583.

Olichney, J.M., Murphy, C., Hofstetter, C.R., Foster, K., Hansen, L.A., Thal, L.J. & Katzman, R. (2005). Anosmia is very common in the Lewy body variant of Alzheimer's disease. J Neurol Neurosurg Psychiatry 76, 1342-1347.

Orimo S., Takahashi A., Uchihara T., Mori F., Kakita A., Wakabayashi K. & Takahashi, H. (2007). Degeneration of cardiac sympathetic nerve begins in the early disease process of Parkinson's disease. Brain Pathol 17, 24-30.

Orimo S., Uchihara T., Nakamura A., Mori F., Kakita A., Wakabayashi K. & Takahashi, H.(2008). Axonal alpha-synuclein aggregates herald centripetal degeneration of cardiac sympathetic nerve in Parkinson's disease. Brain 131, 642-650.

Ponsen, M.M., Stoffers, D., Twisk, J.W., Wolters, ECh. & Berendse, H.W. (2009). Hyposmia and executive dysfunction as predictors of future Parkinson's disease: a prospective study. Mov Disord 24,1060-1065.

Postuma, R.B., Lang, A.E., Massicotte-Marquez, J. & Montplaisir, J. (2006). Potential early markers of Parkinson disease in idiopathic REM sleep behavior disorder. Neurology 66, 845-851.

Postuma, R.B., Gagnon, J.F., Vendette, M., Charland, K. & Montplaisir, J. (2008). Manifestations of Parkinson disease differ in association with REM sleep behavior disorder. Mov Disord 15;23, 1665-1672.

Postuma, R.B., Gagnon, J.F., Vendette, M. & Montplaisir, J.Y. (2009). Markers of neurodegeneration in idiopathic rapid eye movement sleep behaviour disorder and Parkinson's disease. Brain 132, 3298-3307.

Postuma, R.B., Gagnon, J.F., Vendette, M., Fantini, M.L., Massicotte-Marquez, J. & Montplaisir, J. (2009). Quantifying the risk of neurodegenerative disease in idiopathi REM Sleep behavior disorder. Neurology 72, 1296-1300.

Postuma, R.B., Gagnon, J.F., Vendette, M., Desjardins, C. & Montplaisir, J.Y. (2010). Olfaction and color vision identify impending neurodegeneration in rapid eye movement sleep behavior disorder. Ann Neurol. 2010 Oct 28. doi: 10.1002/ana.22282.

Price, M.J., Feldman, R.G., Adelberg, D., Kayne, H. (1992). Abnormalities in color visionand contrast sensitivity in Parkinson's disease. Neurology 42, 887-890.

Ross, G.W., Abbott, R.D., Petrovitch, H., Tanner, C.M., Davis, D.G., Nelson, J., Markesbery, W.R., Hardman, J., Masaki, K., Launer, L. & White, L.R. (2006). Assocoation of olfactory dysfunction with incidental Lewy bodies. Mov Disord 21, 2062-2067.

Ross, G.W., Petrovitch, H., Abbott, R.D., Tanner, C.M., Popper, J., Masaki K., Launer, L. & White, L.R. (2008). Association of olfactory dysfunction with risk for future Parkinson's disease. Ann Neurol 63, 167-173.

Schenck, C.H., Bundlie, S.R., Ettinger, M.G. & Mahowald, M.W. (1986). Chronic behavioral disorders of human REM sleep: a new category of parasomnia. Sleep 9, 293-308.

Schenck, C.H., Bundlie, S.R. & Mahowald, M.W. (1996). Delayed emergence of a parkinsonian disorder in 38% of 29 older men initially diagnosed with idiopathic rapid eye movement sleep behavior disorder. Neurology 46, 388-393.

Schenck, C.H. & Mahowald, M.W. (2002). REM sleep behavior disorder: Clinical, Developmental, and Neuroscience perspectives 16 years after its formal identification in sleep. Sleep 25, 120-138.

Scherfler, C., Frauscher, B., Schocke, M., Iranzo, A., Gschliesser, V., Seppi, K., Santamaria, J., Tolosa, E., Högl, B. & Poewe, W.; SINBAR (Sleep Innsbruck Barcelona) Group. (2011). White and gray matter abnormalities in idiopathic rapid eye movement sleep behavior disorder: a diffusion-tensor imaging and voxel-based morphometry study. Ann Neurol 69, 400-407.

Sengoku, R., Saito, Y., Ikemura, M., Hatsuta, H., Sakiyama, Y., Kanemaru, K., Arai, T., Sawabe, M., Tanaka, N., Mochizuki, H., Inoue, K. & Murayama, S. (2008). Incidence and extent of Lewy body-related alpha-synucleinopathy in aging human olfactory bulb. Neuropathol Exp Neurol 67,1072-1083.

Shirakawa, S., Takeuchi, N., Uchimura, N., Ohyama, T., Maeda, H., Abe, T., Ishibashi, M., Ohshima, Y. & Ohshima,H. (2002). Study of image findings in rapid eye movement sleep behavioural disorder. Psychiatry Clin Neurosci 56, 291-292.

Silveira-Moriyama, L., Mathias, C., Mason, L., Best, C., Quinn, N.P. & Lees, A.J. (2009). Hyposmia in pure autonomic failure. Neurology 72, 1677-1681.

Turner, R.S., D'Amato, C.J., Chervin, R.D. & Blaivas, M. (2000). The pathology of REM sleep behavior disorder with comorbid Lewy body dementia. Neurology 55, 1730-1732.

Uchiyama, M., Isse, K., Tanaka, K., Yokota, N., Hamamoto, M., Aida, S., Ito, Y., Yoshimura, M. & Okawa, M. (1995). Incidental Lewy body disease in a patient with REM sleep behavior disorder. Neurology 45, 709-712.

Unger, M.M., Belke, M., Menzler, K., Heverhagen, J.T., Keil, B., Stiasny-Kolster, K., Rosenow, F., Mazza, S., Soucy, J.P., Gravel, P., Michaud, M., Postuma, R., Massicotte-Marquez, J., Decary, A. & Montplaisir, J. (2006). Assessing whole brain perfusion changes in patients with REM sleep behavior disorder._Neurology 67, 1618-622.

Wenning, G.K., Shephard, B., Hawkes, C., Petruckvitch, A., Lees, A. & Quinn N. (1995). Olfactory function in aptypical parkinsonian syndromes. Acta Neurol Scand 91, 247-250.

Williams, S.S., Williams, J., Combrinck, M., Christie, S., Smith, A.D. & McShane, R. (2009). Olfactory impairment is more marked in patients with mild dementia with Lewy bodies than those with mild Alzheimer disease. J Neurol Neurosurg Psychiatry 80, 667-670.

Yoshita, M., Taki, J., Yokoyama, K., Noguchi-Shinohara, M., Matsumoto, Y., Nakajima, K. & Yamada, M. (2006). Value of 123 I-MIBG radioactivity in the differential diagnosis of DLB from AD. Neurology 66, 1850–1854.

7

Advances in Drug Therapy: Alternative Treatments for the Control of Motor Fluctuations and Dyskinesias

José Matías Arbelo González and Rocío Malo de Molina Zamora
Insular of Gran Canaria University Hospital, Spain

1. Introduction

The treatment of Parkinson´s Disease (PD) remains largely symptomatic and it controls effectively motor symptoms of the disease for some years. This is a treatment that is considered basically substitute, which only acts on the nigrostriatal pathway but does not provide adequate plasma levels 24 hours a day in most cases. As a result, conventional medication, especially levodopa, produces pulsatile stimuli that with the progression of the disease is associated with the development of motor complications (Markham & Diamond, 1986).

In recent years new formulations and alternative therapies (dopamine receptor agonists extended release, rotigotine patch, continuous infusion of apomorphine and continuous duodenal infusion of Duodopa) have been introduced in order to avoid pulsatile stimulation and thus prevent the "peaks " and "valleys" and achieve continuous dopaminergic stimulation to avoid, reduce or control the motor fluctuations and dyskinesias. Thus concept of continuous dopaminergic stimulation is born, which is not intended to restore modulatory physiological role exerted by dopamine on striatal function but to explain the benefits of using drugs that provide a more uniform and consistent dopamine stimulation, which has proven to be most appropriate and in practice more beneficial than traditional treatments. This review focuses on the treatment for symptomatic control of Parkinson's disease and complications from chronic treatment, the usefulness of new dopamine agonists and the beneficial effect of Duodopa as a possible alternative in the treatment of advanced PD compared with subcutaneous apomorphine infusion or deep brain stimulation of the subthalamic nucleus, this latter effective to control of motor complications but applicable to a very selective population with no cognitive or behavioral complications.

It is clear that oral Levodopa combined with peripheral inhibitory amino-acid decarboxylase remains still the gold standard in the treatment of PD 40 years later after their use by Cotzias. However, chronic treatment with levodopa (LD) is related to the onset of motor complications in form of fluctuations in the response with wearing-off phenomenon and dyskinesia, which may occur after 3 to 5 years after the start of the LD (Markham & Diamond, 1986; Marsden, 1994). This variability in motor response is correlated with the fluctuation in plasma concentration of LD (related to oral intermittent delivery and irregular gastric emptying) and consequently with the level of pulsatile stimulation of dopamine receptors in the striatum (De la Fuente-Fernández et al., 2001). As the disease progresses, the therapeutic window is narrowed in such a way that reduces the response time "on" increases the off time and is easily reached the threshold for dyskinesias. Motor complications and the also increasingly important non-motor complications are being accentuated with the worsening of the disease and therefore impacts the quality of life of patients (Dodel et al., 2001; Clarke et al., 2002; Witjas et al., 2002).

2. Medical treatment

2.1 Dopamine agonist

Different strategies have been developed to achieve greater continuous dopaminergic stimulation with the sole purpose of delay, reduce or avoid fluctuations (Holloway et al., 2004; Rascol et al., 2006). These options include the administration of dopamine agonists (DA) which have proven effective in both the early stage of the disease and in the moderately advanced stage, improving motor symptoms and delaying the onset of motor complications resulting from the use of LD (Hauser et al., 2007). However, one of the biggest problems of AD has been the need for a slow titration to ensure good tolerance and therefore a delay in obtaining clinical benefits. The new formulations of extended-release agonists provide the advantage of producing a continuous release ensuring sustained absorption over 24 hours and reducing plasma fluctuations (Tompson & Vearer, 2007). Certainly in the treatment of PD, non-ergot dopamine agonists are considered first-line therapy in a substantial proportion of patients.

2.1.1 Ropinirole prolonged-release (RPR)

Perhaps one of the most interesting contributions was the fact that in a recent study, prolonged release ropinirole has shown good tolerance with higher starting dose that immediate release ropinirole and this results in a faster titration (Stocchi et al., 2008) and better clinical response significantly in a period of 4 weeks compared with placebo (Herh et al., 2010). It has been proven non-inferiority of therapeutic response with respect to the formulation of immediate response in monotherapy and in early stages of the disease (Stocchi et al., 2008). Its effectiveness has also been tested in advanced stage patients which not adequately controlled with levodopa, in a randomized, double-blind, placebo for 24 weeks, with a significant reduction in off time of 2.1 hours against 0.3 hours compared to placebo group, and improved quality of life PDQ (Pahwa et al., 2007). Due to the effect observed for 24 hours with this new formulation, several aspects of sleep and nocturnal symptoms improve. As a side effect, RPR causes sleepiness and fatigue which remain practically the same percentage as the immediate release formulation. Finally it is expected a better adherence to the administration once a day.

2.1.2 Delayed pramipexole

Another interesting alternative in the no ergot-AD group is the new long acting formulation of pramipexole, administered once daily to maintain stable levels 24 hours. It has proven effective in improving parkinsonian symptoms in the early stages of the disease and in advanced patients with motor fluctuations resulting in a decrease in off time compared to placebo. No differences in the tolerance respect the immediate release form and the side effects are also comparable (Poewe, 2008; Schapira, 2007). Perhaps the most important indication when compared to immediate-release pramipexole is the fact that it improves treatment adherence in PD.

2.1.3 Rotigotina

Rotigotina is the only non-ergot D3/D2/D1 AD with a formulation which allows for transdermal administration which is very important when it is necessary to reduce the oral medication. Its bioavailability is 37%, its active ingredient is released into the skin during 24 hours (Chen et al., 2009), reaching concentrations that are stable for 24 hours (Chen et al., 2009; Reichmann, 2009) and it has a low risk of accumulation due to its half-life of about 5-7 hours. It is administered by a transdermal patch of silicon and due to its lipophilic, follicular and eccrine properties rotigotine penetrates the skin by transcellular and intercellular pathways, providing a constant supply. It is rapidly metabolized and eliminated by renal and hepatic via and it avoids first-pass effect.

Studies in early stages of the disease support the efficacy compared with other agonists. In addition there is a better tolerance in relation to classical complications such as drowsiness, orthostatic hypotension and hallucinations, but on the other hand must be taken into account cutaneous reactions (The Parkinson Study Group, 2003; Giladi et al., 2007). It has also shown efficacy in advanced stages compared with oral agonists (Poewe et al., 2007), facilitating its administration when complications occur, such as dysphagia, alteration of intestinal transit and when the patient requires absolute diets such as in preoperative and postoperative situations (Korczyn et al., 2007.) Another interesting aspect is its possible effect on non-motor disorders of PD, mainly on the improvement of quality of sleep by improving other aspects such as akinesia, dystonia, nocturia and nocturnal cramps, without worsening daytime sleepiness (Giladi et al., 2006). RECOVER study results support the improvement of sleep disorders by PDSS scale and UPDRS-III scores on awakening (Trenkwalder et al., 2009).

2.1.4 Apomorphine

Apomorphine was the first dopamine receptor agonist used to treat Parkinson's disease over 60 years ago (Schwab et al., 1951; Cotzias et al., 1970). It is an a short-term agonist dopamine that direct acts on D1 and D2 receptors (Kempster et al., 1990; Colosimo et al., 1996), with clinical antiparkinsonian action very powerful, equivalent to the LD, both qualitatively and quantitatively. Apomorphine has a rapid absorption (C max 20 minutes) and a half-life of 43 minutes, which is consistent with its rapid onset of action with evident effects after 15-20 minutes of subcutaneous administration.

The efficacy of intermittent subcutaneous apomorphine has been confirmed in several studies (Poewe & Wenning, 2000; Pfeiffer et al., 2007). Moreover, the effectiveness of continous subcutaneous apomorphine infusion apomorphine (CSAI) has been evaluated both in monotherapy as in addition to levodopa treatment in advanced PD. Several clinical studies support the CSAI to control motor fluctuations poorly controlled by conventional oral route. Apomorphine generally leads to an improvement on the time off between 50-80% and improves dyskinesias associated with LD (Katzenschlager et al., 2005). While the improvement in off time is constant in all studies, the improvement of dyskinesias is less significant and is related to the reduction of the dose of LD. Moreover apomorphine in monotherapy can be achieved only at very high doses, usually above 100 mg / day, which are poorly tolerated by patients. Therefore most require a combination with oral LD, which in fact does not eliminate the effect of pulsatility and prevent the benefit on dyskinesia (Antonini & Tolosa, 2009). From the practical point of view we recommend pre-medicating the patient with domperidone at least three days before the start to prevent peripheral dopaminergic effects and alleviate or eliminate the effect of nausea and vomiting. Oral AD medication should be discontinued and start the infusion of apomorphine with 1 mg / hour maintaining the same dose of L-Dopa. The dose of apomorphine should be gradually increased depending on tolerance at the same time it should be gradually reduced the dose of L-dopa to reduce dyskinesias and if possible remove it completely.

However, the CSAI is not free of side effects, the most constant are the presentation of subcutaneous nodules (70-80%), sedation and somnolence (23%), nausea and vomiting (10%), renal failure (6%), positive Coombs test (6%) and orthostatic hypotension (5%). The adecuate local hygiene and daily change of subcutaneous injection site are important measures to prevent panniculitis. (Antonini et al., 2009)

There is no clear definition of the best candidates. They are usually advanced PD patients with good motor response to L-dopa but inadequately controlled on oral medication and who have motor fluctuations. Patients with cognitive impairment, elderly, orthostatic hypotension, severe systemic disease and a history of dopaminergic psychosis must be excluded.

In a study of continous subcutaneous apomorphine infusion realized in Spain from 2003 to March 2007 in 35 tertiary care hospital centers with a recruitment of 166 patients of whom 82 patients were selected with on-off fluctuations (96%), dyskinesias (48%), whose main objective was to improve the fluctuations, while the dyskinesias associated with L-dopa was not the main purpose unless very severe dyskinesias, with apomorphine dose continuous infusion between 35 mg and 160 mg/day for an average 14 hours per day the following results were found statistically significant: improvement in total UPDRS and motor UPDRS, reduction in the number of off hour per day and number of off episodes per day, reduction in dyskinesias and improvement in balance of gait, reduction in total dose of oral antiparkinsonian medication. Only 3 patients received CSAI in monotherapy, while only 20 needed oral L-dopa mainly in a morning standard dose or in a controlled release Ldopa at night. Most patients had side effects; the most common were subcutaneous nodules. Neuropsychiatric side effects were frequent and the most common have been hallucinations, hypersexuality, confusional state and other complications such as sedation, drowsiness, nausea, orthostatic hypotension and hemolytic anemia. About duration of the 82 patients studied, 27 had been received CSAI for over two years and 9 patients for at least 4 years (García Ruiz et al., 2008).

In conclusion CSAI is a non aggressive, easy to perform and relatively easy to control technique. Certainly the patient and family should have some skill in handling the device and must maintain scrupulous hygiene. This confirms once again that CSAI is effective for control of advanced PD with severe fluctuations that are not well controlled with conventional oral medication.

However, the real impact of CSAI in advanced PD is still a subject for debate.

2.2 Entacapone

Another option is the use of inhibition of catechol-O-methyltransferase (ICOMT), entacapone. It has been noted that its administration increases the levodopa half-life of over 85% and decreases its metabolite 3-O-methyldopa plasma concentrations (Nutt et al., 1994). However, we must consider that it may have a heterogeneous effect in patients. Thus patients with low COMT activity would obtain a low optimal effect, while patients with high activity would obtain better clinical effect but also increase risk of adverse effects. This is due to the existence of polymorphisms of the COMT, which enzyme activity is variable in the population and is related to the substitution of valine for methionine at codon 158 (Syvanen et al., 1997). In Several randomized controlled trial, in which we evaluated the adjuvant effect of entacapone versus placebo in patients with PD and motor complications, there is a significant reduction in off time, improved on time, decrease the dose of levodopa. Its main side effect is the presentation of nausea, vomiting and diarrhea, as well as dyskinesias that can be easily controlled with levodopa reduction (Pahwa et al., 2006). Their use has led to the hypothesis that if a continuous release of LD is gotten may reduce the risk of motor complications. This could be possible with the combination of LD with entacapone, an inhibitor of catechol-0-methyltransferase. This hypothesis recently led STRIDE-PD (Stalevo Reduction in Dyskinesia Evaluation), a multicenter, double-blind, randomized, flexible dose of levodopa (200-1000 mg), with monitoring between 134 and 208 weeks in 747 patients that require initiation of LD, in four doses per day, establishing two groups (LD and LD + entacapone stratified by use of AD at the beginning), which results did not support the early initiation of LD + entacapone reduces the risk of complications and delays the presentation of dyskinesias. There are an increase the risk and higher frequency of dyskinesias in the subgroup of patients taking AD, whereas in the subgroup not taking agonists there are no difference in the time of onset of this complication. The wearing-off occurs more frequently in the LD group than in the LD + entacapone group, but the start time of wearing-off was similar in both groups. This result was not affected by the use of agonists (Stocchi et al., 2010).

2.3 Duodopa

Duodopa is a recent use drug. It is a suspension of micronized levodopa in a methylcellulose thickener gel, which was initially used as compassionate use, but since 2004 its indication was approved in several European countries in advanced PD. At this stage of the disease, levodopa infusion via the gut is an important alternative because it reduces the fluctuations of plasma LD levels and therefore improves the motor response unresponsive to conventional oral therapy (Nyholm et al., 2008), however it should be subject to selection criteria (table 1).

- PD with disabling motor fluctuations (ON_OFF phenomena) - Lack of efficacy of conventional treatments - Response to levodopa, preferably with some quality ON periods - Preferably with no cognitive impairment or mild cognitive impairment - Without psychiatric or behavioral disorders - No age limit (good condition) - Good family or social support

Table 1. Choosing the right candidate

2.3.1 Infusion intrayeyunal of duodopa: control of motor and non motor symptoms

Intrayeyunal infusion of gel levodopa/carbidopa (Duodopa) may represent the more physiological treatment of motor complications in advanced PD using the concept of continuous dopaminergic stimulation observed LD plasma stability compared with oral therapy. Numerous studies have shown a reduction in off-time, an increase in on-time, reduction the severity of dyskinesias and their duration, including patients with deep brain stimulation therapy whose results have been insufficient or ineffective (Antonini et al., 2008). Compared to other options such as subcutaneous apomorphine infusion and DBS surgery, monotherapy with duodopa is usually achieved, avoiding therefore other pulsatile administration of additional medications (Antonini, 2007). DBS will not be discussed in this chapter.

However in advanced PD, motor symptoms are not the only major disruption but also the existence of non-motor symptoms (NMS) are often refractory to conventional treatment and contributes to a deterioration in the quality of life, stress and hospitalizations (Chaudhuri et al., 2006; Martínez-Martín et al., 2007) so in recent years have gained considerable recognition for the impact of these symptoms on quality of life (Chaudhuri et al., 2008). Non-motor signs of PD can be quantified using the non-motor symptoms scale (NMSS) that has been validated (Global Parkinson´s Disease Survey Steering Committee, 2002). His assessment suggests that quality of life is strongly correlated with NMSS but only modestly with the score of the UPDRS III and IV. This observation has been endorsed by other studies. More recently, the highly significant benefit infusion Duodopa has been demostrated in prospective studies by sleep scale, PDQ-8 and total score of the NMSS (cardiovascular, sleep / fatigue, mood / cognition, perception / hallucination , attention / memory, gastrointestinal, urinary, sexual, and miscellaneous (Honig et al., 2009).

These findings together with the recent publication of PDLIFE study, which shows a worsening of motor symptoms and NMS in patients undertreated, demonstrate the importance of global symptom control over the control of other focal symptoms (Grosset et al., 2007).

The observation of improvement in important domains of NMSS underscores the hypothesis that important aspects of the NMS may in part be related to the pathophysiology of dopamine. This finding is consistent with studies suggesting that depression, aspects of sleep dysfunction such as insomnia, restless leg syndrome, nocturia, pain, sexual dysfunction, apathy, and anhedonia are partly related to dysfunction of the dopaminergic system (Remy et al., 2005; Devos, 2009).

2.3.2 Complications

The infusion system of Duodopa includes infusion pump systems, internal and external connection to the jejunum and percutaneous gastrostomy. Any complications may present in any of these levels, the most common are unintentional disconnection of the tube, obstruction of the tube kinking or migration intestinal. Other complications related to gastrostomy as infection, local inflammation or peritonitis are rare. Complications can also occur due to the Duodopa itself such as psychosis, biphasic dyskinesias, behavioral changes with impaired impulse control, orthostasis, and hallucinations, usually easily controlled (Honig et al., 2009).

Adverse effects in relation to Duodopa (drowsiness, visual hallucinations, psychotic episodes, dizziness, headache) are similar to those seen with conventional levodopa

(Nyholm et al., 2005). There have been case reports of polyneuropathy of the Guillain Barre type (Antonini et al., 2007) and development of vitamin B12 and B6 deficiency polyneuropathy (Onofrj et al., 2009).

2.3.3 Conclusion

Duodopa can be summarized that is effective and safe, with significant benefit for the control of motor and non motor symptoms. Most problems are not serious and generally easy to solve, with favorable risk/benefit ratio. Its indication in patients with advanced PD with severe motor fluctuations and dyskinesias may represent an alternative to surgery and continuous infusion of apomorphine. The candidate selection is not as restrictive as in the other two techniques, so that patients which are not optimal for surgery and apomorphine can be treated successfully with Duodopa (Devos, 2009; Sánchez-Castañeda et al., 2010).
But despite clinical benefits, total number of patients treated with infusions is still limited due to the complexity of the procedure.
The general conclusions are:

1. Infusions provide constant plasma levels preventing the peaks and valleys that are typical of the medication orally.
2. Infusions can reduce dyskinesias and extend the therapeutic window in advanced PD.
3. Apomorphine is effective in reducing off time but improvement of dyskinesias is limited by the need to continue with oral L-dopa in most patients. Its use remains limited in time and its discontinuation is mainly due to the development of skin reactions.
4. Experience with continuous infusion of duodenal L-dopa/carbidopa shows that the benefit is also related to the quality of life and better control of non-motor symptoms such as cardiovascular system, bladder, gastrointestinal function and sleep quality

3. Behavioral disorders and their relationship with dopaminergic medication

In recent years interest has focused on behavioral disorders in Parkinson´s Disease due to their higher prevalence than in the general population and its relation to dopaminergic therapy, primarily to the use of dopamine agonists. It includes impulse control disorders (ICD) such as pathological gambling, buying and compulsive food intake, hypersexuality and repetitive stereotyped behaviors-punding devoid of purpose and dopamine dysregulation syndrome also known as syndrome of addictive behavior, in which there is a progressive, increased and excessive consumption of dopaminergic drugs, higher than needed to control the motor symptoms of the disease despite the occurrence of severe dyskinesias. It develops a tolerance to the euphoric effect of dopaminergic therapy and often produces a state of abstinence because of the reduction or withdrawal of medication in addition to motor worsening, complicating the management of this type of addictive disorder.
The impulse control disorder is characterized by an inability to resist an impulse or temptation to perform an act that can be harmful to other or to themselves. It is very important to identify because it can cause significant distress to patients and caregivers, serious financial and socio-familiar consequences. Its key feature is the participation in a repetitive and compulsive behavior despite adverse consequences, an impulse of appetite or desire before engaging in the problematic behavior and a hedonic quality during the

execution of the act. It shares a conceptual resemblance to the drug addiction in which patients perform compulsive activity despite adverse consequences (Ceravolo et al., 2010).

Addictive behavior syndrome is a neuropsychiatric disorder of behavior associated with excessive use of dopaminergic drugs, more frequently with levodopa and apomorphine. The clinical features met the accepted criteria for addiction: compulsive use of drugs, hypomania, impulsivity, withdrawal symptoms such as anxiety and dysphoria. The psychiatric features include manic, elation, irritability, psychomotor agitation, paranoia towards hospital staff and family. Complusive acts with stereotyped behaviors frecuently occurs in this syndrome. These acts are characterized by an intense fascination for handling technical equipment repetitively and continuously or review and classification of common objects (Ceravolo et al., 2010).

The prevalence of these disorders varies according to the series. They are often underdiagnosed because not all patients are aware of the problem and they do not relate them to the PD. At other times patients are reluctant to admit the existence of these disorders. Recently in a large cross-sectional study of 3090 patients with idiopathic PD has been described the existence of any impulse control disorder in 13.6%, of which pathological gambling 5.0%, compulsive behavior of sex 3.5%, compulsive buying 5.7%, eating disorder 4.3%. Several disorders are often associated in the same individual 3.9%. This disorder occurs more frequently in patients taking AD (17.7%) compared to those who do not take (6.9%), finding no significant difference between Pramipexole 17.7% vs Ropinirole 15.5% (Weintraub et al., 2010).

In addition to individual factors, predisposing factors have been identified such as the duration of the disease, high doses of medication, especially AD unrelated to any specific (class effect) (Ceravolo et al., 2010) but may also occur at low doses, at lower age, at disease onset (Voon et al., 2006), the existence of affective disorders (Pontone et al., 2006) and a ICD before PD (Weintraub et al., 2006) and the presence of motor complications. However, no differences were found in Hoehn and Yahr stage between patients with and without ICD.

Treatment usually involves the reduction/suspension of AD, adjusting the dose of levodopa. If these measures are insufficient alternative pharmacological measures can be employed, though less user experience. Thus selective inhibitors of serotonin reuptake have proven effective in binge eating and stereotyped behaviors (Wolters et al., 2008). Atypical antipsychotics such as quetiapine are useful in pathological gambling and hypersexuality. In the latter case can be used antiandrogens such as cyproterone acetate (Klos et al., 2005).

4. References

Antonini, A. & Odin, P. (2009). Pros and cons of apomorphine and L-dopa continuous infusion in advanced Parkinson´s disease. *Parkinsonism Relat Disord,* Vol.15, Suppl.4, (December 2009), pp. S97-100

Antonini, A. & Tolosa, E. (2009). Apomorphine and levodopa infusion therapies for advanced Parkinson´s disease: selection criteria and patient management. *Expert Rev Neurother,* Vol.9, No.6, (June 2009), pp. 859-867

Antonini, A.; Mancini, F.; Canesi, M.; Zangaglia, R.; Isaias, IU.; Manfredi, L. Pacchetti, C.; Zibetti, M.; Natuzzi, F.; Lopiano, L.; Nappi, G & Pezzoli, G. (2008). Duodenal levodopa infusión improves quality of life in advanced Parkinson´s disease. *Neurodegener Dis,* Vol.5, (March 2008), pp. 244-246

Antonini, A. (2007). Continuous dopaminergic stimulation-from theory to clinical practice. *Parkinsonism Relat Disord,* Vol.13 Suppl, (September 2007), pp. S24-28

Antonini, A.; Isaias, IU; Canesi, M; Zibetti, M.; Manzzini, F; Dal Fonte, M; Lopiano, L & Pezzoli, G. (2007). Duodenal levodopa infusion for advanced Parkinson´s disease: 12-month treatment outcome. *Mov Disord,* Vol.22, No.8, (June 2007), pp. 1145-1149

Ceravolo, R.; Frosini, D.; Rossi, C. & Bonuccelli, U. (2010). Spectrum of addictions in Parkinson´s disease:from dopamine dysregulation syndrome to impulse control disorders. *J Neurol,* Vol.257, Suppl.2, (November 2010), pp S276-283

Chaudhuri, KR. & Martínez Martín, P. (2008). The quantitation of non motor symptoms of Parkinson´s disease. *European J Neurol,* Vol.15, Suppl.2, (August 2008), pp. 2-8

Chaudhuri, KR.; Healy, DG. & Shapira, AH. (2006). Non-motor symptoms of Parkinson´s disease: diagnosis and management. *Lancet Neurol,* Vol.5, (March 2006), pp. 235-245

Chen, JJ.; Swope, DM.; Dashtipour, K. & Lyons, KE. (2009). Transdermal rotigotine: A clinically innovative dopamine-receptor agonist for the management of parkinson´s disease. *Pharmacotherap,* Vol.29 No.12, (December 2009), pp. 1452-1467.

Clarke, CB.; Vieregge, P.; Ziegler, M.; Voinet, C. & Pechevis, M. (2002). The impact of L-dopa-induced dyskinesias on patients quality of life in Parkinson´s disease: a prospective European study. *Neurology* Vol.58, Suppl.3, pp. A469.

Colosimo, C.; Merello; M.; Hughes, AJ.; Sieradzan, K. & Lees, AJ.(1996). Motor response to acute dopaminergic challenge with apomorphine and levodopa in Parkinson´s disease: implications for the pathogenesis of the on-off phenomenon. *J Neurol, Neurosurg Psychiatry.* Vol.60, No.6, (June 1996), pp. 634-637

Cotzias, GC.; Papavasiliou, PS.; Fehling, C.; Kaufman, B. & Mena, I. (1970). Similarities between neurologic effects of L-dopa and apomorphine. *N Engl J Med,* Vol.282, pp. 31-33

De la Fuente-Fernández, R.; Lu, JQ.; Sossi V, Jivan, S.; Schulzer, M.; Holden, JE.; Lee, CS.; Ruth, TJ.; Calne, DB. & Stoessl, AJ. (2001). Biochemical variations in the synaptic level of dopamine precede motor fluctuations in Parkinson´s disease: PET evidence of increased dopamine turnover. *Ann Neurol,* Vol.49, (March 2001), pp. 298-303.

Devos, D. French Duodopa Study Group. (2009). Patient profile, indications, efficacy and safety of duodenal levodopa infusion in advanced Parkinson's disease. *Mov Disord., 2009.* Vol.24, pp. 993-1000

Dodel, RC.; Berger, K. & Oertel, WH. (2001). Health-related quality of life and healthcare utilisation in patients with Parkinson´s disease: impact of motor fluctuations and dyskinesias: *Pharmacoeconomics,* Vol.19, No.10, (December 2001), pp. 1013-1038

García Ruiz, P.; Sesar, A.; Ares, B. & al. Efficacy of Long-Term Continous Subcutaneous Apomorphine Infusion in Advanced Parkinson´s disease with Motor Fluctuations: A Multicenter Study. *Mov Disord.,* Vol 23, No.8, (April 2008), pp. 1130-1136

Giladi, N.; Boroojerdi, B.; Korczyn, AD.; Burn, DJ.; Clarke, CE. & Schapira, AH. (2007). Rotigotine transdermal patch in early stage Parkinson´s disease: a randomized, double-blind, controlled study versus placebo and ropinirole. *Mov Disord,* Vol.22, No.16, (December 2007), pp. 2398-2404

Giladi, N. & al. (2006). Effects of rotigotine transdermal path on early morning motor function, sleep quality and daytime sleepiness in patients with idiopathic Parkinson´s disease. Results of a multicenter, multinational trial. *Proceeding of The 10th Congress of the EFNS,* Glasgow, September 2006

Global Parkinson´s Disease Survey Steering Committee. (2002). Factors impacting on quality of life in Parkinson´s disease: results from an international survey. *Mov Disord*, Vol.17, No.1, (Jan 2002), pp. 60-67

Grosset, D.; Taurah, L.; Burn, DJ. & al. (2007). A multicentre longitudinal observational study of changes in self reported health status in people with Parkinson´s disease left untreated at diagnosis. *J Neurol Neurosurg Psychiatry*, Vol.78, No.5, (May 2007), pp. 465-469

Hauser, RA.; Rascol, O.; Korczyn, AD. & al. (2007). Ten-Year follow-up of Parkinson´s disease patients randomized to initial therapy with ropinirole or levodopa. *Mov Disord*, Vol.22, No.16, (December 2007), pp: 2409-2417.

Herh, BP.; Earl, NL.; Hauser, RA. & Stacy, M. (2010). Early treatment benefits of ropinirole prolongued release in Parkinson´s disease patients with motor fluctuations. *Mov Disord*, Vol.25, No.7, (May 2010), pp. 927-931

Holloway, RG.; Shoulson, I.; Fahn, S. & al. (2004). Pramipexole vs levodopa as initial treatment for Parkinson´s disease: a 4 year randomized controlled trial. *Arch Neurol*, Vol.61, No.7, (July 2004), pp. 1044-1053

Honig, H.; Antonini A.; Martínez- Martín P. & al. (2009). Intrajejunal levodopa infusion in Parkinson´s disease: a pilot multicenter study of effects on nonmotor symptoms and quality of life. *Mov Disord*, Vol.24, No.10, (July 2009), pp. 1468-1474

Katzenschlager, R.; Hughes, A.; Evans, A. & al. (2005). Continuous subcutaneuous apomorphine therapy improves dyskinesias in Parkinson´s disease: a prospective study using single-dose challenges. *Mov Disord*, Vol.20, No.2, (February 2005), pp. 151-157

Kempster, PA.; Frankel, JP.; Stern, GM. & Lees, AJ. (1990). Comparison of motor response to apomorphine and levodopa in Parkinson´s disease. *J Neurol Neurosurg Psychiatry*, Vol.53, No.11, (November 1990), pp. 1004-1007

Klos, KJ.; Bower, JH.; Josephs, KA.; Matsumoto, JY. & Ahlskog, JE. (2005). Pathological hypersexuality predominantly linked to adjuvant dopamine agonist therapy en Parkinson´s disease and multiple system atrophy. *Parkinsonism Relat Disord*, Vol.11, No.6, (September 2005), pp. 381-386

Korczyn, AD.; Reichmann, H.; Boroojerdi, B. & Häck, J. (2007). Rotigotine transdermal system for periopertive administration. *J Neural Transm*, vol.112, No.2, pp. 219-221

Markham, CH. & Diamond, SG. (1986). Long term follow-up of early dopa treatment in Parkinson´s disease. *Ann Neurol*, Vol.19, No.4, pp. 365-372

Marsden, C. (1994). Problems with long-term levodopa therapy for Parkinson´s disease. *Clin Neuropharmacol*, Vol17, Suppl.2, pp. S32-44

Martínez-Martín, P.; Schapira, AH.; Stocchi, F. & al. (2007). Prevalence of non-motor symptoms in Parkinson´s disease in an international setting: Study using nonmotor symptoms questionnaire in 545 patients. *Mov Disord*, Vol.22, No.11, (August 2007), pp. 1623-1629

Nutt, JG.; Woodward, WR.; Beckner, RM. & al. (1994). Effect of peripheral catechol-O-methyltransferase inhibition on the pharmacokinetics and pharmacodynamics of levodopa in patients with Parkinson´s disease. *Neurology*, Vol.44, No.5, (May 1994), pp. 913-919.

Nyholm, D. ; Lewander, T. ; Johansson, A. & al. (2008). Enteral levodopa/carbidopa infusion in advanced Parkinson´s disease : long-term exposure. *Clin Neuropharmacol*, Vol.31, No.2, (March-April 2008), pp. 63-77

Nyholm, D.; Nilsson, R.; Dizdar, N. & al. (2005). Duodenal levodopa infusión monotherapy vs oral polypharmacy in advanced Parkinson´s disease. *Neurology*, Vol.64, No.2, (January 2005), PP. 216-223

Onofrj, M.; Bonanni, L.; Cossu, G. & al. (2009). Emergencies in parkinsonism:akinetic crisis, life-threatening dyskinesias, and polyneuropathy during L-dopa gel treatment. *Parkinsonism Relat Disord*, Vol.15, Suppl.3, (December 2009), pp. S233-236

Pahwa, R. ; Stacy, MA. ; Factor, SA. & al. (2007). Ropinirole 24-hour prolonged release: randomized, controlled study in advanced Parkinson disease. *Neurology*, Vol.68, No.14, (April 2007), pp. 1108-1115

Pahwa, R. ; Factor, SA. ; Lyons, KE. ; Ondo, WG. & al. Quality standars subcomittee of the American Academy of Neurology. (2006). Practice parameters: treatment of Parkinson´s disease with motor fluctuations and dyskinesia (an evidence-based review): report of the quality standards subcommittee of the American Academy of Neurology. *Neurology*, Vol.66, No.7, (April 2006), pp. 983-995

Pfeiffer, RF.; Gutmann, L.; Hull, KL. & al. APO302 Study Investigator. (2007). Continued efficacy and safety of subcutaneous apomorphine in patients with advanced Parkinson´s disease. *Parkinsonism Relat Disord*, Vol.13, No.2, (March 2007), pp. 93-100

Poewe, W. (2008). Non-motor symptoms in Parkinson's disease. *Eur J Neurol*, Vol.15, Suppl.1, (April 2008), pp. S14-20

Poewe, W.; Rascoll, O.; Quinn, N.; Tolosa, E. & al. (2007). Efficacy of pramipexole and transdermal rotigotine in advanced Parkinson´s disease: a double-blind, double-dummy, randomised controlled trial. *Lancet Neurol*, Vol.6, No.6, (June 2007), pp. 513-520

Poewe, W. & Wenning, GK. (2000). Apomorphine: an underutilized therapy for Parkinson´s disease. *Mov Disord*, Vol.15, No.5, (September 2000), pp. 789-794

Pontone, G.; Williams, JR.; Basset, SS. & Marsh, L. (2006). Clinical features associated with impulse control disorders in Parkinson disease. *Neurology*, Vol.67, No.7, (October 2006), pp. 1258-61

Rascol, O.; Brooks, DJ.; Korczyn, AD. & al. (2006). Development of dyskinesias in a 5-year trial of ropinirole and L-dopa. *Mov Disord*, Vol.21, No.11, (November 2006), pp. 1844-1850

Reichmann, H. (2009). Transdermal delivery of dopamine receptor agonists. *Parkinsonism relat disord*, Vol.15, Suppl.4, (December 2009), pp. S93-96

Remy, P. ; Doder, M. ; Lees, A. & al. (2005). Depression in Parkinson´s disease. Loss of dopamine and noradrenaline innervations in the limbic system. *Brain*, Vol.128, No.6, (February 2005), pp. 1314-1322

Sánchez-Castañeda, C.; Campdelacreu, J.; Miró, J. & al. (2010). Cognitive improvement after duodenal levodopa infusion in cognitively impaired Parkinsonn´s disease patients. *Prog Neuropsychopharmacol Biol Psychiatry*, Vol.34, No.1, (February 2010), pp. 250-251

Schapira, AH. (2007). Future directions in the treatment of Parkinson's disease. *Mov Disord*, Vol.22, Suppl.17, (September 2007), pp. S385-391

Schwab, RS.; Amador, LV. & Lettvin, JY. (1951). Apomorphine in Parkinson´s disease. *Trans Am Med Assoc*, vol.56, (1951), pp. 251-253

Stocchi, F.; Rascol, O.; Kieburtz, K. & al. (2010). Initiating levodopa/carbidopa therapy with and without entacapone in early Parkinson disease: the STRIDE-PD study. *Ann Neurol*, Vol.68, No.1, (July 2010), pp. 18-27

Stocchi, F.; Hersh, BP.; Scott, BL. & al. (2008). Ropinirole 24 hour prolonged release and ropinirole inmediate release in early Parkinson´s disease: a randomized, double-blind, non-inferiority crossover study. *Curr Med Res Opin*, Vol.24, No.10, (October 2008), pp. 2883-2895

Syvanen,AC.; Tilgmann, C.; Rinne, J. & Ulmanen, I. (1997). Genetic polymorphism of catechol-O-methyl-transferase (COMT): correlation of genotype with individual variation of S-COMT activity and comparison of the allele frequencies in the normal population and parkinsonian patients in Finland. *Pharmacogenetics*, Vol.7, No.1, (February 1997), pp. 65-71

The Parkinson Study Group. (2003). A controlled trial of rotigotine monotherapy in early Parkinson´s disease. *Arch Neurol*, Vol.60, No.12, (December 2003), pp. 1721-1728

Tompson, D. & Vearer, D. (2007). Steady-state pharmacokinetic properties of a 24-hour prolonged-release formulation of ropinirole: results of two randomized studies in patients with Parkinson´s disease. *Clin Ther*, Vol.29, No.12, (December 2007), pp. 2654-2666

Trenkwalder C, Chaudhuri, KR. Anderson, T. & al. (2009). Effect of rotigotine on control of early morning motor function and sleep quality in subjects with idiopathic Parkinson´s disease. *Proceedings of XVIII WFN World Congress on Parkinson´s Disease and Related Disorders*. (December 2009), pp. 15S2: S136

Voon, V; Hassan, K.; Zurowski, M. & al. (2006). Prevalence of repetitive and reward-seeking behaviors in Parkinson disease. *Neurology*, Vol.67, No.7, (October 2006), pp. 1254-1257

Weintraub, D.; Koester, J.; Potenza, MN.; Siderowf, AD. & al. (2010). Impulse control disorders in Parkinson´s disease: A cross-sectional study of 3090 patients. *Arch Neurol*, Vol.67, No.5, (May 2010), pp. 589-595

Weintraub, D.; Siderowf, AD.; Potenza, MN.; Goveas, J.; Morales, KH.; Duda, JE. & al. (2006). Association of dopamine agonist use with impulse control disorders in Parkinson disease. *Arch Neurol*, Vol.63, No.7, (July 2006), pp. 969-73

Witjas, T.; Kaphan, E.; Azulay, JP. & al. (2002). Nonmotor fluctuations in Parkinson´s disease: frequent and disabling. *Neurology*, Vol.59, No.3, (August 2002), pp. 408-413

Wolters, EC.; Van der Werf, YD. & Van der Heuvel, OA. (2008). Parkinson disease-related disorders in the impulsive compulsive spectrum. J. Neurol Vol.255, Suppl.5, (September 2008), pp. 48-56

8

The Role of Feedback in Decision Making

Magda Osman
Queen Mary University of London
United Kingdom

1. Introduction

To date there has been no comprehensive review of the kinds of decision making tasks and their requirements with respect to investigating preserved and impaired behavior in patients with Parkinson's (PD). The aim of this chapter is to address this by examining recent work in this domain. The chapter is divided into three mains sections. The first will discuss tasks which have been typically used to study decision making in patients with PD. The aim here is to present an over view of critical features that are common to them along with the associated findings. The second section then focuses on decision making behavior when patients are studied on dopaminergic medication, and when examined off medication. The concluding section discusses reinforcement learning models that have been used to account for differences in cognitive impairments in PD patients. The main claim that will be expounded is that some of the discrepancies found in the literature concerning impairments in decision making activities may be due to the structure of the task rather than the dopamine overdosing hypothesis *per se*.

2. Different flavours of decision making

To what extent does Parkinson's disease (PD) impair core cognitive functions such as decision making? The vast literature that has amassed in attempt to answer this question has spawned a diverse range of tasks, loosely classed as decision making tasks. These include, but are not limited to the follow: the Iowa Gambling Task (Mimura et al, 2006; Poletti, et al, 2010), Game of Dice Task (Brand et al, 2004; Lubudda et al, 2010), Probabilistic Classification task (Bodi et al, 2009; Jahanshahi et al, 2010; Shohamy et al, 2004), Procedural learning transitive inference task (Frank et al, 2004), Conditional associative learning task (Gotham et al, 1988; Jahanshahi et al, 2000), Probabilistic reversal learning (Cools et al, 2006), and Dynamic decision making task (Osman et al, 2008; Witt et al, 2006).

To shed some light on the various approaches to understanding decision making in the clinical domain, Gleichgerrcht et al's (2010) recent review of decision making in patients with PD and Huntington's Disease, offered the following description of decision making "Decision-making is a complex mental function influenced by multiple cognitive and behavioral processes" (p 612). This clearly recognizes the multifaceted nature of decision making and its involvement with other functions and though this is a popular characterization (Brand et al, 2004; Delazer et al, 2009; Mimura et al, 2006), it fails to describe the types of activities associated with decision making; it simply established that there are many of them.

Therefore, one might well do to ask the following question, if we strip the aforementioned decision making tasks to their essential features, what is it that constitutes a decision making task? More to the point, what are the types of processes that are under investigations when patients with Parkinson's are required to undertake one of these aforementioned decision making task? If the general findings from studies on PD patients performing the decision making tasks converge on the same general conclusions, which could be that performance is poor relative to healthy age matched controls (HCs), then that could be used to imply that some general aspect of decision making is affected. In actual fact, the evidence suggests that PD patients' performance is impaired under specific conditions (e.g., depending on feedback) but this is not consistently the case for all decision making tasks. Unless we understand what behaviors are engaged in these various tasks, and unless we can be sure that they are essentially tapping the same facets of decision making behavior, our conclusions are somewhat limited. All we can be sure of is that, at best, a broad class of tasks labeled as decision making tasks reveal impaired performance when carried out by patients with PD. At worst, we can are left concluding that a collection of tasks that are thought to involve decision making may actually be examining entirely different processes.

At a minimum then, we need to begin with some basic description of decision making. Most commonly, decision making needs to be thought of as a goal-directed pursuit that involves the ability to predict and manage outcomes (Osman, 2010). Without a goal we cannot direct our actions towards anything. Without a goal we cannot assess the relative success of our actions because we don't have a target by which to evaluate our behaviors against. To assist with the evaluation, interpreting the effects of actions on outcomes can come about through intrinsically driven or externally determined feedback (i.e. gains, losses; reward, punishment). This can often inform us of how much closer or further away we are from attaining our goal, but more often it will serve as an additional source of motivation. From this, we can outline the following three component parts of decision making: 1) sensitivity to the situation in terms of the rates at which rewards and punishments are experienced, (i.e. the amount of reward/punishment received, and the probabilities with which rewards and punishments occur), 2) evaluation of actions in relation to a desired goal (e.g., via rewards and punishments that our actions generate), 3) evaluation of future actions based on the outcome that we have achieved in trying to reach a desire goal (Doya, 2008, Schultz, 2006; Yu, 2007).

All of these components point to the fact that decision making is a sequential processes. In fact rarely is it the case that we make a one shot decision, we choose an action, that in turn has an effect, and shortly after we need to follow that up with yet another decision (Brehmer, 1992). Thus, decision making is often a sequential process. It involves inter-dependent decisions (e.g., choosing where to eat out, choosing where to sit in the restaurant, choosing what to eat and what to drink etc...), and the effects of our actions are inter-dependent (e.g., we invited 5 people to join us for dinner, instead, 7 people came, so we now need to find somewhere to accommodate 7 people instead of 5). Importantly, what should be stressed is that as a goal directed pursuit, decision making typically involves more than one step.

Having established the critical components of decision making, it is important to also outline the general conditions under which decision making takes place. Trepel, Fox, and Poldrack (2005) draw on a broad distinction between two situations that those in the decision making sciences will recognize as "*Decisions under risk*" and "*Decision under uncertainty*". In the former, people are engaged in planning actions against knowledge of the probabilities of the outcomes following their actions. For instance, betting on the roll of a dice, or placing money on a roulette wheel. Some estimation of the outcome can be calculated (e.g., the likelihood of the ball landing on black) and an action from it then follows. The estimation is a prediction of the outcome, and along with that we attach some value to it (e.g., betting money), or else there is some inherent value to it (e.g., the intrinsic value of correctly guessing that the roll of the dice would land a 4). The latter decision making scenario is a case in which people plan their actions from limited available knowledge of the possible outcomes, and in which the probabilities of the outcomes following actions is not known, or cannot be known. For example, deciding on when in the financial year to sell the house, or whether to make an investment by buying stocks in a major clothing company. Again, some estimation of the outcome is needed (i.e. how much of a profit will I make if I sell now/buy shares now rather than later). In the same way as decisions under risk, actions are informed by the estimation of the outcome occurring, and there are different values attached to the different possible outcomes that could follow. Similarly, the success of the decision is evaluated according to the eventual outcome. In sum, the simple distinction draw between risk and uncertainty is that, either we can decide what actions to take in the face of knowing the probability of the desirable and undesirable outcomes, or we make a decision to act in situations in which the probabilities of outcomes are not known to us.

For the remainder of this section the focus will be on three types of tasks, two of which are commonly used to investigate decision making behavior in patients with PD, and one which is currently gaining in interest in the clinical field: the Probabilistic Classification task - alternatively known as the Weather prediction task (WPT), IOWA Gambling Task (IGT), and Dynamic decision making tasks (DDM). For each task, the aim is to examine the components of decision making, and the conditions under which decisions are being made. PD patient studies that are reported in this section refer to findings from patients on L-dopa medication.

2.1 Weather prediction task (WPT)

The original motivation behind the WPT was to examine habit learning independently from the development of explicit reportable knowledge (i.e. declarative knowledge). To achieve this Knowlton et al (1994) designed a task in which stimuli and responses were associated probabilistically. Importantly, as with habit learning, this task was designed to encourage the incremental acquisition of knowledge of associations between stimuli and responses, because no one single encounter with a stimulus would reliably predict the outcome. So, when faced with the WPT task (See Fig. 1), a decision maker is shown one of 14 (15 - if all four cards are presented) possible combinations of four cards (Card 1= Triangles, Card 2 = Circles, Card 3 = Diamonds, Card 4 = Squares). So, on a single trial, Card 1 and Card 3 could be shown, and on the next trial you might see Card 1, Card 3 and Card 4. The presentation of cards is psuedo-randomized, so that people are unable to experience runs of trials in which the same combinations of cards is presented in succession. Each individual card is associated with an outcome with a fixed independent probability, though card combinations do not appear with equal frequency, in fact some are more common than others. Importantly, the four cards have different cue validities. That is, one card is highly predictive (i.e. Card 4), and another card only weakly predictive of rain (i.e. Card 3), and similarly one card is highly predictive (Card 1) and weakly predictive (Card 2) of sun. In the course of the experiment which may involve between 100 - 350 trials, the two outcomes are equally likely to be correct.

What you are told when you are performing this task is that the different cards predict the weather, which can either be one of two states, sunny or rainy. What you have to do is work out on each trial based on the combination of cards presented, if it will rain or if it will be sunny by selecting one of the two options.

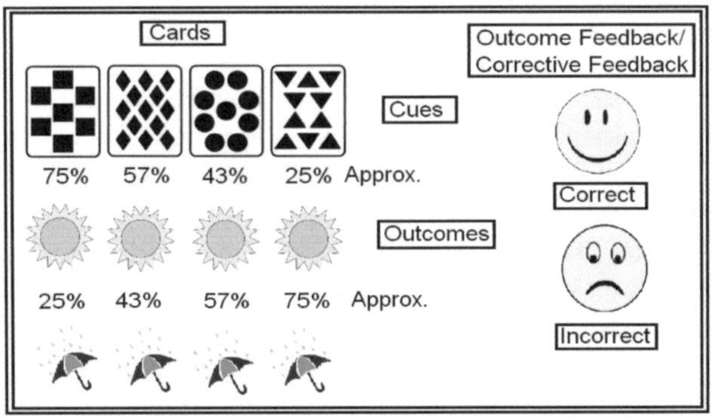

Fig. 1. Details of the Weather Prediction Task (WPT)

Typically, after your choice is made, your only way of knowing if you are correct is either seeing a smiley face, or a sad face; there is no presentation of labels to indicate what the outcome is. In this case corrective feedback and outcome feedback are presented as one and the same. In the task, our action/response is choosing what we think the outcome will be, and we can only do this based on limited knowledge - given that we are unaware of the precise probabilities of the outcomes associated with each card/card combinations. On a given trial, you can only infer from the correspondence of the feedback to your own prediction what the actual outcome is; where positive feedback is simply confirmation of our predictions, and negative feedback indicates that the basis of our predictions is incorrect.

So, what constitutes a decision in this task, what are the conditions in which decisions are being made, and how do PD patients perform in it? This task, and other variants like it, are referred to as probabilistic category learning tasks (Jahanshahi et al, 2010; Shohamy et al, 2004), predictive learning tasks (Knowlton et al, 1994), or multiple cue probability tasks (Lagnado et al, 2006). In actual fact, they are all aspects of decision making, and so subject to evaluation of the three components outlined earlier. 1) In the WPT people are required to learn the rates at which rewards and punishments are experienced, because this indicates the success of learning the probabilistic relationship between the cues and outcomes. The findings are mixed with respect to this. Some show that impaired performance in PDs is localized to this component of decision making (Poldrack et al, 2001; Shohamy et al, 2004; Witt et al, 2002), whereas other have shown that the impairments are more general (Jahanshahi et al, 2010; Wilkinson et al, 2008). In one case, there was no overall difference in performance between PDs and HCs (Moody et al, 2004). 2) In the WPT actions are evaluated in relation to a general goal which is to learn cue-outcome associations in order to successfully predict the outcome on each trial. 3) Future performance is based on evaluating the rate of success of past predictions, as well as the usefulness of strategies from which cue-outcome knowledge informs actions taken. Both HCS and PDs show better performance when learning cue-outcome associations when they are given (i.e. presenting the cue pattern and the corresponding outcome) and then applied, compared with when they are acquired through corrective feedback (Shohamy et al, 2004; Wilkinson et al, 2008). This could be taken to suggest that in general, corrective feedback interferes or competes with goal directed learning of cue-outcome associations in a probabilistic environment. This may be because learning probabilistic cue-outcome associations is demanding of executive functions, and so integrating corrective feedback requires additional resources that are simply not available. However, Wilkinson et al (2008) demonstrated that when removing the response deadline from the feedback and the no-feedback version, PD's showed equivalent learning in both conditions. Thus suggesting that actual feedback processing *per se* is not the reason for decrements in WPT performance. 4) Finally, because the probabilistic relationship between cues and outcomes is unknown, decision making in the WPT is under uncertainty. When compared with Amnesics, or patients with frontal lesions, PD's show poorer performance on the WPT task. Some have taken these findings to suggest that it is impairments to the striatum, and not the Medial temporal lobe or frontal lobes that are associated with impaired decision making under uncertainty in PDs (Knowlton, et al, 1996; Witt et al, 2002).

2.2 IOWA Gambling Task (IGT)

Bechara et al, (1994) devised a task that examined decision making under uncertainty in which the goal was obvious. People have to make advantageous decisions in order to make a profit, or else pay a penalty for a poor decision and lose money.

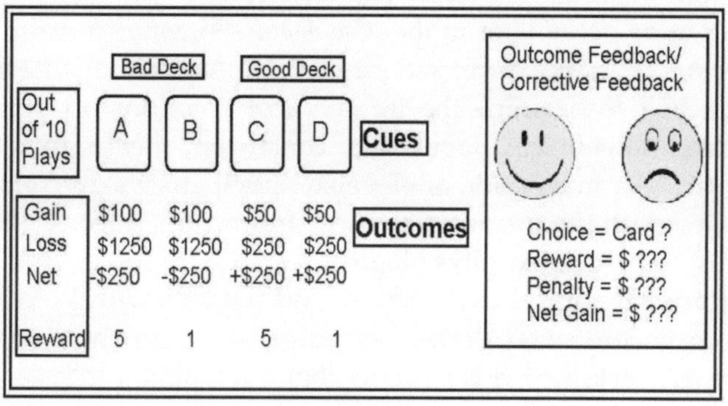

Fig. 2. Details of the IOWA Gambling task (IGT)

The IGT is highly motivating because it presents people with a situation in which at the start of the game they are given a fictional loan of $2000 loan to play with. Not only is the task designed to examine decision making with gains and losses, it is designed to invoke emotions that could guide decision making in uncertain situations. In this sense the IOWA gambling task is not a risky decision making situation. Unlike other gambling tasks (Roulette, Poker) in which the probabilities of outcome can be estimated, in this task the decision maker is unaware of the probabilities of wins and losses associated with each deck. When presented with the task (see Fig 2), the decision maker is simply told that for each play (trial), they are to select a card from one of four decks A-D; which will not be placed back in the deck after selection. Two cards (A and B) have high rewards, and two cards have low rewards (C and D). However, they are unaware that over the course of 10 plays, cards selected consistently from a deck will result in a penalty that is high (Deck A or B, $1250) or low (Deck C or D, $250), with the difference between the two sets of decks based on the frequency of losses (5, or 1). The problem for the decision maker is that they are not told in advance how many plays (actually 100) they will have, so they have to proceed cautiously by learning that two decks have high pays-outs and high penalties, and so to maximize their overall wins, they ought to go for decks with lower pay-outs and low penalties.

A combination of outcome and corrective feedback is often used in the IGT. That is, on each trial, decision makers will know how much they gained/or lost (outcome feedback), and this is often accompanied by a smiley face or sad face depending on the outcome (corrective feedback). In addition, progress bars are presented on screen after a decision is made in order for people to see their cumulative wins and losses over the successive trials they have played. In sum, in the IGT, an action/response is reflected in the choice of deck that will help maximize wins and minimize losses. This is done in the absence of knowledge of the cue (decks)-outcome (wins and losses) associations, as well as the magnitude (high/low wins/losses) associated with each card selection. The experience of uncertainty is compounded because the decision maker does not know how to incorporate feedback from their choice of decks, because they are unaware of how many total plays they are required to make. Given this fact, it may be the case that decision makers focus on the gain-loss frequency, rather than learning to make decisions that will contribute to a good final outcome (Chui & Lin, 2007).

It is clear from the outset that the condition under which decisions are made is an uncertain one for two reasons: 1) not knowing the probabilities associated with the outcomes, 2) not knowing how to distribute one's choices because of being unaware of the length of the game. For this reason, this makes the IGT rather different from the WPT task, though we will consider this in more detail later in the discussion. So, what constitutes a decision here and what other factors influence performance in PDs? As mentioned earlier, Bechara et al (1994) designed the IGT to examine the influence of emotions on decision making, and reported that in their non-clinical population, concurrent measurement of galvanic skin responses showed that the magnitude of elevated anticipatory skin conductance responses (SCRs) was associated with the magnitude of loss from cards selected (Bechara et al, 1997). However, there was no associated physiological response to losses from card selections in patients with orbitofrontal cortical dysfunction, and patients with Prefrontal damage were unable to shift from bad to good decks. The implications of these findings fit with the general function of this task, which is to show that autonomic processes may underlie our ability to interpret feedback in order to make decisions that maximize our outcome.

The IGT can also be evaluated with respect to the three proposed components of decision making. 1) In the IGT the rates at which rewards and punishments are experienced is critical to learning how to maximize one's earnings and at the same time avoid extreme losses. This is because over successive trials the decision maker learns the probabilistic relationship between cue and the magnitude of the outcome value. The findings are mixed with respect to this. Thiel et al (2003) showed that the distribution of choices for advantageous and disadvantageous decks was no different in PDs as HCs. Though it is important to note that their sample size was small, and the data was not presented in such a way as to determine any incremental improvements over successive trials. With respect to this, there are contradictory reports that over all trials PDs show improved card selection and equivalent rates of learning to HCs (Euteneuer et al, 2010), whereas there is also evidence suggesting that over blocks of trials practice only marginally improves performance as compared to HCs (Czerneki et al, 2002). However, in Czerneki et al (2002) participants performed the IGT twice, and only in the second repetition was there evidence of advantageous card selection even in HCs. This is unusual, since advantageous card selection typically emerges after 20 trials (Bechera et al, 1994; 1997), which suggests that the way in which Czerneki et al (2002) present the task slowed learning rates for both HCs and PDs. There is a range of information that a participant can receive as feedback (as shown in Fig 2), and not all studies report the exact presentation format or the actual range of information that is provided as feedback. Given that this can vary from one study to another, this appears to be one of the only main differences between any of the studies discussed here, with exception of the method of analysis of card selection behavior.

2) The goal of the IGT is unambiguous, and is made obvious to the decision maker from the start, so that each decision on each trial is an incremental step towards, or away from the target - i.e. maximize one's profits. Some have shown that PDs' overall winnings are substantially less than HCs, as indicated by failure to select the advantageous deck (Czerneki et al, 2002; Kobayakawa et al, 2008; Mimura et al, 2006). But, others have shown that the overall success in maximizing earnings is equivalent in both HCs and PDs (Euteneuer et al., 2010; Poletti, et al, 2010; Thiel et al, 2003). While Euteneuer et al (2010) showed that behavioral performance was the same, when comparing PDs with HCs on electrodermal response (EDRs) which indexes emotional/stress responses, they found that HCs showed higher anticipatory EDRs before choosing disadvantageous decks, whereas PDs showed lower anticipatory responses. 3) In the IGT future performance is based on evaluating the rate of success of past choices of the winning or losing deck, and this in turn indicates to the decision maker the usefulness of the strategies designed to reach the goal. Rossi et al (2010) compared IGT decision making behavior of PDs diagnosed as pathological gamblers (PG), with a group of non-gambling PDs. They showed that over successive trials, PDs that were PG tended to select deck B most often, preferring to opt for a high reward high loss strategy compared with PDs (non-PG) that showed a shift in strategy away from disadvantageous decks towards advantageous decks.

The implications here are that future decision making behavior under uncertainty is strongly influenced by sensitivity to previously rewarding outcomes. It maybe that PDs tend to base their strategies on large short term gains, while ignoring big losses, but over time can flexibly adapt their strategies. However, PDs with associated pathological gambling show inflexibility in adapting their strategies over time.

Despite the IGT being labeled as a gambling task, for reasons already discussed, excessive card selection of high gain/high loss decks does not reveal exceptional risk seeking behavior, because decisions are not made under risk. However, findings from a variant of the IGT task, do suggest that actually PDs are highly risk seeking. In the Game of Dice Task (GDT) the structure is transparent to the participant. They are aware of the probabilities and the rules for gains and losses. In GDT decision makers are required to improve on their initial loan of fictional money ($1000), by rolling a virtual dice. The decision maker has to guess what number will come up by choosing a single number or a combination of numbers (2, 3, or 4). As the combination of numbers increases, the winnings and losses incrementally decrease. PD's tended to show that when experiencing high losses they often failed to shift to a better strategy compared to HCs (Brand et al, 2004). Moreover, when directly comparing the IGT with the GDT, PD's showed poorer performance on the GDT than the IGT (Euteneuer et al, 2010). However, the proportion of occasions in which they shifted strategies after experiencing losses was equivalent in both tasks, and EDRs for both tasks were lower after losses, but were at comparable levels to HCs after gains. Unfortunately, these studies do not include recall tests in which participants record the proportion of trials in which they estimate their experienced high wins, high losses, low wins, and low losses. This measure would give some insight as to whether the low physiological responses to losses are also accompanied by poorer encoding of, and memory of losses. More to the point, it would help elucidate the reasons for the similar patterns of behavior in the IGT and the GDT.

2.3 Dynamic Decision Making tasks (DDMs)

Dynamic decision making tasks are designed to transpose problems faced in applied contexts into experimentally controlled situations in which the decision maker is faced with complex dynamic situations (Brehmer, 1992). However, participants are typically naïve to the context, and so decision making is not based on established expertise, but developing expertise. In these tasks skill is defined as the ability to systematically choose cue values that will change the outcome value in order to reach a target criteria and maintain it. The decision maker is told from the outset that they need to learn the relationship between the cues and outcomes. This is because either after a period of training (Osman, et al, 2008) or right from the outset (Witt et al, 2006) they make interventions on the cues in order to control an outcome in a dynamic environment. In this sense, the goal of the task is explicit and there is no uncertainty about the length of the decision making period. However, the conditions under which decisions are made is uncertain because people are unaware of the associated probabilities or noisy functions that describe the cue-outcome relationship.
The process by which a decision maker learns about the task is revealed by the values of the cue that they change and the corresponding changes to the outcome value. Also, by directly manipulating the cues via changing their values, the decision maker is able to acquire knowledge about the underlying structure or rule that connects cues to outcomes.

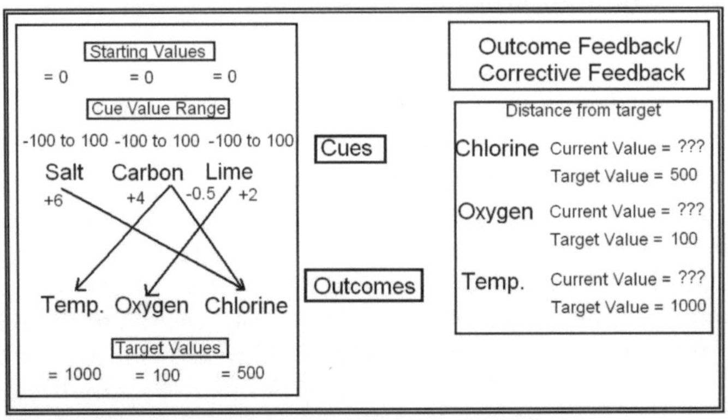

Fig. 3. Details of the Dynamic Decision Making task (DDM)

In the example presented in Fig. 3 the relationships between the cues (Salt, Carbon and Lime) and outcomes (Temperature, Oxygen, Chlorine) is based on a causal structure, in which the cue-outcome associations are linear but noisy (e.g. increasing the value of Lime by 100, will increase Oxygen by 102). The context for the example in Fig. 3 is based around a water purification plant in which participants and asked to imagine that they are trainee operators, and that they need to work out what levels of salt, carbon and lime are needed to purify the water. Their goal is to reach and maintain specific outcome values which indicate the safest purity levels (Oxygen = 100, Temperature = 1000, Chlorine = 500) (Burns &

Vollmeyer, 2002; Osman et al, 2008). At the start of the task all values are set to 0. So, manipulating the cue values will change the outcome values directly, which are observed on every trial. More importantly, the changes to the outcome value are cumulative over trials. That is, while the cue values are reset to 0 the outcome values are retained from the previous trial. In this sense, a poor decision on Trial 2 will need to be corrected on Trial 3 and possibly Trial 4 in order to bring the outcome values back on target, and keep them there.

Not all DDM tasks precisely follow the cue-outcome structure as described here. For instance, some DDM tasks only involve one cue and one outcome, but the functional relationship between the two is still complex (Berry & Broadbent, 1988). Nevertheless, the basic features of the tasks are consistently the same. Cue-outcome relations are opaque to the decision maker and through direct manipulations of the cues (which are typically continuous values) changes to the outcome occur, and the goal is to reach and maintain specific outcome states. Moreover, the type of feedback presented in DDM tasks usually involves presentation of the target value, which is the residing goal throughout the task, and the outcome values directly following from cue manipulations. In so doing, the decision maker is alerted to the discrepancy between the achieved outcome values and the target outcome values.

The same criteria for evaluating the WPT and the IGT as decision making tasks will now be applied to DDM tasks. To begin, given that the DDM task includes a number of features that are unknown to the decision maker at the start, decision making proceeds under uncertainty just as with the IGT and the WPT. So, what constitutes a decision in this task and how do PD patients perform? 1) DDM task requires people to track the rates at which rewards and punishments are experienced, because this indicates the success of learning the relationship (e.g., probabilistic, dynamic, non-linear, linear) between the cues and outcomes. A positive outcome is reflected in a decrease between achieved and target outcome, and a negative outcome is reflected in an increase between achieved and target outcome. Thus, rates of rewards and punishments are experienced in a manner that is different from the IGT or the WPT; this point will be discussed in more detail later in this section. In the main, there is consensus that PDs show intact goal directed decision making when compared to HCs (Osman et al, 2008; Witt et al, 2006). PDs are able to consistently reach and maintain a specific goal by making interventions that involve selecting appropriate cue values.

2) DDM tasks are principally goal directed decision making tasks. In fact, accuracy in decision making and outcome and corrective feedback are all based on the success of reaching and maintaining a specific goal. The task is set up to inform the decision maker precisely about their status in the task with respect to a given goal. The difficulty of the task is determining the right cue interventions that are needed when the outcomes deviate from the target. The evidence suggests that this component of decision making is also intact in PDs (Osman et al, 2008; Witt et al, 2006). To complement this, similar findings have also been reported with amnesic patients performing DDM tasks (Squire & Frambach, 1990), and PD patients performing a predictive task in which the reward structure of the task is dynamic (Rutledge et al, 2009). While successful control behaviors have been demonstrated in PD patients, there is evidence to suggest that structural knowledge (i.e. causal cue-outcome associations, or functional relationship between cue-outcomes) of the task is impaired (Osman et al, 2008; Witt et al, 2006). This has led some to suggest that complex planning behaviors are needed to decide on which cues to intervene on. But, given that PDs are unable to provide accurate verbal reports of their cue-outcome knowledge, planning is

based on knowledge that is not consciously accessible (Witt et al, 2006). In contrast to Witt el al's proposals, McKinlay et al. (2010) presented PDs with a test battery including decision making and problem solving tasks designed to engage executive functions. PDs showed preserved goal directed behaviors, though the authors suggest that performance reflected conscious access to knowledge in their tasks.

3) In DDM tasks future performance is based on evaluating the rate of success of past predictions, as well as the usefulness of strategies from which cue-outcome knowledge informs actions taken. Using previous strategies to make future decision has been examined in DDM tasks, however the evidence is mixed. Osman et al (2008) found that PDs were no different to HCs, and both were able to successfully transfer their decision making strategies from one version of a DDM task to a similar version in which the cover story differed. This is all the more notable given that the training phase of each DDM task performed was different. Some first experienced trials in which they directly manipulated cues (active learning) while others experienced trials much like Wilkinson et al's (2008) WPT. In their task learning cue-outcome associations was observational based, in which all trial information was presented (i.e., Cue Values, Outcome Values and Target values) without the decision maker making any decisions. However, Witt et al (2006) failed to show transfer of decision making skills in PDs. Despite the fact that both tasks were structurally identical and only differed with respect to the cover story, there was no benefit in performance following initial exposure to the first version. However, Witt et al (2006) found that HCs also failed to show transfer, and this same finding has been found with amnesic patients (Squire & Frambach, 1990) and young healthy controls (Berry & Broadbent, 1988). The main reason for the mixed findings is that the DDM task used by Osman et al (2008) and those used by Witt et al (2006) are structurally different. In the former case, there is a complex structure that may be intuitively easier to learn because it is causal, whereas in the latter study the structure is a non-causal rule, and therefore transfer may in fact be facilitated as a result of causal reasoning.

2.4 Summing up: Different flavours of decision making

2.4.1 What are the similarities between the WPT, IGT and the DDM?

The WGT, IGT and DDM require the decision maker to examine events (cues) that probabilistically predict an outcome. By accruing knowledge of the associations between cues and outcomes they can utilize it in such a way as to predict or control an outcome. When a response is made in which an outcome is predicted, feedback directly related to the outcome (outcome feedback) is presented given after the response is made. Finally, correct responses may in principle be taken to be rewarding outcomes, that is, a correct response serves as a reward in and of itself, or a reward structure is in place in the task in which virtual money can be gained or lost. However, from the discussion thus far it is clear that whilst they share a number of fundamentally similar features, the WPT, IGT and DDM tasks differ in a number of important ways.

2.4.2 Are there differences between the WPT, IGT and DDM based on the brain systems they engage?

Overall, compared to HCs, PDs tend to show poorer performance in the WPT. Some have argued that this is because the task engages the striatum and medial temporal lobes (MTL), which are regions that are impaired in PDs (Poldrack et al, 2001; Shohamy et al, 2004). In contrast, the IGT has generated mixed findings, and so it is unclear what can be inferred. Euteneuer et al (2010) claimed that the IGT and its close cousin the GDT engage the limbic-orbitofrontal striatal loop because both tasks involve some emotional processing because of their reward structures. Given that in PDs there are impairments to this system, this candidate explanation could account for why it is that in both tasks, PDs show lower physiological responses to emotional outcomes, albeit specific to negative outcomes. The DDM poses somewhat of a problem in understanding what brain systems are engaged because PD's performance is comparable to that of HCs. Moreover, this has been shown in two entirely different versions (structurally, contextually, perceptually): the water purification system (Osman et al, 2008) and the sugar factory task (Witt et al, 2006). The general claim has been that DDM tasks engage neocortical structures that are recruited when binding complex information. The problem is however, that the DDM task is likely to engage more than just neocortical structures, but which other structures is as yet not clearly specified. An alternative route that has been taken is to focus on the regions that are unlikely to be engaging. Given that PD is associated with neurodegeneration in the striatum, particularly the posterior putamen, the implication is that DDM tasks do not engage midbrain regions, and so processes associated with them, such as incremental error-corrective learning and reward/feedback learning aren't necessary to perform the task (Witt et al, 2006). However, this simply cannot be the case for DDM tasks given the task analysis covered earlier in this section.

Goal directed processes tend to be preserved in PDs, but incremental acquisition of cue-outcome knowledge which enables the quick execution of highly practiced knowledge (i.e. habits) is impaired (McKinlay et al, 2010; Redgrave et al, 2010; Shohamy et al, 2006). But, Redgrave et al (2010) propose that some of the impairments observed in decision making may reflect intact goal directed learning (e.g., rostromedial striatum) that cannot be expressed autonomically because of a dysfunctioning habit learning systems (e.g., midbrain). In other words the acquisition of information (e.g., WPT- cue patterns that predict rain, IGT -cues that predict High gain/High loss) is not severely affected by PD, but what is severely affected is the speed up that would typically occur through repeated application of this information. In PDs the rate at which knowledge can be expressed is affected because the mechanism that forms habits is impaired. For example, there is evidence that PDs can learn probabilistic information in an incremental way in a sequence learning task (Wilkinson & Jahanshahi, 2007), but that the magnitude of learning is reduced as compared with HCs. In their goal directed task, Wilkinson and Jahanshahi (2007) showed that PD's learning involved acquisition of the probabilistic cue (stimulus) - outcome (response) associations, but expression of this knowledge through speed up of responses was impaired (Wilkinson & Jahanshahi, 2007).

To bring these points to bear more specifically to PD performance in the decision making tasks, some have claimed that failure to exhibit incremental cue-outcome learning (as in the WPT, or in some cases the IGT) is the result of slower rates of learning (McKinlay et al, 2010; Redgrave et al, 2010; Rutledge et al, 2009). Indeed, the most consistent core cognitive deficits reported in PDs are speed of processing, along with visuo-spatial ability and some components of executive functioning (McKinlay et al, 2010). McKinlay et al (2010) propose that deficits in general memory, planning, and attention are much more variable, and one reason for this could be as a result of the particular methodology used to study these processes. Similarly then, decision making may also be included in this latter category of processes in which methodology plays a big role in explaining the mixed findings. Alternatively, poor performance in decision making tasks may reflect a more profound problem that begins with deficits in encoding cue-outcome knowledge as well as later problems in expressing it (Poldrack et al, 2001). If one accepts this claim, then failing to encode cue-outcome knowledge is as a result of impairments to processing feedback (Poldrack et al, 2001; Shohamy et al, 2004, 2006). However, one problem with this view is that, with exception of the WPT, which can be accounted for on this basis, studies using the IGT revealed mixed findings with respect to impaired performance in PDs, and the DDM actually shows intact decision making in PDs.

2.4.3 Where do the differences lie between the WPT, IGT and DDM?

Goals: Each of the three decision making tasks involve a goal, but the tasks differ with respect to the specificity of the goal. In the WPT the goal is general, and that is to simply learn to accurately predict the outcome from the cue patterns. The goal of the IGT is more specific and requires the decision maker to maximize their earnings and minimize their losses. But, the decision maker isn't told what the maximum earnings are that they can achieve. In the DDM task, the goal is often specified from the outset, so the decision maker is aware what the precise target is. Thus, the goal of the task, or rather the specificity of the goal may be a contributing factor to the differences in performance in the WPT, IGT and DDM. Planning behaviors are not thought to be severely affected in PD, and one reason for this is that tasks used to examine and successfully show unimpaired performance involve problem solving tasks with an obvious specific goal (McKinlay et al, 2008). McKinlay et al (2008) deconstructed the components of the tower of London task which is a problem solving tasks that involves following specific rules that state how a series of discs can be moved from one peg to another. They found that so long as the goal isn't ambiguous - more to the point, if the actual hierarchy of goals/sub-goals is made clear, then goal directed processes remain intact in PDs. In contrast, PD's failure to encode or re-organize representations, and their lack of flexibility and poor incremental learning has been extended to account for impaired decision making in general (Owen, 2004; Poldrack et al, 2001; Shohamy et al, 2004, 2006). However, it may well be the case that the goal structure of the tasks in these studies interferes with PD's ability to perform decision making well; this says more about the task than the nature of the cognitive impairments in decision making.

Uncertainty: The discussion of the WPT, IGT and the DDM suggest that they are tasks that induce uncertainty. A decision maker in the WPT is unaware of the probability of cue-outcome associations (i.e. how often certain cue patterns will appear) and the cue-outcome probabilities (the association between cues and certain outcomes). In the IGT the decision maker is unaware of the cue-outcome probabilities, and also how many opportunities they have to make decisions. In the DDM the cue-outcome probabilities are unknown, and also the structural features or functional relationships between cues and outcomes (causal associations between cue-outcomes, rules describing cue-outcome associations). In general it seems that three tasks generate uncertainty about the cue-outcome associations, but they differ markedly with respect to other sources of uncertainty.

Outcome/Reward/Feedback: The tasks can also be differentiated on the basis of the outcomes and their rewards. In the WPT, the decision maker predicts an event (i.e. sunny, rainy) from a given cue pattern, and then the accuracy of the prediction is indicated either by positive or negative feedback (i.e. smiley face, sad face). In the IGT, the decision maker selects a deck and the outcome is either positive (a gain of $50 or $100) or negative (loss of $1250 or $250), and in either case they differ in magnitudes. In the DDM, the decision maker manipulates a cue by selecting a cue value, and this changes the outcome value. Based on the manipulation, the outcome value will either be closer to target as compared to the previous trial (Positive outcome), or the outcome can deviate further away from target as compared with the previous trial (Negative outcome). The IGT and the DDM are similar to each than with the WPT. First, a decision has a direct consequence on the outcome, given that for both the IGT and DDM the outcome value is dependent on the choice of cue selected. In fact in the DDM, this is even more pronounced, because in this task the decision maker can directly change the cue value. Second, for both the IGT and the DDM a good decision is in itself the reward (i.e. IGT - increasing outcome value; DDM -closer to target). Third, the magnitude of the reward can vary in both the IGT and the DDM (i.e. IGT - high/low, DDM - closer to target/exactly on target). For the WPT a decision has no consequence on the outcome itself. This is an important matter because the decision maker doesn't choose the cues and so cannot influence the outcome. Their decision making simply involves a prediction, the status of which is indicated through feedback.

3. The effects of medication on decision making

As mentioned, the core cognitive impairments associated with PD's are speed of processing, visuo-spatial processing, and also executive functioning (Cools et al, 2001; Muslimovic et al, 2005; Owen, 2004). The problem is that, executive functioning is not one thing, it involves a combination of activities that are used to different degrees for different tasks. Similarly, as we have considered thus far, decision making has many components, and tasks that are designed to engage decision making processes reveal mixed findings in terms of the extent of impairments found in patients with PD. For this reason it is hard to infer what role medication plays in alleviating or impairing components of the decision making process. As mentioned, the findings from all reported studies discussed thus far involve patients on medication, typically Levadopa (L-Dopa). Dopamine deficiency in the (e.g., putamen and dorsal caudate) midbrain is the hallmark of PD (Hornykiewicz & Kish, 1984), and so dopamine replacement therapy with L-Dopa or dopamine agonists is the most affective method of alleviating motor symptoms (e.g., tremors, rigidity, bradykinesia, akinesia, balance and walking) associated with PD.

As well as mobility, dopamine replacement therapy improves cognitive functioning associated with brain areas which have depleted levels of dopamine (e.g., putamen and dorsal caudate). For instance, improvements have been reported in tasks involving object and spatial recall (Cooper et al., 1992), fluency in generating semantically associated words (Gotham et al, 1988) and task switching between letter naming and digit naming tasks (Cools et al, 2001). However, dopamine replacement therapy also increases dopamine levels in unaffected areas (e.g., prefrontal cortex and ventral striatum). The prefrontal cortex is speculated to be involved in processing probabilistic cue information (Forstman et al, 2010; van Veen et al., 2008) and the ventral striatum has been associated with classification of probabilistic cue-outcome associations (Cools, et al, 2006). In support, dysfunction of cognitive processes include deterministic cue-outcome learning (Gotham et al., 1988) and probabilistic cue-outcome learning (Cools, et al, 2006; Cools et al., 2001; Shohamy et al, 2006; Swainson et al, 2000; Swainson et al, 2006). Findings of this kind have been used to support the dopamine overdosing hypothesis, which proposes that dopamine levels in unaffected brain regions are "overdosed" and this then leads to dysfunction of processes such as cue-outcome learning (e.g., Cools et al, 2001; Gotham et al, 1988). Recall, the features of cue-outcome learning are the basic building blocks of the three main decision making tasks (WPT, IGT, DDM) discussed in this chapter. Therefore, by implication, decrements in performance on these tasks while on medication may be explained by the overdosing hypothesis.

3.1 The effects of on vs. off L-Dopa medication in the WPT

One might predict that if impairments to decision making performance in PDs is observed while on L-Dopa medication, as is the case with the WPT, then if the overdosing hypothesis bears out, PDs off L-Dopa medication should show improvements in the WPT performance. This is exactly what has been shown (Shohamy et al, 2002; Jahanshahi et al, 2010). Jahanshahi et al (2010) found that the same patients on medication, then performed the task after having withdrawn from medication, showed equivalent predictive accuracy to HCs. However, patients tested off and on medication were able to discriminate between strong and weak cards as well as HCs. Importantly, critical behavioral differences between those off and on medication were found to be the result of the types of strategies that were implemented (Speekenbrink et al, 2010). HCs and PDs off medication showed hypothesis testing type behavior, partly resulting in more flexibility in switching strategies when experiencing poor outcome feedback, where as PDs on medication switched to poorer strategies. This strongly implies that the impairments in performing the task are not located at an encoding level, given that all participants learnt which cues strongly and weakly predicted a particular outcome.

In two analogous probabilistic cue-outcome learning tasks (Probabilistic Selection task, Probabilistic Discrimination task) which share many similarities with the WPT, similar improvements in predictive accuracy have been reported while PDs are off medication (Frank et al, 2004; Shohamy et al, 2006). The facilatory effects of withdrawing from medication are thought to improve feedback processing, in particular negative feedback (Frank et al, 2004; Shohamy et al, 2006). In support, in WPTs or equivalent tasks, PD patients on medication show impaired performance, whereas when no feedback is presented in identical tasks, there is no reported impairment in performance (Shohamy et al, 2004; Shohamy et al, 2006); though some have speculated that this result is because the time limit to respond was removed in the no feedback version (Wilkinson et al, 2008). From this, Shohamy et al (2006) proposed that the overdosing hypothesis can be used to explain the discrepant effects of feedback on performance because midbrain dopamine systems are implicated in reward-related error-correcting incremental learning processes. Thus, increasing dopamine levels interferes with error processing in tasks that provide feedback, whereas presenting PD patients with versions without feedback eliminates error corrective processing and in turn the detrimental effects of overdosing on incremental learning. To complement this, Frank (Frank et al, 2004; Frank, 2005) has claimed that positive and negative feedback have differential effects on dopamine release. In sum, it is not clear whether probabilistic cue-outcome learning is impaired in PDs on medication because of critical features of the task that require flexibility in strategy application, or failure to process negative feedback. PDs on medication may perseverate on poorer strategies, or have greater difficulty switching to better strategies, which indirectly suggest failure to process negative feedback.

3.2 The effects of on vs. off L-Dopa medication in the IGT

Despite the popularity of the task, only Czerneki et al (2002) examined the effects on decision making while patients were medicated on L-Dopa and when they had withdrawn from it for 24hrs. Recall that in Czerneki et al's (2002) study all groups (PDs on medication, PDs off medication, HCs) performed the IGT twice. While HCs showed a net improvement across repetitions, PDs showed no relative improvement in selecting from the advantageous decks more often. These findings strongly suggest that increasing dopamine levels in the midbrain as well as unaffected regions doesn't have any adverse effects on IGT performance any more than restoring levels of dopamine in unaffected regions through withdrawal of dopaminergic medication. To add to this, while Czerneki et al's (2002) is the only study that has contrasted the effects of on vs. off medication on IGT performance, while Pagonabarraga et al (2007) examined the effects of different levels of dosage of L-Dopa on IGT performance. They compared PDs on medication that were receiving L-Dopa on a daily basis (405 +/- 300 mg) and showed stable responses to medication, and PDs on medication also receiving L-Dopa but showing a fluctuating responses to medication, or wearing-off responses which involve increases in L-Dopa dosage (930 +/- 411 mg). Pagonabarraga et al (2007) found that there was no influence of type of dosage on IGT performance, although they found that in general PDs performed worse than HCs. Nevertheless, this too is an example in which medication, and more to the point, the overdosing hypothesis cannot exclusively explain PD's performance in the IGT.

Finally, Perratta et al (2005) compared PDs with early stages of the disease (i.e. less than a score of 3 on the Hoehn and Yahr Scale score), and those with late stages of the disease (i.e. more than a score of 3 on the Hoehn and Yahr Scale score) on the WPT and the IGT. They found that on the WPT, HCs and the early PD group showed equivalent performance on 100 blocks of trials they carried out, but that late PDs showed worse performance than both other groups, and accuracy decreased in the last 30 trials. It is important to note that it is rather atypical to only present participants 100 trials, however, even in Jahanshahi et al (2010) study they used 200 trials. However, in line with Perratta et al's findings, they only reported a marginal negative correlation between performance and Hoehn and Yahr stage of illness and performance on the WPT. When focusing on the IGT, Perratta et al (2005) found that stage of illness made no difference in performance, and that for early and late PDs, performance was equivalent. With the exception of one block of trials, PDs also showed equivalent performance to HCs. While Perrratta et al's (2005) manipulation did not include an on vs. off medication manipulation, one could argue that those in early stages of PD would be more susceptible to overdosing in regions such as the ventral striatum and orbitorfrontal cortex which remains relatively spared in early stages of PD. Given that the ventral striatum has been associated with probabilistic cue-outcome associations, then one might predict that both the WPT and the IGT would be affected. However, only performance in the WPT was in fact impaired. Moreover, the location of impairments was against what would be predicted by the overdosing hypothesis. Those in late stages of PD were affected rather than those in early stages of PD. Clearly then, across these different studies, there is a strong indication that L-Dopa medication does not impair performance on the IGT, and that withdrawing from medication does not improve performance above baseline.

3.3 The effects of on vs. off L-Dopa medication in the DDM

The use of DDM tasks in clinical populations is in its infancy, and so only two studies can potentially inform the debate concerning the effects on vs. off medication on performance in these tasks. Osman et al (in preparation) have shown that comparing PDs on L-Dopa medication and off L-Dopa medication while performing a DDM did not differentially affect performance, and that both groups performed as well as HCs. However, they did find that those off medication and HCs adopted similar strategies when choosing how many cues to intervene on in order to control the outcome. Both these groups tended to manipulate one cue at a time and observe the effects of their manipulation on the outcome. This is a more effective strategy for acquiring cue-outcome knowledge in a dynamic environment, because it is hard to isolate which factors may contribute to changing the outcome value (Osman, 2010). In contrast, PDs on medication tended to manipulate all the cues most of the time in order to control the outcome, which makes learning the association between cues and outcomes harder depending on the cue values that are selected. That is, all three cues may be manipulated, but cue 1 could be set at 75, cue 2 set at 50 and cue 3 set at 50. If on trial two cue 1 is set to 100, and cue 2 and cue 3 are set to 50, then this is the same strategy as varying one cue at a time. In general, performance, as indicated by consistently achieving and maintaining a specific outcome for a course of trials was not differentially affected by the presence or absence of dopaminergic medication.

Though not a DDM task, Rutledge et al's (2009) study involved a dynamic environment in which the rewards associated with certain cues would change throughout the course of the task. Participants were told they were on a fishing vessel and that they were required to choose between one of two crab traps to send into the water. They received real monetary rewards for each successful decision they made. The relative reward rates would change in blocks of 70-90 trials (i.e., 6:1, 3:1, 1:3, 1:6), and the identity of the high reward option alternated between blocks of trials. The task essentially involves making a prediction about which crab trap will yield the highest catch which will in turn lead to high rewards. They found that PDs on as well as off medication earned as much as HCs that were aged matched, though younger HCs earned the most money and more than PDs from either group. When examining rates of learning and sensitivity to transitions in rewards over trials, they found that PDs on medication showed different rates of learning to those off medication. Moreover, Rutledge et al's (2009) reported that when comparing learning rates when receiving positive outcomes, PDs on medication showed higher learning rates than PDs off medication. For negative outcomes, learning rates were lower than for positive outcomes, and for both groups learning rates were the same.

3.4 Summing up: The effects of medication on decision making

In line with the general pattern of findings discussed in the previous section, the effects of withdrawing from medication seem to impact most reliably on performance in the WPT. For the IGT and the DDM the implications are that brain regions that would be overdosed with dopamine through drug treatment are not engaged in these tasks. Alternatively, it may be that the way in which the tasks are structured enable patients to exhibit more robust aspects of decision making which may well be preserved in PD, or at least, less affected than other cognitive functions that consistently reveal decrements in performance. The examination of the different tasks in the previous section reveal that both the IGT and the DDM are more clearly defined in their goals than the WPT is. Also, the feedback presented in the IGT and the DDM share more features in common, than with the feedback presented in the WPT. However, this is largely because of one critical factor. The decisions that are made in the IGT and the DDM affect the outcome and rewards/punishments, whereas in the WPT, the decision only affects rewards/punishments. If one is making choices that have direct consequences for the outcome, then predictions about the effects that those choices will bring, could in turn lead to differences in processing feedback as compared to when the outcome is already predetermined. In addition, feedback indicates the effects of incremental changes in positive and negative outcomes in the IGT and DDM. While Shohamy et al (2004) and Shohamy et al (2006) claim that the WPT is an incremental cue-outcome learning task, in actual fact feedback in this task does not revealing incremental changes in the outcome or rewards or punishments. Rather, the WPT reveals the success of a decision on a discrete trial basis. The concluding section of this chapter will consider these points in more detail.

4. Reinforcement learning models and feedback

The effects of dopamine replacement therapy on decision making provides important clues as to the components of decision making that are impaired and spared. From what we know of the way dopamine neurons behave, they tend to show different activity associated with different outcomes. If one is expecting an outcome and receives it, then there is tonic activity in dopamine neurons. However, there is short phasic activation in the presence of unexpected rewarding outcomes (e.g. presentation of money), which over time shifts towards the predictor of the reward (e.g., cards from a particular deck). Activation tends to decrease in the presence of negative outcomes (e.g., loss of money) or when there is a discrepancy between the expected reward and the actual reward (Hollerman & Schultz, 1998; Schultz, Apicella, & Ljungberg, 1993).

There are currently two reinforcement learning models that are used to account for the differential activation patterns in dopaminergic neurons. The Reward Prediction Error (RPE) model (Montague et al, 2004; Rangel, et al, 2008; Rutledge et al, 2009; Shultz et al, 1997) claims that learning about cue-outcome associations comes about through the generation of expectations about future events; these expectancies influence the rate of learning of the associations. By developing expectancies, one can gain information about the accuracy of one's prediction in the form of prediction errors. If one sees a combination of tarot cards and predicts rain, but the actual outcome is sun, then the expectancy of rain receives a negative prediction error through outcome feedback. Thus, the outcome itself can either positively or negatively deviate from one's expectancies. In each state (positive error, negative error) there is a corresponding pattern of activation in dopamine neurons. The Response-Selection model (Frank et al, 2004; Frank, 2005) instead proposes that choices become associated with relevant predictive cues. Receiving positive feedback from one's actions increases activity in dopamine neurons and this reinforces the selected response (go signal). Negative feedback decreases activity in dopamine neurons and this reinforces an inhibition of the selected response (no-go signal). The critical difference between the two models is that in the former updated cue-outcome knowledge is based on prediction errors, whereas in the latter model it is based on response errors. Both reinforcement models have incorporated the overdosing hypothesis into their accounts. The RS model proposes that intact brain networks have a greater baseline of dopamine which decreases the dynamic range of phasic peaks and dips. This is thought to specifically impair processing negative feedback, and as a result there is less suppression of no-go signals. The RPE model claims that increase in dopamine though L-dopa modulate RPE magnitude, to the extent that the RPE is amplified, and in turn increases the rate of learning of cue-outcome associations, which in turn can be detrimental because of hypersenitvity to rewarding outcomes. This perspective does not place specific deficits on processing of particular forms of feedback, but rather different forms of reward.

4.1 Impaired feedback processing may not be the answer

Dopaminergic neurons have been associated with reward processing, and the striatum is thought to play an important role in reinforcement learning, which is why presenting PDs with decision making tasks that involve rewards structures and incremental feedback reveals important clues about cognitive dysfunction associated with the disease. However, surveying the findings from three different decision making tasks, in which all involve incremental learning of cue-outcome associations, and processing feedback - sometimes with rewards attached, the picture that emerges is not in obvious support of impaired feedback processing in PD.

A task like the WPT does not involve continuous incremental choice-outcome behavior, because there aren't any choices made that would lead to outcome changes; in fact, this applies to Cool et al's (2001) probabilistic reversal learning task, and Franks et al's (2004) Probabilistic selection task. It may be the case that in tasks of these kinds, settling on a consistent decision strategy to start with is one of the most important ways of performing well in them. Maintaining a consistent strategy enables the decision maker to accurately interpret the feedback from each discrete prediction made. Of course, this is less of a concern when the decisions and their effects can be tracked easily over trials, as in the case of the IGT and DDM. Thus, either because the decisions made in these tasks have consequences on the outcomes, or because one can observe the cumulative effects on ones decisions, learning to make decision from cue-outcome associations is facilitated regardless of whether PDs are on or off medication. PDs on medication tend to show hypersenitivity to novel outcomes (Bodi et al, 2009) and an amplified PRE (Rutledge et al, 2009), both of which become relaxed while off medication. Paying special attention to novel changes and having an enlarged error signal when estimating changes in an outcome in combination could explain the fact that performance is poorer in the WPT while on medication, because both contribute to poor strategy selection. That is, PDs would be more susceptible to changing their strategies or even show random responding while on medication because they are acting on each discrete change that they experience from trial to trial, and prompted to do so from an amplified error signal. In fact, PDs on medication show more random guessing early in the WPT task (Speekenbrink et al, 2010), and take considerably longer to switch to a single strategy that they can test which enables them to better track cue-outcome associations over trials (Jahanshahi et al, 2010; Speekenbrink et al, 2010).

Overall, the studies reviewed suggest that cue-outcome association learning is preserved in spite of stage of PD, level of medication, and withdrawal from medication. Thus, acquisition of probabilistic cue-outcome knowledge in PD is not impaired, but rather the implementation of cue-outcome knowledge may in fact be facilitated or hampered by the nature of the task. It may be the case that implementing cue-outcome knowledge is facilitated in tasks in which the effects of one's decisions are cumulative, either through direct manipulation of the cue values (DDM) or selecting cues in order to achieve a specific goal (IGT). As a result, midbrain regions are still needed in order to perform the task, but the IGT and the DDM may not show disrupted performance when PDs are on or off medication, because the observed cumulative effects of one's decisions are enough to facilitate incremental learning via the continuous updating of action effects on rewards/punishments.

One might ask: Why is actual choice so important? The Pre-supplimentary motor area (Pre-sma) has been associated with action-effect bindings and control of voluntary actions, and has projections to the striatum (Potsuma & Dagher, 2006), which we know is disrupted in PD. Pre-sma is associated with binding of actions to their effects. Intentional action-effect binding involves forming an association between an action (i.e. choosing which cue to manipulate and by which value) and the effect of that action (i.e. the corresponding change in the outcome value) is fed back and this reveals changes in the outcome. This process is an important basis for which to incrementally learning cue-outcome associations (Moore et al, 2010). Therefore, agency is an important aspect of decision making (Osman, 2010), which is why perhaps PDs benefit from tasks in which they are required to make choices, and can adjust their strategies because they incrementally observe the effects of their own decisions.

5. Conclusion

At a more general level, stage of PD, level of medication, and medicated vs. non-medicated do not substantially impair the basic incremental cue-outcome learning mechanism that decision making activities are reliant on. Even in cases in which PD patients on medication are shown to have deficits in decision making, with extended exposure to the decision making task, they are able to eventually switch their strategies to better ones. Unless a detailed analysis of the task and its requirements is conducted, and compared with other existing decision making tasks, little progress will be made in understanding the extent of impairments in decision making in patients with PD. The studied reviewed here suggest that tasks with a dynamic element to them reveal intact complex decision making. This in turn provides greater impetus to improve on the kinds of assessments used to determine the range of abilities that are still preserved in patients with PD.

6. Acknowledgment

Preparation for this research project was supported by the Engineering and Physical Sciences Research Council, EPSRC grant - EP/F069421/1. I would also like to thank Prof Jahanshahi for her insights throughout the many illuminating discussions we have had.

7. References

Bechara A, Damasio, A, Damasio, H, & Anderson, S. (1994). Insensitivity to future consequences following damage to human prefrontal cortex. *Cognition, 50*, 7–15.

Bechara A, Damasio, H, Tranel, D, & Damasio, A. (1997). Deciding Advantageously Before Knowing the Advantageous Strategy. *Nature*, 275, 1293-1295.

Berry, D. C., & Broadbent, D. E. (1988). Interactive tasks and the implicit-explicit distinction. *British Journal of Psychology, 79*, 251-272.

Bodi, N., Keri, S., Nagy, H., Moustafa, A., Myers,C., Daw, N., Dibo, G., Takats, A., Bereczki, D., & Gluck, M. (2009). Reward-learning and the novelty-seeking personality: a between- and within-subjects study of the effects of dopamine agonists on young Parkinson's patients. Brain, 132, 2385–2395

Brand, M., Labudda, K., Kalbe, E., Hilker, R., Emmans, D., Fuchs, G., Kessler, J., & Markowitsch, H. J. (2004). Decision making impairments in patients with Parkinson's disease, *Behavioural Neurology, 15,* 77–85.

Brehmer, B. (1992). Dynamic decision making: Human control of complex systems. *Acta Psychologica, 81,* 211–241.

Burns, B. D., & Vollmeyer, R. (2002). Goal specificity effects on hypothesis testing in problem solving. *Quarterly Journal of Experimental Psychology, 55,* 241-261.

Chui, Y-U, & Lin, C-H. (2007). Is deck C an advantageous deck in the Iowa Gambling Task? *Behavioral and Brain Functions,* 3, 37.

Cooper, J. A., Sagar, H. J., Doherty, S. M., Jordan, N., Tidswell, P.,&Sullivan, E. V. (1992).Different effects of dopaminergic and anticholinergic therapies on cognitive and motor function in Parkinson's disease—A follow up study of untreated patients. *Brain, 115,* 1701–1725.

Cools, R., Altamirano, L., & D'Esposito, M. (2006). Reversal learning in Parkinson's disease depends on medication status and outcome valence. Neuropsychologia, 44, 1663–1673.

Cools, R., Barker, R. A., Sahakian, B. J., & Robbins, T. W. (2001). Enhanced or impaired cognitive function in Parkinson's disease as a function of dopaminergic medication and task demands. *Cerebral Cortex, 11,* 1136–1143.

Czernecki, V., Pillion, B., Houeto, J., Pochon, J., Levy, R., & Dubois, B. *(2002).* Motivation, reward, and Parkinson's disease: influence of dopatherapy. *Neuropsychologia, 40,* 2257–2267.

Delazer, M., Sinz, H., Zamarian,L., Stockner, H., Seppi, K., Wenning, G., Benke, T., Poewe, W. (2009). Decision making under risk and under ambiguity in Parkinson's disease. Neuropsychologia, 47, 1901–1908

Doya, K. (2008). Modulators of decision making. *Nature Neuroscience, 11,* 410-416.

Euteneuer, F., Schaefer, F., Stuermer, R., Boucsein W., Timmermann, L., Barbe, T., Ebersbach, G., Otto, J., Kessler, J., & Kalbe, E. (2010). Dissociation of decision-making under ambiguity and decision-making under risk in patients with Parkinson's disease: A neuropsychological and psychophysiological study. . Neuropsychologia, 47, 2882-2890.

Forstmann,B., Brown, S., Dutilh, G., Neumann, J., & Wagenmakers, E. (2010). The neural substrate of prior information in perceptual decision making: a model-based analysis. *Fronteirs in Human Neuroscience,4,* 1-12.

Frank, M. J. (2005). Dynamic dopamine modulation in the basal ganglia: A neurocomputational account of cognitive deficits in medicated and nonmedicated Parkinsonism. *Journal of Cognitive Neuroscience, 17,* 51–72.

Frank, M. J., Seeberger, L. C., & O'Reilly, R. C. (2004). By carrot or by stick: Cognitive reinforcement learning in Parkinsonism. Science, 306, 1940–1943.

Gleichgerrcht, E., Ibáñez, A., Roca, M., Torralva, T., & Manes, F. (2010). Decision- making cognition in neurodegenerative diseases. *Nature Reviews, 6,* 611-623.

Gotham, A. M., Brown, R. G., & Marsden, C. D. (1988). Frontal cognitive function in patients with Parkinson's disease on and off levodopa. *Brain, 111,* 299–321.

Hollerman, J. R., & Schultz, W. (1998). Dopamine neurons report an error in the temporalprediction of reward during learning. *Nature Neuroscience, 1,* 304–309.

Hornykiewicz, O.,& Kish, S. J. (1984). Neurochemical basis of dementia in Parkinson's disease. *Canadian Journal of Neurological Sciences, 11,* 185–190.

Jahanshahi, M, Ardouin C, M. A., Brown, R. G., Rothwell, J. C., Obeso, J, Albanese, A, Rodriguez-Oroz, M. C., Moro, E.,Benabid, A L, Pollak, P, & Limousin-Dowsey, P.(2000). The impact of deep brain stimulation on executive function in Parkinson's disease. *Brain, 123,* 1142–1154.

Jahanshahi,M., Wilkinson, L., Gahir, H., Dharmindra,A., & Lagnado,D.A. (2010). Medication impairs probabilistic classification learning in Parkinson's disease. *Neuropsychologia, 48,* 1096–1103

Kobayakawa, M., Koyama, S., Mimura, M., & Kawamura, M. (2008). Decision making in Parkinson's disease: Analysis of behavioral and physiological patterns in the Iowa Gambling Task. *Movement Disorders, 23,* 547–552.

Knowlton, B. J., Mangels, J. A. & Squire, L. R. (1996). A neostriatal habit learning system in humans. *Science, 273,* 1399-1402.

Knowlton, B. J., Squires, L. R., & Gluck, M. A. (1994). Probabilistic category learning in amnesia. *Learning and Memory, 1,* 106-120.

Labudda, L., Brand, M., Mertens, M., Ollech, I., Markowitsch, H. J., & Woermann F. G., (2010). Decision making under risk condition in patients with Parkinson's disease: A behavioural and fMRI study. *Behavioural Neurology, 21,* 131-143.

Lagnado, D., Newell, B. R., Kahan, S., & Shanks, D. R. (2006). Insight and strategy in multiple cue learning. *Journal of Experimental Psychology : General, 135,* 162-183.

McKinlay, A., Grace, R., Dalrymple-Alford, J., & Roger, D. (2010). Characteristics of executive function impairement in Parkinson's disease patients without dementia. *Journa of the International Neurospsychological Society, 6,* 268-277.

McKinlay, A., Kaller, C., Grace, R., Dalrymple-Alford, J., Anderson, T., Fink, J., & Roger, D. (2008). Planning in Parkinson's disease: a matter of problem structure? *Neuropsychologia, 46,* 384–389.

Mimura, M, Oeda, R., & Kawamura, M. (2006) Impaired decision-making inParkinson's disease. *Parkinsonism and Related Disorders, 12,* 169–175

Montague, P. R., Hyman, S. E., & Cohen, J. D. (2004). Computational roles for dopamine in behavioural control. *Nature, 431,* 760–767.

Moody, T. D., Bookheimer, S. Y., Vanek, Z., & Knowlton, B. J. (2004). An implicit learning task activates medial temporal lobe in patients with Parkinson's disease. *Behavioral Neuroscience, 118,* 438_442.

Moore, J., Ruge, D., Wenke, D., Rothwell, J., & Haggard, P. (2010). Disrupting the experience of control in the human brain: Pre-Supplementary motor area contributes to the sense of agency. *Proceedings of the Royal Society, 277,* 2503-2509

Muslimovic , D. , Post , B. , Speelman , J.D. , & Schmand , B . (2005). Cognitive profile of patients with newly diagnosed Parkinson disease . *Neurology, 65,* 1239 - 1245

Osman, M. (2010). Controlling Uncertainty: Learning and Decision Making in complex worlds. Wiley-Blackwell Publishers, Oxford.

Osman, M., Ryterska, A., Karimi, K., Tu, L., Obeso, I., Speekenbrink, M, Jahanshahi, M. (in preparation). Provision of gradual feedback overrides the effects of medication on prediction and control -based decision making in Parkinson's disease.

Osman, M., Wilkinson, L., Beigi, M., Parvez, C., & Jahanshahi, M. (2008). The striatum and learning to control a complex system? Neuropsychologia, 46, 2355–2363.

Owen, A. M. (2004). Cognitive dysfunction in Parkinson's disease: The role of frontostriatal circuitry. *Neuroscientist, 10,* 525–537.

Pagonabarraga, J., Garcia-Sanchez, C., Llebaria, G., Pascual-Sedano, B., Gironell, A., & Kulisevsky, J. (2007). Controlled study of decision-making and cognitive impairment in Parkinson's disease. *Movement Disorders, 22,* 1430–1435.

Perretta, J. G., Pari, G., & Beninger, R. J. (2005). Effects of Parkinson disease on two putative nondeclarative learning tasks: Probabilistic classification and gambling. *Cognitive and Behavioral Neurology, 18,* 185–192.

Poldrack, R. A., Clark, J., Pare-Blagoev, E. J., Shohamy, D., Moyano, J. C., Myers, C., & Gluck, M. (2001). Interactive memory systems in the human brain. *Nature, 414,*546–550.

Poletti, M., Frosini, D., Lucetti, C., Del Dotto, P., Ceravolo R., & Bonuccelli, U. (2010). Decision making in De Novo Parkinson's Disease. *Movement Disorders, 25,* 1432-1436.

Potsuma, R., & Dagher, A. (2006). Basal Ganglia Functional Connectivity Based on a Meta-Analysis of 126 Positron Emission Tomography and Functional Magnetic Resonance Imaging Publications. *Cerebral Cortex, 16I,* 1508--1521

Rangel, A., Camerer, C., & Montague, P. R. (2009). A framework for studying the neurobiology of value-based decision making. *Nature Neuroscience, 9,* 545-556.

Redgrave, P., Rodriguez, M., Smith, Y., Rodriguez-Oroz, Lehericy, S., Bergman, H., Agid, Y., DeLong, M., & Obeso, J. (2010). Goal-directed and habitual control in the basal ganglia: implication for Parkinson's disease. *Nature Reviews Neuroscience, 11,* 760-772.

Rossi,M., Gerschcovich, E., de Achaval, D., Perez-Lloret, S., Cerquetti, D., Cammarota, A., Ine´s Nouzeilles, M., Fahrer, R., Merello, M., & Leiguarda, R. (2010). Decision-making in Parkinson_s disease patients with and without pathological gambling. *European Journal of Neurology, 17,* 97-102.

Rutledge, B., Lazzaro, S Lau, B., Myers, C., Gluck, M., & Glimcher, P. (2009). Dopaminergic Drugs Modulate Learning Rates and Perseveration in Parkinson's Patients in a Dynamic Foraging Task. *The Journal of Neuroscience, 29,* 15104 –15114.

Schultz, W. (2006). Behavioral theories and the neurophysiology of reward. *Annual Review of Psychology, 57*, 87-115.

Schultz, W., Apicella, P., & Ljungberg, T. (1993). Responses of monkey dopamine neurons to reward and conditioned-stimuli during successive steps of learning a delayed-response task. *Journal of Neuroscience, 13*, 900–913.

Shultz, W., Dayan, P., & Montague, R. (1997). A Neural Substrate of Prediction and Reward. *Science, 275*, 1593 - 1599.

Shohamy, D., Myers, C. E., & Gluck, M. A. (2002). The effect of L-Dopa on category learning in Parkinson's Disease. 32nd Annual Meeting of the Society for Neuroscience, 2002, 777.3.

Shohamy, D., Myers, C. E., Grossman, S., Sage, J., Gluck, M. A., & Poldrack, R. A. (2004). Cortico-striatal contributions to feedback-based learning: Converging data from neuroimaging and neuropsychology. *Brain, 127*, 851–859.

Shohamy, D., Myers, C. E., Geghman, K. D., Sage, J., & Gluck, M. A. (2006). L-dopa impairs learning, but spares generalization, in Parkinson's disease. *Neuropsychologia, 44*, 774–784.

Speekenbrink, M., Lagnado, D., Wilkinson, L., Jahanshahi, M, & Shanks, D. (2010). Models of probabilistic category learning in Parkinson's disease: Strategy use and the effects of L-dopa. *Journal of Mathematical Psychology, 54*, 123-136.

Squire, L. R., & Frambach, M. (1990). Cognitive skill learning in amnesia. *Psychobiology, 18*, 109–117.

Swainson, R., Rogers, R. D., Sahakian, B. J., Summers, B. A., Polkey, C. E., & Robbins, T. W. (2000). Probabilistic learning and reversal deficits in patients with Parkinson's Disease or frontal or temporal lobe lesions: Possible adverse effects of dopaminergic medication. *Neuropsychologia, 38*, 596–612.

Swainson, R., SenGupta, D., Shetty, T., Watkins, L. H. A., Summers, B. A., Sahakian, B. J., Polkey, C. E., Barker, R., & Robbins, T. W. (2006). Impaired dimensional selection but intact use of reward feedback during visual discrimination learning in Parkinson's disease. *Neuropsychologia, 44*, 1290–1304.

Thiel, A. Hilker, R., Kessler, J., Habedank, B., Herholz, K., & Heiss, W-D. (2003). Activation of basal ganglia loops in idiopathic Parkinson's disease: a PET study. *Journal of Neural Transmission*, 110, 1289–1301.

Trepel, C., Fox, C. R., & Poldrack, R. A. (2005). Prospect theory on the brain? Toward a cognitive neuroscience of decision under risk. *Cognitive Brain Research, 23*, 34–50.

Wilkinson, L., Lagnado, D. A., Quallo, M., & Jahanshahi, M. (2008). The effect of feedbackon non-motor probabilistic classification learning in Parkinson's disease. *Neuropsychologia, 46*, 2683–2695.

Witt, K., Daniels, C., Daniel, V., Schmitt-Eliassen, J., Volkmann, J., & Deuschl, G. (2006). Patients with Parkinson's disease learn to control complex systems: An indication for intact implicit cognitive skill learning. *Neuropsychologia, 44*, 2445–2451.

van Veen, V., Krug, M. K., and Carter, C. S. (2008). The neural and computational basis of controlled speed-accuracy tradeoff during task performance. *Journal of Cognitive Neuroscience, 20,* 1952–1965.

Witt, K., Nuhsman, A., & Deuschl, G. (2002). Dissociation of habit-learning in Parkinson's and cerebellar disease. *Journal of Cognitive Neuroscience, 14,* 493–499.

Witt, K., Nuhsman, A., & Deuschl, G. (2002). Dissociation of habit-learning in Parkinson's and cerebellar disease, *Journal of Cognitive Neuroscience , 14,* 493–499

Yu, A. (2007) Adaptive behavior: Humans act as Bayesian learners. *Current Biology, 17,* 977-980.

9

Balance and Gait Rehabilitation in Patients with Parkinson's Disease

Nicola Smania, Alessandro Picelli, Christian Geroin, Patrizia Ianes, Elisabetta La Marchina, Andrea Zenorini and Marialuisa Gandolfi
Neuromotor and Cognitive Rehabilitation Research Centre
Department of Neurological, Neuropsychological, Morphological and Movement Sciences, University of Verona
Italy

1. Introduction

Parkinson's disease (PD) is a neurodegenerative disorder characterized by cardinal features - resting tremor, rigidity, bradykinesia, and postural difficulties - which are thought to arise primarily from the loss of dopamine producing neurons and subsequent dysfunction of the basal ganglia-thalamo-cortical pathway (Konczak et al., 2009). Patients with PD have difficulties in performing various motor tasks, such as walking, writing and speaking. Furthermore, PD leads to abnormalities in two main components of postural control: orientation (maintaining a normal postural arrangement and alignment) and stabilization (maintaining equilibrium) (Vaugoyeau & Azulay, 2010). Postural instability (PI) is a disabling disorder, which is associated with sudden falls, progressive loss of independence, immobility and high costs for healthcare systems (Grimbergen et al., 2004). It usually occurs at the later stages of the disease and, unlike gait disorders, responds poorly to medication. Marked alteration of gait is common in advanced PD, although there is evidence suggesting that initial impairment in gait can be detected even early in the course of the disease (Stolze et al., 2005; Baltadjieva et al., 2006). Gait disorders, along with turning and balance disturbances, are the most important determinants of falls, which are recognized to be a major problem among people with PD. Falls occur despite maximal treatment with levodopa, confirming that axial disability in late stage PD is largely dopa-resistant (likely due to extranigral and non-dopaminergic brain lesions). Falls often have dramatic consequences, such as traumas and fractures. The high risk of fractures was demonstrated in a large case control study (Vestergaard et al., 2007), which showed that patients with parkinsonism (not just PD) had a more than two-fold increased risk of sustaining a fall-related fracture. It has been established that PD has a negative impact on the quality of life (QoL) of patients (Diamond & Jankovic, 2005). Interestingly, in PD, non-motor symptoms such as depression and cognitive impairment are major predictors of QoL (Martinez-Martin, 1998). Although investigators have examined the effect of specific PD symptoms such as tremor, rigidity and bradykinesia (Peto et al., 1995), medication-related complications (Chapuis et al., 2005), insomnia (Caap-Ahlgren & Dehlin, 2001), fatigue (Herlofson & Larsen, 2003) and sweating (Swinn et al., 2003), their relative contributions to the patient's QoL have not been assessed. The negative impact of gait disorders on QoL is related to immobility (causing loss of independence) and increased risk of falling. 'Episodic' gait disorders, which are only intermittently present, are particularly incapacitating because patients cannot easily adjust their behaviour to these paroxysmal walking difficulties (Snijders et al., 2007). A textbook example is freezing of gait (FoG), in which patients with PD experience debilitating episodes during which they are unable to start walking, or while walking suddenly fail to continue moving forward. Because of its sudden and unpredictable nature, FoG is an important cause of falls and injuries. Perhaps not surprisingly, a recent study showed that FoG was independently associated with a decreased QoL (Moore et al., 2007). In the last 2 decades research studies focusing on the rehabilitation of patients with PD have progressively increased. Most of the rehabilitation studies have focused on the treatment of balance and gait disorders. It has been shown that exercise is beneficial to physical functioning, health related QoL, strength, balance and gait speed. Current models of rehabilitation often use compensatory strategies as the basis of therapeutic management. However, there is a growing body of evidence regarding the benefit of exercise in terms of neuroplasticity and the ability of the brain to self-repair. Animal models have found that exercise has protective benefits against the onset of symptoms in PD (Faherty et al., 2005). In PD, it has been found that exercise stimulates dopamine synthesis in the remaining dopaminergic cells, thus reducing symptoms. Fox et al. (Fox et al., 2006) suggest that there are five key principles of exercise that enhance neuroplasticity in PD: intensive activity maximizes synaptic plasticity; complex activities promote greater structural adaptation; activities that are rewarding increase dopamine levels and therefore promote learning/relearning; dopaminergic neurons are highly responsive to exercise and inactivity ("use it or lose it"); and if exercise is introduced at an early stage of the disease, progression can be slowed. In this chapter we aim to discuss several issues related to balance and gait rehabilitation in PD. First, we will describe the mechanism of balance and gait control in humans. Then, we will focus on the pathophysiology of balance and gait impairment in PD. In particular, we will discuss the role of defects in the processing of afferent inputs from the vestibular, proprioceptive and visual systems, in the pathogenesis of the postural orientation and stabilization disorders in PD. Furthermore, we will describe the relationship between the postural control deficit and the abnormal choice of postural strategies. A section will be dedicated to the dramatic problem of falls. As to gait disturbances, central nervous system (CNS) circuits involved in controlling automatic repetitive movement such as gait will be described. The role of the basal ganglia in enabling movement sequences and the role of sensory cues in compensating for the deficit of internal rhythm generation by the basal ganglia in PD will be discussed. Subsequently, a section will be dedicated to the usefulness and limitations of common clinical and instrumental assessments of balance and gait disturbances. Then, rehabilitation approaches to balance and gait impairment in PD will be reviewed. Advantages and limits of the rehabilitation approaches described will be discussed.

2. Human postural and gait control

2.1 Mechanisms of postural control

Postural control is a complex function, which is particularly evolved in humans. Postural control is important as it allows a person to maintain a stable position in different postural conditions (i.e. sitting, standing). Furthermore, it is essential to the stability of axial body segments during the execution of voluntary movements (arms or whole body movements). The ability to stand upright, while standing still or moving, allows humans to have control over their environment. Maintaining this position is a challenging task because of the narrow base of support (feet) of bipeds. This task (maintaining the body upright) is even more difficult when a person has to move around the environment following straight or more complex trajectories. Nonetheless, by supporting themselves on one or both feet, humans perform various activities such as walking, going from sit to stand, turning etc. These activities may be further complicated by various environmental conditions such as in the case of uneven ground, climbing stairs, going downhill, carrying heavy or big objects etc. How can our postural and movement control systems accomplish all these challenging tasks, despite the perturbing effects of gravity and other external forces? Amblard et al. (Amblard et al., 1985) suggested the existence of a dual postural control system, part of which deals with body orientation with respect to gravity, and part of which deals with body stabilization. The first system allows a proper arrangement of body segments (i.e. erect axial segments aligned with gravitational coordinates and limbs positioned in such a way that the involvement of the muscles for joint stabilization is minimized). The second system, body stabilization, is aimed at maintaining the centre of the body mass within the limits imposed by the base of support (equilibrium). These two postural control systems do not operate independently, but most likely interact, providing a stable physical basis for perception and action (Vaugoyeau et al., 2007; Vaugoyeau & Azulay, 2010). When organizing a given movement, the CNS has to coordinate the control of body equilibrium and body orientation. In order to achieve this complicated organization, the CNS relies on three main distinct processes: 1) sensory organization, in which one or more of the orientational senses (somatosensory, visual and vestibular) are involved and integrated in the CNS; 2) a motor adjustment process involved with executing coordinated and properly scaled neuromuscular responses; 3) the background tone of the muscles, through which the changes in balance are affected (Horak et al., 1992).

2.2 Sensory organization

Erect human postural control (orientation and stabilization) is known to depend on vestibular, visual and somatosensory information, arising from sensory sources such as muscle, skin, and joints (Vaugoyeau et al., 2007). A recent work by Kuo (Kuo, 2005) describes how all these senses interact in human balance control. There are two types of vestibular organs. First, semicircular canals, which are fluid-filled canals in the inner ear, and detect the angular velocity of the head by sensing viscous motion of the fluid. Second, otoliths, which are crystal-like masses mounted on hair cells, and act as linear accelerometers. Thus, vestibular organs are able to detect motion and the position of the head with respect to gravitational coordinates. Vision is similarly sensitive to self-motion of the head. In order to maintain posture, the relevant signals are processed by motion detection circuitry, not only in the retina but also in the visual cortex, so that the vestibular nuclei receive signals proportional to rotational and translational motion of the visual field (Young, 1981). The somatosensors are also important receptors subserving postural control. They are responsible for proprioception—the sensing of joint motion and limb position. Proprioception is subserved by muscle spindles, joint and coutaneuous receptors. These sensory signals are fed back to a series of hierarchical feedback loops to generate stabilizing motor commands.

2.3 Postural adjustments

In order to maintain balance, humans bring into play two types of postural responses, feedback and feedforward. The type of response activated depends on the postural task. Feedback postural responses have been well depicted in studies where subjects were submitted to unexpected disturbances of balance by means of controlled destabilizations. When the surface on which humans are standing unexpectedly moves, the body is destabilized in the direction opposite to that of the surface displacement (Leonard et al., 2009). To regain balance, humans produce medium-latency automatic postural responses in the supporting limbs that oppose the perturbation and drive the centre of mass (CoM) back toward its initial position relative to the support surface (Horak & Nashner, 1986). The latency from the initiation of the support surface movement to the onset of the evoked electromyographic (EMG) response is in the order of 80–120 ms in humans (Ting & Macpherson, 2004). These compensatory automatic postural responses are triggered by somatosensory feedback from the feet and legs (Bloem et al., 2000a, 2002), and unless prior warning of the upcoming perturbation is given (Jacobs & Horak, 2007) they are produced entirely using a feedback mode of neural control. Studies in animals and humans have examined feedback-based automatic postural responses to unexpected translations of the support surface in multiple directions with the aim of identifying strategies that the CNS may adopt to simplify the control of perturbed stance (Fung et al., 1995). These feedback responses may involve various levels of the CNS, depending on the complexity of the required response (Kuo, 2005). The route for all movement signals is the spinal cord, which also produces the lowest level of neural feedback. This feedback is in the form of local reflexes, in which stretch signals from a muscle are relayed to the spinal cord, passed across one or a few intermediate neural connections, and then fed directly back to the muscle, commanding a compensatory contraction. This short feedback loop has fast latency, in the range of 30–60 ms. However, the speed of such a loop comes with a disadvantage: local reflexes are the least integrative of postural responses, and are limited to relatively simple behaviours (Nashner, 1977). The second and most important level of feedback for balance control involves signals travelling up to the mid-brain. The brainstem serves as a relay and integration centre, receiving and sending great numbers of sensory and motor command signals. The mid-level feedback loop involves longer conduction paths and greater numbers of neural synapses, and consequently has a longer latency than spinal reflexes (often 90 ms and greater). However, the convergence of many signals and complexity of the connections allows the brain stem to generate much more complex movements, mostly of an automatic nature. The brainstem modulates the behaviour of lower level reflexes, and is itself modulated by the higher levels. The cerebral cortex and related structures generate highly complex movements, mostly of a voluntary nature, with longer latencies than the two lower feedback loops. The longer latencies suggest that the cerebral cortex has a modulatory, rather than a direct role in posture control. Unlike the condition of unexpected perturbation of balance, during daily life, most postural perturbations are caused by an individual's own movement (i.e. reaching forward). In this case, postural adjustments occur prior to movement onset, to prevent the CoM from shifting outside the base of support (Bouisset & Zattara, 1987; Commissaris et al., 2001). To ensure a controlled transition from one postural configuration to another, these adjustments of posture must be planned by the CNS in advance, and a feedforward mode of neural control sends commands to both focal and postural muscles to initiate and stabilize posture.

2.4 Background tone of the muscles

In the absence of external support, tonic activation of skeletal muscles is necessary to maintain the relative positions of body segments and to prevent the body from collapsing against gravity. Such ongoing subconscious muscular activity is referred to as "postural tone" (Cacciatore et al., 2010). Tonic muscular activity is assessed clinically as the resistance to passive joint rotation, typically in the limbs (Foster, 1892). However, because a clinician commonly supports the limb being examined, resistance to joint rotation does not explicitly reflect the state of postural tone, as skeletal muscles must be engaged in anti-gravity postural support for postural tone to manifest. While postural tone consists, in part, of low-level stable activity—typically a few percent of maximal voluntary contraction (Masani et al., 2009)—this baseline activity can be modulated dynamically to adapt to changes in joint position and load. Any time one part of the body moves, postural tone in both that and other parts of the body must be modulated to prevent resisting the movement and to maintain static equilibrium. Thus, modulation of postural tone can provide the body with both mechanical and operational flexibility for different types of movements.

2.5 Mechanisms of gait control

The coordination of limb rhythmic activities is one of the main features of locomotion (Dietz, 2002). Locomotor activity is driven by particular neural circuits located in the upper and lower spinal cord, called central pattern generators, which organize lower and upper limb movement respectively (Grillner, 1981). These circuits are coordinated by long propriospinal neurons, which couple the cervical and lumbar enlargements of the spinal cord (Dietz & Michel, 2009). It has been proposed that a flexible coupling of thoracolumbar and cervical centres allows humans to use the upper limbs for manipulative and skilled movements or, alternatively, for locomotor tasks. This implicates a functional, task-dependent gating of neuronal pathways between the neuronal circuits controlling lower and upper limb muscles during walking, which would stabilize the body during walking (Dietz & Michel, 2009). In fact, during gait the swing of the arms serves to regulate the rotation of the body. Therefore, swinging of the arms can be seen as an integral part of the dynamics of progression. Regulation of human locomotion requires a close coordination of muscle activation between the two legs. This pattern of interlimb coordination is in line with the presence of central pattern generators and the half-centre model proposed for generation of locomotor movements (Dietz, 2002). In this model, the neuronal circuits that coordinate the leg flexor activity of both sides during the swing phase of locomotion (i.e. the flexor half-centres) mutually inhibit one another. On the contrary, the extensor half-centres on each side have no mutual inhibitory connections, according with the coexistence of the stance phase on the two sides. There is also interlimb coordination of the arms, that appears to be organized in a similar way to that of the legs during rhythmic movements. This implicates similar control mechanisms of the upper and lower limbs (Zehr & Kido, 2001). There is some evidence that interlimb coordination is organized similarly in the lower and upper limbs during cyclic movements of humans. This indicates that the neuronal coordination is conserved within the human lumbar and cervical spinal cord (Dietz, 2002). A linkage between the cervical and lumbar enlargement of the spinal cord by propriospinal neuronal circuits with long axons has been inferred on the basis of H-reflex studies. For example, during rhythmic movements of one foot, a cyclic H-reflex modulation was observed in the upper limbs (Baldissera et al., 1998). According to previous studies using functional magnetic resonance imaging (Debaere et al., 2001), the supplementary motor area might be involved in the supraspinal control of this coupling between upper and lower limbs movements. These observations indicate a flexible task-dependent neuronal coupling between upper and lower limbs (Dietz, 2002). The pathway that couples upper and lower-limb movements seems to become gated by the activity of the central pattern generators during walking. The stronger impact of leg flexors in interlimb coordination is in line with the increasing evidence that leg flexor and leg extensor muscles are differentially controlled in humans (Cazalets & Bertrand, 2000). It has been shown that arm and leg muscle activity is well coordinated during walking or swimming (Wannier et al., 2001). This indicates a coupling of the neuronal circuits controlling arm and leg movements, which is again under supraspinal control.

2.6 Differential control of upper-limb movements

The task-dependency of the neuronal coupling between upper and lower limbs might be based on a differential neuronal control of upper limbs during skilled hand movements and during locomotion. Direct cortico-motoneuronal connections to hand muscles are thought to determine the degree of dexterity in humans (Dietz, 2002). It has been suggested that these phylogenetically new components are integrated into pre-existing neuronal circuits (Maier et al., 1998). As a result of previous studies, there has been speculation that the greater influence of the direct cortico-motoneuronal system that parallels increased dexterity is accompanied by a decline in the indirect transmission of corticospinal excitation by propriospinal neurons in the upper cervical spinal cord (Nakajima et al., 2000). The strong direct cortico-motoneuronal input from the cortex enhances the possibility of selective activation of hand muscles during skilled voluntary hand movements. However, indirect evidence obtained by different experimental approaches indicates that propriospinal neuronal circuits persist, and most likely remain involved in the control of arm movement (Nicolas et al., 2001). It is possible that there is an indirect corticospinal pathway to upper limb motoneuron pools, in addition to the well-documented direct cortico-motoneuronal pathway (Dietz, 2002). Efficient corticospinal excitation of upper-limb motoneurons via propriospinal neurons might occur during automatically performed movements, such as locomotion. On the contrary, during skilled hand movements, strong cortico-motoneuronal input dominates and transmission through the propriospinal system becomes suppressed. This might explain why stimulating the pyramidal tract or the motor cortex fails to demonstrate the indirect corticospinal projection in humans (de Noordhout et al., 1999).

3. Pathophysiology of postural and gait abnormalities in Parkinson's disease

3.1 Postural control abnormalities

Patients with PD are typically impaired in both components of postural control: orientation and stabilization (Benatru, 2008; Vaugoyeau & Azulay, 2010). Clinical findings and experimental studies both in patients with PD and in animals provide evidence that the control of the axial orientation is markedly impaired in PD. Nevertheless, the postural orientation component has been poorly investigated. Indeed, most studies dealing with the postural disturbances of patients with PD have been devoted to research on pathophysiological mechanisms of the deficit of postural stabilization. The greater attention to the equilibrium component of posture is probably due to the fact that PI may frequently lead to falls, and thus worsening outcome of the later stages of PD.

3.2 Impairment of axial orientation

Clinical evidence shows that patients postural orientation abnormalities can be considered a hallmark of PD. Patients with PD may present several types of orientation difficulties, the most frequent being the presence of a stooped posture with a moderate flexion of the knees and trunk, with elbows bent and arms adducted. Other postural abnormalities include extreme neck flexion (antecoli), Pisa syndrome and Camptocormia. Camptocormia is characterized by an abnormal posture of the trunk in the antero-posterior plane with marked flexion of the thoracolumbar spine (Azher & Jankovick, 2005). Pisa syndrome (Gambarin et al., 2006) is characterized by a tilting of the trunk in the lateral plane, particularly when sitting or standing (see Benatru et al., 2008, for a review). Impairment of body orientation control has also been reported in animal experiments. Indeed, in rats and cats, unilateral lesions of the Substantia Nigra, performed by a local injection of 6 hydroxydopamine, provoke forced rotations, indicating a specific role of the basal ganglia in body rotation (Marshall & Ungerstedt, 1997). Lesions of a single caudate nucleus also influence the ability to orient the body towards the side opposite to the lesion. These results suggest a specific role of the basal ganglia in the control of axial posture. Although little attention has been geared towards body verticality control in PD (compared to balance control), a recent study by Vaugoyeau & Azulay (Vaugoyeau & Azulay, 2010) investigated the hypothesis that an impaired integration of proprioceptive signals may be a main cause of the deficit of postural orientation in PD. Authors used an original procedure, consisting in applying slow oscillations to the platform on which the subjects were standing. The perturbation was delivered at an amplitude and frequency kept below the semicircular canal perception threshold. The specific contribution of somesthetic cues (arising from sensory sources such as muscle, skin, and joints), possibly along with otholitic information, was tested in subjects who performed the task with their eyes closed. This paradigm was first tested on a group of young healthy subjects (Vaugoyeau et al., 2008). It was demonstrated that these subjects tend to align their bodies with the space vertical, despite the absence of vestibular and visual information. These data obtained with young healthy subjects confirm the predominance of proprioceptive information in the control of postural orientation in a quasi-static condition, and shows that the vestibular system requires large postural change to detect any change in body orientation. In a second experiment using the same experimental paradigm, authors compared the postural performances of patients with PD with those of control subjects. In this condition, the performances of patients with PD were much less efficient than those of the control group. They were unable to maintain the vertical trunk orientation without vision and they followed the oscillations of the supporting platform, whereas the control subjects kept their body upright when deprived of visual cues and vestibular information. These results demonstrated for the first time that patients with PD present a major deficit of postural orientation and that these deficits develop earlier than equilibrium impairment. Moreover, the patients were unable to properly control their postural orientation on the basis of the sensory information, probably due to a deficit of proprioceptive function. The comparison of the parkinsonian patients' postural performances with and without vision provides further evidence that visual inputs contribute to maintaining upright posture in patients with PD. The presence of an abnormal processing of sensory inputs in PD has been emphasized in many previous studies (see Abbruzzese & Berardelli, 2003 for a review). Authors have suggested that not only is proprioceptive guidance during voluntary movements impaired in PD, but the sensory scaling of kinesthesia is also impaired. Kinesthetic deficit, and in particular deficit in axial kinesthesia, may thus be a mayor determinant of abnormal posturing in PD (Carpenter & Bloem, 2011). With regards to the pathogenesis of the stooped posture, some experiments suggest that an abnormality of the trunk alignment perception may have a causal role. For example, in situations where the support surface is shifted from a purely horizontal position, PD patients have difficulty in re-orienting themselves to a vertical position without the aid of visual cues (Vaugoyeau et al., 2007; Proctor et al., 1964). Because of their defective axial kinaesthesia, patients might also falsely perceive their subjective vertical to be shifted backward, forcing them to adopt a stooped posture (Kitamura et al., 1993). Some evidence supports this concept of incorrect trunk perception. In one experiment, patients were confronted with line drawings showing varying degrees of stoop and lateral deviation (Moore et al., 2000). When asked to identify the drawing that best resembled their self-perceived posture, patients were likely to underestimate the severity of their abnormalities. This suggests that patients have lost their normal sense of trunk position in space. This finding supplements clinical experience that many patients are surprised to observe their own posture in a mirror. The deficit of integration of somatosensory inputs may also be associated with body schema abnormalities, which may explain why patients with PD are often unaware of their stooped posture. It is worth noting that the possible role of body schema abnormalities in the pathogenesis of axial disturbances has been also emphasized in some studies dealing with other trunk deformities, such as adolescent idiopathic scoliosis (see Smania et al., 2008 for a review).

3.3 Postural instability

Postural instability is a common feature of PD that usually occurs after the onset of non-motor symptoms and becomes a clinical concern in the middle-later stages of the illness (Jankovick, 2008). Postural instability consists of alterations in postural control strategies during standing tasks, when responding to an unexpected destabilizing perturbation, or when performing voluntary movements (Adkin et al., 2003). This is a highly disabling disturbance that is difficult to treat, and predisposes patients with PD to a loss of equilibrium and unexpected falls (Marchese et al., 2003). Postural instability has been widely studied at both the overall (Marchese et al., 2003; Pastor et al., 1993), and segmental levels (Bronstein et al. 1990), probably because falling has such serious effects on the daily life of patients with PD. The mechanisms of PI in PD are not well known, however it is speculated that they possibly involve dysfunction at the level of several neural subsystems. Studies on the pathophysiology of postural control in PD have found abnormalities in the processing of afferent inputs from vestibular, proprioceptive and visual systems. Deficiencies in postural control have also been found to be related to an abnormal choice of postural strategies under different surface conditions (Horak et al., 1992). Overall, PI in PD may involve changes in both anticipatory (feedforward) and compensatory (feedback) postural reactions (Lee et al., 1995; Schieppati et al., 1991). Based on the available evidence, it actually seems unlikely that axial kinaesthetic deficits contribute to the abnormalities in automatic postural reactions previously observed in PD. If balance impairment in patients with PD could be related to a global loss in proprioception, then their postural responses would be expected to be attenuated, and potentially delayed if proximal deficits are involved. However, patients with PD have normal timing of postural reactions, and in fact show excessive muscle activity in their automatic balance reactions (Carpenter et al., 2004). Furthermore, unlike kinaesthetic abnormalities, which appear to be worsened by dopaminergic medication (Wright et al., 2007), postural reactions are typically not responsive to dopaminergic medications (Carpenter et al., 2011; Bloem et al., 1996). Similarly, deep brain stimulation can improve kinaesthesia in PD (Maschke et al., 2005), but provides a less convincing improvement in postural reactions of PD patients (Visser et al., 2008). Therefore, deficits in the timing and modulation of postural reactions in PD are unlikely to be caused by abnormalities in kinaesthesia. Another significant issue related to PI regards the tendency to retropulsion in patients with PD. Indeed, in spite of their forward inclination in upright posture, patients with PD tend to fall backwards very easily, with only a slight push, resulting in retropulsion (Grimbergen et al. 2004). Both axial rigidity and poor trunk coordination contribute to the poor stability of patients with PD in response to backward body sway. Horak et al. (Horak et al., 2005) studied patients with PD in their off-state and showed different stability margins for different directions of body sway. The smallest stability margin occurred for backward body sway in both narrow and wide stance, suggesting that patients with PD are more vulnerable to falls in the backward direction. The reduced stability margin in patients with PD was due to a slower rise and a smaller peak of their centre of pressure, when compared to control subjects. Therefore, widening the sustentation base is unlikely to help patients with PD to prevent backward falls. Previous studies suggested that a disturbance of the central integration of sensory inputs may partly account for the PI of patients with PD (Bronte-Stewart et al., 2002). Kitamura et al. (Kitamura et al., 1993) reported that in the absence of visual cues, the position of the CoP shifted significantly backward in patients with PD, whereas it shifted significantly forward in age-matched control subjects. This provides further evidence that visual inputs contribute to maintaining upright posture in PD patients. Similar results were obtained by Bronstein et al. (Bronstein et al., 1990), who studied the postural responses to slow displacements of the visual environment. In this situation, patients with PD produced exaggerated responses, probably due to hyperactivity of the visuo-postural loop. Concerning the proprioceptive contribution to postural control in PD, Smiley-Oyen et al. (Smiley-Oyen et al., 2002) showed that a similar adaptation to vibration occurred in both patients with PD and control subjects. The authors suggested that, in patients with PD, proprioceptive impairments might affect kinesthetic abilities more than their postural control. Vaugoyeau et al. (Vaugoyeau et al., 2007) assessed the proprioceptive contribution to postural control in PD by using particular perturbation of the supporting platform and showed that proprioceptive impairments contribute to disturb postural orientation control. They suggested that, in patients with PD, increased visual dependence might reflect the adaptive strategy to compensate their proprioceptive deficits. As the disease progresses and the proprioceptive deficits increase, the strategy consisting of re-weighting sensory inputs in favor of the visual sensory mode may no longer suffice. In regards to the neural subsystems involved in PI pathogenesis, studies of automatic leg responses to sudden platform movements have partially clarified that, unlike the situation in bradychinesia, PD postural abnormalities may not be related to a dysfunction of the dopamine systems (Beckley et al. 1993). This accounts for the fact that some studies have shown that dopaminergic medications lead to a limited improvement of PI in PD (Bloem et al., 1994; Visser et al., 2008). In particular, the velocity of postural movements is not improved by drugs (Bronte-Stewart et al., 2002), and early automatic postural responses are only partially corrected, while later occurring postural corrections do not improve at all (et al., 1996).

3.4 Gait disturbances in Parkinson's disease

In PD dopamine depletion has been observed to be associated with increased synchronization of neuronal activity throughout the basal ganglia (Obeso et al., 2008). Thus, the balance of basal ganglia activity is shifted toward the indirect circuit that increases output from the globus pallidus pars interna and inhibits the thalamocortical projection with a consequent reduction of cortical activation associated with movement initiation. Moreover, the basal ganglia activity is shifted toward inhibiting cortically aided movements by an increased gain of the subthalamic nucleus-globus pallidus pars interna network and reduced excitability in the direct circuit (Obeso et al., 2008). Finally, the movements mediated by the brainstem are also functionally impaired by excessive basal ganglia inhibitory outputs. Other essential characteristic motor abnormalities in PD, such as difficulty in performing simultaneous and sequential movements and a progressive reduction in amplitude while performing a repetitive movement, do not find an adequate explanation in the current understanding of basal ganglia physiopathology (Obeso et al., 2008). Another known mechanism contributing to the locomotor disorder in patients with PD is the insufficient activation of leg extensor muscles and the poor adaptation to environmental influences as a consequence of a deficit in proprioceptive feedback. Also, an impaired quadrupedal neuronal coordination of lower and upper limbs has been described to contribute to the locomotor disorder (Dietz & Michel, 2008). Gait disturbances in PD can be divided into episodic and continuous disturbances. The episodic disturbances may occur randomly or intermittently and include start hesitation, festination and FoG. Festination is a feature of PD where patients take rapid small steps in an attempt to maintain their feet beneath their forward moving trunk. It is associated with involuntary shortening of steps and hastening of cadence part way through a task. In patients with gait festination, consecutive footsteps become progressively shorter with an accompanying reduction in walking speed. This has been hypothesized to be related with an insufficient motor cue production in the globus pallidus (Morris et al., 2008). In particular, in the presence of progressive delays in the timing of phasic firing from the globus pallidus pars interna to the cortex (supplementary motor area and pre-motor cortex), footsteps become shorter and the gait speed decreases. When the phasic firing is slow or absent, freezing occurs because the motor cortical regions are not able to generate force for the next step in the sequence. Gait festination is progressive, whereby each step in a long gait sequence becomes progressively shorter, eventually leading to blocking. Freezing of gait is defined as an inability to initiate walking sequences, a sudden cessation of stepping part-way through a locomotor task, or difficulty igniting subsequent steps in the sequence once motor block as occurred. On the contrary, the continuous alterations of gait are persistent and apparent all the time (Hausdorff, 2009). These disturbances include slowed ambulation (in part as a consequence of bradykinesia) with decreased or absent arm swing. The key element of these disturbances is the inability of patients with PD to generate adequate amplitude of movement and in particular a sufficient stride length (Morris et al., 1994). Thus, the shortened stride length may explain other typical features of continuous gait disturbances in PD such as reduced walking speed, increased cadence and double support duration (i.e. more time with both feet spent on the ground during ambulation). In addition, increased left-right gait asymmetry and diminished bilateral coordination have to be included together with a loss of ability to produce a steady gait rhythm (Hausdorff, 2009). On the contrary, the base of support is typically normal in patients with PD (it is often widened in patients with atypical parkinsonism) (Snijders et al., 2007). As a whole, gait disturbances contribute to the increased risk of falls as the disease progresses (Hausdorff, 2009).

4. Falls in Parkinson's disease

It is well known that PI (Bronte-Stewart et al., 2002; Morris, 2000; Smania et al., 2010) predisposes patients with PD to unexpected falls (Marchese et al., 2003). Balance is certainly needed within the context of many functional tasks of everyday living to keep the body oriented appropriately while performing voluntary activities, during external perturbations and when the support surface or environment changes (Bronte-Stewart et al., 2002). Thus, impaired balance and PI occur mainly during walking, while maintaining upright stance and stability in, or when transferring from one position to another.

4.1 Epidemiology of falls

Patients with PD experience falls and suffer fall-related injuries, including fractures and head traumas, more often than age-matched people (Melton et al., 2006; Pickering et al., 2007). In particular, a study by Bloem et al. showed that patients with PD had a 9-fold increased risk of sustaining recurrent falls when compared to age-matched people without PD (Bloem et al., 2001). It has been emphasized that the incidence of falls in PD is high. In the past few years, six prospective studies have examined fall rates and consequently falls among community-dwelling patients with PD living in Canada, Netherlands, Australia and United Kingdom (Ashburn et al., 2001; Bloem et al., 2001; Bloem & Bathia, 2004; Hely et al., 1999; Temlett & Thompson, 2006; Morris, 2000). All these studies included patients suffering from Idiopathic PD who were able to walk and had no other causes for falls. The duration of follow-up ranged from 3 to 12 months and falls were ascertained by means of a falls diary or by phone calls made weekly/monthly. Results showed that 70% of patients reported at least one fall (Wood et al., 2002) in the previous months. A recent meta-analysis by Pickering and colleagues addressed an important point on the incidence of falls in PD (Pickering et al., 2007). For the first time, the potential predictors of falling for patients who had never fallen before was studied. The authors provide a large sample size (473 patients) by pooling the six prospective studies previously mentioned. Each of these studies involved sufficiently similar methods, allowing the data to be pooled. The prospective follow-up data were therefore recalculated for a comparable 3-month period in order to determine the actual number of falls over the first 3 months. Results underscore the high frequency of falling in PD during a relatively brief follow-up of only 3 months, as the fall rate was 46% (95% confidence interval: 38-54%) and 21% (95% confidence interval: 12-35%) among patients with or without prior falls, respectively. Another study determined the frequency of falls in a group of 350 ambulatory people with PD. They reported that 46% of people with PD fell at least one time per week and 33% fell at least 2 or more times per week (Balash et al., 2005). High fall rate was also observed in the Sydney multicentre study (Hely et al., 2008), in which 136 newly diagnosed patients with PD were followed for 20 years. Of the 36 survivors, 87% had experienced falls and 35% had sustained multiple fractures. Hip fractures are associated with considerable morbidity and even an increased mortality in patients with PD, and are a leading reason for nursing home admission (Idjadi et al., 2005; Coughlin & Templeton, 1980).

4.2 Falls phenomenology

A fall is "an event that results in a person coming to rest unintentionally on the ground or other lower level, not as a result of a major intrinsic event or overwhelming hazard" (Clarke et al., 1993). Another phenomena that has been taken into account in outcome studies in PD is near-falls. A near-fall is defined as the feeling that an individual feels/thinks that they were going to fall but do not actually do so (Steinberg et al., 2000).

4.3 Pathogenesis of falls in Parkinson's disease

The pathogenesis of falls in PD has more than one determinant. Obviously, PI is perhaps the main cause of the loss of balance leading to a fall in PD. However, several other manifestations of PD have shown to have a potential role in falls pathogenesis. One of these manifestations is difficulty in turning. This difficulty is clinically evident at the early stages of the disease, when individuals with PD have trouble turning in bed. In addition, they have difficulties turning in the seated position, and in particular in the standing position, even when straight walking is unaffected (Crenna et al., 2007). Turning whilst walking is a challenging component of locomotor ability, due to the need of complex integration between functionally different control mechanisms. These include neural commands for redirecting the cyclical motion of the lower limbs by asymmetric tuning step lengths and ground reaction forces (Hase & Stein, 1999; Orendurff et al., 2006), controlled rotation and bending of the axial segments aimed at coping with a curved path and preserving dynamic stability (Patla et al., 1991; Imai et al., 2001), and anticipatory orientation of gaze toward the intended direction of travel (Grasso et al., 1998; Hollands et al., 2002). These turning movements while standing are performed slowly (Visser et al., 2007), with small and abnormally timed steps (Huxham et al., 2008; Stack et al., 2004) and 'en bloc' (i.e. without the normal multi-segmented axial flexibility) (Crenna et al., 2007; Vaugoyeau et al., 2006). Turning problems may result from inability to adequately maintain an interlimb coordination (Baltadjieva et al., 2006; Hausdorff et al., 2003; Plotnik et al., 2007). This is especially difficult during turning when -by necessity- the two legs have to move more "in phase" rather than "out of phase," as is usual during over ground straight walking. Another important factor is axial "stiffness" and loss of intersegmental flexibility (Boonstra et al., 2008). One study (Wright et al., 2007) measured trunk resistance to passive axial rotations and found an increased axial rigidity in PD. Most importantly, patients who took levodopa showed no improvement, again suggesting that axial disability is largely dopa-resistant, unlike the appendicular movements, which appear to be controlled by separate dopaminergic neural systems (Boonstra et al., 2008). The great relevance of these findings lies within the relation to falls and injuries. Turning around the body's axis is the most important cause for FoG in PD (Schaafsma et al., 2003; Snijders et al., 2008). During turning, FoG is an important risk factor for falls in PD (Latt et al., 2009; Kerr et al., 2010). Falls occurring while turning cause the subject to fall sideways, and this is commonly associated with hip fractures (Greenspan et al., 1998). It would be helpful to have simple tools to detect turning difficulties, to estimate the risk of falling, and to record the outcome of therapeutic interventions. Several recent studies (Boonstra et al., 2008) have shown that simply timing a patient's performance and counting the number of steps during a 180 degree axial turn may suffice, as patients with PD require more steps and turns lower than controls. Another relevant disturbance that may have an influence on falls is FoG (Brichetto et al., 2006). The freezing phenomenon indicates sudden and short-lasting breaks in voluntary motor activity that interrupts the execution of a complex movement or switching from one movement to another (Giladi et al., 1992). Freezing of gait is frequent in patients with advanced PD and is characterized by a large variability of manifestations. Patients may freeze when starting to walk (start-hesitation), during turning, or when approaching a narrow space such as doorways (Giladi et al., 1992; Schaafsma et al., 2003). Freezing of gait seems mainly related to disease progression and is influenced by cognitive and emotional factors (attention, anxiety and stress), but its definite pathophysiology is still uncertain (Brichetto et al., 2006). In recent years, some studies have recognized that walking and postural stability are not purely automatic tasks regulated by subcortical control mechanisms, but also require some conscious attention (Boonstra et al., 2008). Under particular circumstances gait and maintenance of equilibrium may also involve higher-order attentional processes. For example, when challenged with multiple simultaneous tasks, patients with PD may decrease their postural control, predisposing themselves to the risk of falling (Bloem et al., 2006). Stepping responses are effective strategies aimed at correcting balance and preventing falls in case of a great displacement of the centre of body mass. Forward stepping responses have reduced magnitudes in patients with PD. Recent studies (Jacobs & Horak, 2006; King & Horak, 2008) have shown that patients with PD have difficulties initiating a compensatory step. It is worth noting that patients showed significant more PI and falls when stepping was required for postural correction in response to lateral disequilibrium. This bradykinetic characteristic of the stepping responses helps to explain the greater rate of falls in subjects with PD.

4.4 Fear of falling

Patients with PD often develop a fear of falling while performing daily activities, resulting in a progressive loss of mobility (Adkin et al., 2003; Bloem et al., 2001; Morris, 2000; Pickering et al., 2007). This reduced mobility is associated with a host of negative consequences, including muscle weakness, promotion of osteoporosis and an overall deterioration of fitness, leading to cardiovascular disease and reduced survival (Pickering et al., 2007).

5. Evaluation of motor functions in Parkinson's disease

In the last decades some clinical scales have been developed in order to evaluate motor function in PD (i.e. gait, freezing, turning), while others have been designed to evaluate the impact of disease in activities of daily living. Recently, some instrumental devices that carry out quantitative and qualitative testing of specific motor functions (i.e. gait) have been introduced into clinical practice. All these testing procedures may be used to evaluate the effectiveness of rehabilitation treatment in patients with PD.

5.1 Clinical methods

A wide range of clinical tests have been used to assess balance and gait in elderly people and in people with neurological disorders. Smithson et al. (Smithson et al., 1998) have identified five main groups of tests: (1) tests that measure the ability to maintain steady standing in different foot positions; (2) tests that measure the ability to maintain stability in standing while coping with perturbations to balance by self-initiated movements such as arm raises, lifting a foot up and down onto a step, or reaching forward; (3) tests of postural responses to expected and unexpected external perturbation; (4) functional tests of balance during activities such as walking, standing up, and turning; (5) tests to evaluate the ability to integrate visual, somatosensory, proprioceptive, and vestibular input in order to maintain stability in standing (sensory organization). Many of these tests correlate with frequency of falls in elderly people (Smithson et al., 1998).

5.1.1 Balance in steady standing

The assessment of balance in steady standing can be tested by determining an individual's ability to maintain various stance positions, with eyes open and with no hand support. There are various stance positions. For example, feet 10 cm apart, feet together, and stride stance, with the subject's feet placed 10 cm apart and with the heel of the front foot in line with the toes of the rear foot (Goldie et al., 1990). Another stance position is tandem stance, in which the subject stands with one foot directly in front of the other foot and with the toes of the rear foot contacting the heel of the front foot. Finally, there is the single-limb stance, in which the individual stands on one foot with the opposite knee held at 45 degrees of flexion and both hips in the anatomical position. During this stance both feet should be tested. During feet apart, stride stance, and tandem stance conditions, the individual should be requested to stand on footprint templates, and stride stance and tandem stance should be tested with each of the feet in the front position. The tests are completed if the individual changes their stance position, if the examiner provides assistance to the individual with external support, or if the individual maintains the position for the maximum testing period of 30 seconds. In order to control for the effect of fatigue and other variables, the best of 3 scores should be recorded if all scores are less than 10 seconds. If the score exceeds 10 seconds in any trial, that time must be recorded without further trials (Goldie et al., 1990).

5.2 Perturbation of standing balance by self-initiated movements

5.2.1 Arm raise test

This test requires an individual to stand with their feet placed 10 cm apart and is instructed to lift their arm up and down to shoulder height as many times they can in 15 seconds. The individual begins when the examiner says go. Prior to the start of the test, the examiner demonstrates the required action by passively moving the individual's arm up to 90 degrees of flexion and down again twice. Performance for one trial of the right and left arms should be recorded (Goldie et al., 1990).

5.2.2 Step test

This test involves an individual standing with their feet 10 cm apart, with a 15-cm-high step positioned 5 cm in front of their toes. The examiner delivers the following instructions: "When I say go, step your foot onto then off the step as many times as you can until I say stop. Make sure that all of your foot contacts the step each time". The number of times the individual can successfully place the foot onto the step in 15 seconds is recorded. This procedure must be completed for both feet (Hill et al., 1996).

5.2.3 Functional reach test

The test measures the maximal distance that an individual is able to reach while maintaining a fixed base of support in standing. The individual is asked to stand with their right side close to, but not touching a wall, and with their feet set 10 cm apart. The first position requires the individual to raise their right arm to 90 degrees with the hand outstretched and the position of the third digit is recorded on the wall with removable adhesive tape. The second position requires the individual to reach as far forward as they can without moving their feet, and the position of the third digit is again recorded. The difference between the first and second position is recorded using a tape measure. To reduce fatigue and the duration of testing, only one trial of this test should be performed (Duncan et al., 1990).

5.2.4 Bend-reach test

This test measures the maximal distance that each subject can bend and reach to pick up an object from the ground. The individual is asked to stand on footprint templates and the target object is placed at 5-cm intervals in a straight line from the templates. The maximum distance that the individual can successfully reach to retrieve an object without touching down on the ground with their hands, requiring external support from the examiner, or changing foot position must be recorded for one trial. This test has not been validated, however it has been used in research as patients with PD have demonstrated difficulty retrieving objects from the ground (Smithson et al., 1998).

5.3 Balance in response to an externally generated perturbation

This test consists in giving the individual an external perturbation (shoulder tug) and recording his response. The individual is positioned in a steady stance with their feet 10 cm apart. The examiner stands directly behind the individual and delivers the following instruction: "I am going to tap you off balance, and I won't let you fall". Without giving any information regarding the direction and timing of the perturbation, the examiner delivers a brief and quick tug to the individual's shoulders in a posterior direction with sufficient force to destabilize the individual. The amount of the destabilizing force is determined by the examiner, based on the individual's weight. Postural reactions in response to the shoulder tug is recorded by the examiner using the 5-point clinical rating scale described by Pastor et al. (Pastor et al., 1993): (1) the individual stays upright without taking a step, (2) the individual takes one step backward but remains steady, (3) the individual takes more than one step backward but remains steady, (4) the individual takes one or more steps backward, followed by the need to be caught and (5) the individual falls backward without attempting to step. Bloem et al. (Bloem et al., 2000) have a similar balance evaluation, however the individuals are not informed of the shoulder pull. Thus, the individual's reaction to an unexpected shoulder pull is scored on a 4-point scale, including the speed of restoring balance.

5.4 Functional tests of balance

5.4.1 Berg Balance Scale

The Berg Balance Scale is a 14-item (0-4 points per task; high=best performance) validated scale that evaluates balance abilities during sitting, standing and positional changes. Total scores are indicative of overall balance abilities, with a score of 0 to 20 indicating wheelchair bound; a score of 21 to 40 indicating walking with assistance, and 41 to 56 indicating independent. A score of 43.5 or below suggests risk of falls. It is simple to administer in approximately 15 to 20 minutes and uses a quantitative scale format that has strong internal consistency and good inter and intra-rater reliability with patients with PD (Qutubuddin et al., 2005).

5.4.2 Time 'Up & Go'

The "Get-up and Go" test measures mobility in elderly people and is considered a useful tool for quantifying locomotor performance in individuals with PD. This test requires an individual to stand up from a chair, walk 3 m, turn around, walk back to the chair, and sit down again. The individual is videotaped, and then mobility is rated on a 5-point scale, ranging from "normal" to "severely abnormal" (Morris et al., 2001).

5.4.3 Tinetti mobility scale

The Tinetti Performance-Oriented Mobility Assessment, also referred to as the Tinetti Mobility Test (TMT), is a reliable and valid clinical test used to measure balance and gait in elderly people and patients with neurological disease. The TMT is easily administered in less than 5 minutes and provides information regarding an individual's ability to ambulate and transfer safely. The TMT assesses tasks that reportedly most often lead to falls and predict balance confidence in individuals with PD, such as turning, initiating gait, and slowing to sit down (Kegelmeyer et al., 2007).

5.4.4 Six-minute walk test

This test assesses walking capacity during a 6 minute period. Individuals are instructed to walk back and forth along a 20-m corridor and to cover the maximum distance possible in 6 minutes, taking rests as needed. The maximum distance covered is recorded. Examiners provide standardized encouragement every 30 seconds, by telling individuals "you're doing well, keep up the good work." Two trials should be performed at baseline, approximately 30 minutes apart. During the rest interval, participants can sit down. If an assistive device is used, the type of device is recorded (Falvo & Earhart, 2009).

5.4.5 Ten-meter walk test

This test assesses gait speed performance by requesting an individual to walk 10 m. A distance of 10 m must be marked on the floor with coloured tape, with subsequent marks placed 2 m from the starting point and 2 m from the ending point, thus creating a 6-m timed middle section for the test. The individual may be instructed to walk at a comfortable speed and is provided the following instructions "Walk all the way to the last piece of tape at your comfortable walking speed; you can start when I say 'go'". Alternatively, the individual may be requested to walk fast and is provided with the following instructions: "Walk all the way to the last piece of tape as fast as you can safely walk; you can start when I say 'go'. Timing begins when the individual crosses the initial 2-m mark and ends when the subject crosses the final 2-m mark. Time is measured in seconds and converted to meters per second. Four trials are performed, 2 at a comfortable walking speed and 2 at a fast walking speed (Brusse et al., 2005).

5.4.6 Fall efficacy scale

This test was designed to operationalize fear of falling based on Bandura's theory of self-efficacy. According to this theory, self-efficacy refers to a person's perception of his or her own capabilities within a particular domain of activities. The Fall Efficacy Scale assesses the degree of perceived confidence at avoiding a fall in various situations and has been shown to be useful in assessing fear of falling in elderly communities, as well as subgroups of patients with PD (Thomas et al., 2010).

5.4.7 Freezing of gait questionnaire

This questionnaire constructed by Giladi et al. (Giladi et al., 2000) evaluates the FoG in patients with PD. This detailed gait and falls questionnaire consists of 16 items that assess gait in daily living, frequency and severity of FoG, frequency of festinating gait and its relation to falls, and finally frequency and severity of falls. Responses to each item are on 5-point scales where a score of 0 indicates absence of the symptom, while 4 indicates the most severe stage (Giladi et al., 2000).

5.5 Tests to evaluate the ability to integrate visual, somatosensory, proprioceptive, and vestibular input

5.5.1 Sensory organization balance test (SOT)

The SOT is a validated timed balance test that evaluates somatosensory, visual and vestibular function for maintenance of upright posture. This test requires that patients maintain standing balance during a combination of three visual and two support surface conditions. Tasks are performed with the eyes open and with the eyes closed; a visual conflict dome is used to produce inaccurate visual and vestibular inputs. The support surface conditions include a hard, flat floor and an 8 cm section of 20.4 kg firm density foam rubber that reduces the quality of the surface orientation input. During the test, subjects stand barefoot in the upright position with their arms alongside the body and their feet on the pre-designated site. If the subject activates any postural reaction, the test is stopped immediately and the number of seconds standing prior to the violation constitutes the trial score. The test is performed under six conditions: (1) eyes open - stable surface; (2) eyes open - compliant surface; (3) eyes closed - stable surface; (4) eyes closed - compliant surface; (5) visual and vestibular conflict (wearing visual dome) - stable surface; (6) visual and vestibular conflict (wearing visual dome) - compliant surface. Five trials are carried out for each test condition. Each trial lasts 30 seconds. Total scores for each condition are the sums of the scores of each trial (maximum score for each test condition: 30 x 5 = 150) (Cohen et al., 1996; Di Fabio & Badke, 1990).

5.6 Instrumental methods

5.6.1 GAITRite™ system (CIR Systems, Inc, Clifton, NJ)

The GAITRite System was developed to measure and record temporal and spatial parameters of gait by using a walkway approximately 3 or more meters long with grids of embedded, pressure-sensitive sensors connected to a personal computer (Nelson et al., 2002). While the individual walks across an instrumented mat, electronic recordings of each footfall are made and stored as a computer file. The computer records components of locomotion, including cadence, step time, step length, mean normalized velocity, step length ratio, heel to heel base of support, single support and double percentage and stance percentage. Temporal and spatial parameters of gait are automatically calculated and displayed and can be printed after the individual completes a trial (Nelson et al., 2002).

5.6.2 Gait analysis

Gait analysis is an instrumental method for gait measurement in the clinical setting. Markers (either reflective or light emitting) are placed on the patient's skin and aligned with bony landmarks and/or particular axes of joint rotation. The primary technology that underpins gait analysis includes optica-electronic video camera-based systems that measure the displacement of the markers. Multiple cameras are configured around a calibrated measurement volume. Three-dimensional (3-D) marker trajectory paths are then stereometrically reconstructed from the two-dimensional (2-D) camera image data. Gait analysis is becoming a main system in research on movement disorders in humans (Davis, 1997).

5.6.3 Posturography

Static posturography is an instrumental method to measure postural sway. Individuals stand on a dual force plate platform, with one foot on each force plate. They are instructed to maintain an upright standing position, with arms at their sides, eyes open with their gaze straight ahead at an art poster, and feet shoulder width apart. The centre of the foot pressure (CoP) of each foot (CoPleft and CoPright) and the total body CoP are computed from the vertical forces. The CoP is the point location of the ground reaction force vector and reflects the sway of the body (biological noise) and the forces used to maintain the centre of gravity within the support base. Computerized dynamic posturography is another quantitative method for assessing upright balance function under a variety of conditions that simulate conditions encountered in daily life. Subjects stand on a moveable platform in a loosely fitting harness. Their feet are aligned over defined axes on force plates measuring vertical forces. These measures along with the height and the weight of the patient are used to calculate the centre of gravity (CoG) position and the CoG sway (Nardone & Schieppati, 2010).

5.6.4 Equitest system (NeuroCom International, Inc, Clackamas, OR, USA)

This device determines the COP displacement as well as the sway of COM in different conditions. It can be used to determine the equilibrium score (ES) and postural stability index (PSI). A key assessment of the Equitest device is that it provides information about the integration of the visual, proprioceptive and vestibular components of balance which leads to an outcome measure called the ES, reflecting the overall coordination of these systems to maintain standing posture (Chaudhry et al., 2011). The Equitest System consists of a support surface (platform), a visual surround, and a harness to prevent falls during testing. The device performs a SOT with six conditions: conditions 1, 2 and 3 with the platform fixed and conditions 4, 5 and 6 with the platform moving. When the platform moves, it is referenced to the subject's sway such that as the individual leans forward, the platform tilts forward to minimize the degree of changed proprioceptive input from the self-generated sway. This platform adjustment is called "sway-referenced motion". Similarly, in conditions where the visual surround moves, the surround is referenced to the person's sway so as to minimize the ability to obtain visually relevant information about how far the individual is from the vertical. In other conditions, visual input is removed instead by asking the subject to close his or her eyes. Participants are asked to stand quietly and steadily for 3 trials in each of the following 6 conditions: (1) eyes open, surround and platform stable, (2) eyes closed, surround and platform stable, (3) eyes open, sway- referenced surround, (4) eyes open, sway-referenced platform, (5) eyes closed, sway-referenced platform and (6) eyes open, sway-referenced surround and platform (Chaudhry et al., 2011).

6. Rehabilitation of postural and gait disturbances in Parkinson's disease

6.1 Rehabilitation of postural instability and strategies to prevent falling

Despite gains made in the field of pharmacotherapy and deep brain stimulation in PD, dopaminergic medications may produce a limited improvement in PI (Bloem et al., 1994; Visser et al., 2008). Thus, physiotherapy is the most commonly used procedure as an adjunct to drug therapy to treat PD movement disorders (Deane, 2001a, 2001b). At the moment, there is no uniformity of approaches for physiotherapy in PD. Rehabilitation for PD covers a number of different treatment techniques, largely centered on active exercises and re-education of mobility (Morris, 2000), mainly aimed at maximizing functional ability and minimizing secondary complications within a context of education and support for the person. Two Cochrane reviews on the general physical management of patients with PD (Deane, 2001a, 2001b) underlied that there is insufficient evidence to support or refute the efficacy of physiotherapy or one form of physiotherapy over another. Most of the trials included in these systematic reviews recruited small sample size (less than 20 patients) and were performed with poor research design and methodology. In light of this, the authors highlighted the need for more randomized control trials involving a large sample size to support or refute the efficacy of physiotherapy in patients with PD. In regards to rehabilitation of PI, only recently have a number of studies assessed the effect of specific training (Smania et al., 2010; Ashburn et al., 2007; Ebersbach et al., 2008; Hirsch et al., 2003; Protas et al., 2005; Qutubuddin et al., 2007; Toole et al., 2000; Jöbges et al., 2004; Cakit et al., 2007). It is interesting to note that as the pathophysiology of PI is multifaceted, the different rehabilitative approaches proposed are also very different. Moreover, the dosage of rehabilitation therapy was an inconsistent parameter among the various studies. Different approaches can be identified: exercises aimed at improving sensorimotor integration; balance training; a combination of strengthening and balance exercises; balance training with stepping; treadmill training; training for reducing falls. Studies have reported promising results regarding these different approaches, as well as demonstrated that specific rehabilitation programs can improve PI in patients with PD.

6.2 Sensorimotor integration training

As previously mentioned, increasing evidence suggests that patients with PD have abnormalities in both the peripheral afferent input and in the brain response to this sensory input, leading to a defect in the sensorimotor integration process. Among the different potential causes, it has been suggested that patients with PD usually have disturbances of proprioceptive regulation, possibly related to the abnormal muscle stretch reflexes in the upper and lower limbs (Abbruzzese & Berardelli, 2003). Because of this deficit in proprioceptive perception and processing, muscle vibration has been proposed to excite primary muscle spindles, as well as activate proprioceptors during voluntary movements in patients with PD. Previous neurophysiological findings have shown that the experimental stimulation of proprioceptors using muscle vibration can improve the trajectory of the voluntary movements of the ankle joint in patients with PD (Khudados et al., 1999). This finding suggests that PD may produce a general impairment of proprioceptive guidance and that muscle vibration could be a tool for improving sensorimotor processing. Whole body vibration (WBV) has been demonstrated to be a possible tool to improve balance by enhancing sensorimotor processing in both elderly subjects (Bruyere et al., 2005) and patients with neurological impairment (cerebral palsy, Multiple Sclerosis and stroke) (Ahlborg et al., 2006; Schuhfried et al., 2005; Van Nes et al., 2006). Bruyere et al. investigated the effectiveness of WBV intervention in improving gait and balance in a group of forty-two elderly volunteers by means of the Tinetti test, Time Up&Go and the health related QoL (SF-36) (Bruyere et al., 2005). Patients were randomized in two groups. Both groups received physiotherapy as maintenance therapy, consisting of a standard exercise program (gait and balance exercises, training in transfer skill, strengthening exercises with resistive mobilization of the lower limbs) administered for 10 minutes, 3 times weekly over 6 weeks. In addition to the standard physiotherapy, the experimental group underwent WBV intervention. During the WBV intervention the patient was required to stand on a vertical vibrating platform for 4 series of 1 minute of vibration alternated with 90 seconds of rest. After treatment, patients who underwent WBV plus physiotherapy showed a significant improvement on all outcome measures. As to PD, it has been suggested that the WBV intervention could have beneficial effects on motor symptoms assessed by the UPDRS. In particular, in the study performed by Haas et al., promising effects have been reported, showing that this approach can improve UPDRS score as follows: gait and PI items showed 15% improvement on average, bradykinesia scores were reduced by 12% on average, and tremor and rigidity scores improved 25% and 24% respectively (Haas et al., 2006). Since the UPDRS was the only outcome measure used to evaluate the WBV post-treatment effects, a detailed discussion on the influence of this intervention on balance is not possible. Furthermore, no follow-up evaluation was performed, and hence long lasting effects were not documented. All these drawbacks were partially overcame in the study by Ebersbach et al. (2008). The study was undertaken in order to identify the influence of WBV on balance and gait in 27 inpatients with PD and clinical evidence for PI. Patients were randomized to receive 30 sessions of either WBV on an oscillating platform or conventional balance training. The former consisted of two 15 minute sessions a day, 5 days a week, with intervention on a vibrating platform that thrusts the right and left leg upward alternately with a frequency of 25Hz and an amplitude of 7 to 14mm. The conventional balance training consisted of standard therapy comprising three 40-minute sessions a day (5 days a week), which mainly included relaxation techniques (i.e. muscle stretching, relaxation, body perception) and occupational therapy. During intervention, the daily schedule for all patients enrolled in the study included 150 minutes of exercise, with 30 minutes being exclusively dedicated to balance. Patients were assessed before and after treatment by means of a broad multiple testing procedure for evaluating balance (Tinetti Balance Scale, stand-walk-sit test, pull test, dynamic posturography) and gait (10-meter walking test). A final follow-up assessment was repeated 4 weeks post treatment. In contrast to the previous studies, WBV was found to have no significant effects on equilibrium and gait when compared to conventional balance exercises. Both treatments were associated with improvements on all clinical assessments of mobility and postural strategy. In regards to dynamic posturography, a non significant effect in lower sway was reported at the end of the treatment and at follow-up, even though it was the only parameter that was differentially influenced by type of treatment. Another type of training aimed at stressing sensory motor integration function was proposed by Qutubuddin et al. (2007). Patients were trained to maintain balance under different sensory conditions by using the Computerized Dynamic Posturography (CDP). In this pilot study, fifteen patients with mild-moderate PD were randomized to receive CDP therapy or standard physical therapy treatment. The main aim of the study was to evaluate the feasibility of this new approach in the treatment of balance disorders in PD. Data demonstrated that treatment was tolerated by a high percentage of patients (68%). In regard to the results recorded on the selected outcome measures, results failed to reveal any differences between the two groups.

6.3 Balance exercises

It is well known that pharmacological treatment is insufficient to improve non-dopaminergic symptoms such as lack of balance control and resulting falls. Therefore, rehabilitation programs are warranted for improving PI in patients with PD. Smania et al. (Smania et al., 2010) performed a randomized controlled trial in order to evaluate the effectiveness of a specific training aimed at improving balance control in patients with PD, Hoehn and Yahr (H&Y) stage III-IV. The training consisted of three different predetermined categories of exercises aimed at improving both feedforward and feedback postural reactions: 1) Exercises of self-destabilization of the center-of-body mass involving mainly feedforward control. For instance, patients were required to perform voluntary actions in both static and dynamic conditions such as transferring her/his body weight onto the tips of the toes and onto the heels or bouncing a ball during gait with their 2 hands alternating to the right and to the left side. 2) Exercises of externally induced destabilization of the CoM involving mainly feedback control. During these tasks the patient was required to maintain balance while standing on foam support bases of different consistency, on moveable platforms with different degrees of stability, or while the therapist was applying sternal or dorsal pulling. 3) Exercises emphasizing coordination between leg and arm movement during walking as well as locomotor dexterity over an obstacle course. These types of exercises required continuous feedback and feedforward postural adjustment. Each exercise was individualized to the patient's balance ability documented before training. During the course of the training the complexity of the tasks was progressively increased as the patient improved. The effects of the experimental training were compared with the effects of a training given to a control group, which consisted of exercises not specifically aimed at improving postural reactions (i.e. active joint mobilization, muscle stretching and motor coordination exercises carried out in supine, prone and sitting positions). Both trainings were performed as individual treatment in an outpatient setting with the same duration and frequency as follows: 21 treatment sessions of 50 minutes each, 3 days a week, for 7 consecutive weeks. Outcome measures, consisting of clinical and instrumental assessments, were delivered by a blinded rater before, after, as well as 1 month post-treatment. Results showed that specific balance training could improve postural stability and the level of confidence perceived while performing daily activities that required balance, as evaluated by the Activities Balance Confidence Scale. Furthermore, patients who underwent the balance training, which was not specifically designed to teach strategies to prevent falls, reduced the frequency of falls. Improvements were maintained at the 1-month follow-up. In contrast, patients undergoing the non-specific rehabilitation training (control group) showed no significant changes in any of outcome measures. The authors discussed that the balance training allowed the patient to improve postural control and the ability to plan an appropriate postural strategy, as demonstrated by the center of foot pressure (CFP) self-destabilization and control test (Smania et al., 2010). The CFP self-destabilization and control test is a tool for assessment of balance control ability in PD, porposed for the first time in this study (Smania et al., 2010). In particular, this test could be suitable to evaluate both "corrective" and "protective" postural responses, which are normally impaired in PD (Jöbges et al., 2004; Horak et al., 1992, 1996). After the balance training, patients showed a significant improvement on the CFP self-destabilization and control test. In contrast, no significant changes were seen in the control group. A few recent reports have assessed the effect of specific rehabilitation programs aimed at improving balance, but most of them included a wide variety of treatment approaches and have differences in methodology, and thus a comparison of the different studies cannot be performed. However, it is worth noting that the training proposed by Smania et al. (Smania et al., 2010) showed that the effects on balance abilities acquired after treatment can potentially extend to untrained activities, such as strategies to prevent falls. These results were strengthened by the fact that the study was a randomized controlled trial conducted on a considerable sample of patients (N=64). Moreover, the methods used to assess balance included multiple tests that provided a comprehensive picture of the different aspects of PI (Hirsch et al., 2003; Jacobs & Horak, 2006).

6.4 Combined training: Strengthening and balance exercises

It has been well documented that patients with PD have a reduced level of physical activity compared to healthy individuals, and that they have a lower level of strength and functional ability. However, it has been shown that muscle weakness is not simply a secondary consequence of ageing and inactivity, but is also an elementary symptom of PD (Goodwin et al., 2008). Some studies have reported significantly lower muscles torque values in patients with early stage Parkinsonism, compared to age-matched healthy controls in both upper and lower limbs (Koller, W. & Kase, 1986; Toole et al., 2000; Goodwin et al., 2008). Furthermore, a number of studies on older adults free of pathology have found that PI and an increased tendency to sway result from decreased ankle, quadriceps and hamstring strength. It has been shown that a specific approach, which combines strength and balance exercises, may be useful in improving PI in older adults (Orr, 2010; Keus et al., 2007). A recent review by Orr et al. examined the relationship between muscle strength, power and balance performance in healthy older adults (Orr, 2010). Findings from this review indicate that there is substantial evidence for the contribution of muscle strength and muscle power to balance performance in older adults (more than 60 years). An overall examination of the literature showed that 54% of studies reported significantly improved strength and balance measures and 73% showed improved power and balance following resistance/power training intervention. However, 84% and 86% of cross sectional studies observed significant associations between balance and strength/power outcomes respectively (Orr, 2010). Although the studies reviewed varied in regards to muscle groups trained and tested, including not only those muscle groups specific to balance (ankle plantiflexor and dorsiflexor, hip abductor and adductor, knee extensor and flexor) but also those that have little bearing on postural control (i.e. hand grip strength), most showed that strengthening the quadriceps and hip muscles is essential for improving static balance in older subjects (Orr, 2010). In contrast, increasing ankle plantarflexion strength in balance impaired older adults demonstrated greater protection against backward slips by enhancing ankle postural control strategies (Hess et al., 2006). The use of strength training in patients with PD has been recently explored (Toole et al., 2000; Hirsch et al., 2003). Toole et al. (Toole et al., 2000) evaluated whether a combined strength and balance training program could improve both lower limb strength and PI in patients with PD (H&Y Stage 1-3) (Toole et al., 2000). Patients were randomized in an experimental or control group. The experimental group underwent 10 weeks of lower limb strength training and balance exercises, three times per week, for 1 hour each session. Patients trained the knee flexor and extensor muscle groups bilaterally, using leg extension and side lying leg flexion machines at 60% of a four-repetition maximum force test. The strength assessment included peak torque during ankle inversion, knee extension and knee flexion evaluated by Biodex. The peak torque was defined as the maximal rotational tendency of a joint and it was chosen because of its ecological validity. The peak torque, in fact, relates to when the body starts to fall and the maximal peak torque is produced by lower limb muscles to centre the body back over the base of support, thus preventing loss of balance. The authors measured the ankle inversion instead of dorsiflexion because it has been demonstrated that it is highly correlated with balance. The training load for each muscle was adjusted weekly to keep the stimulus on 60% of the patients'maximum force. Patients were required to perform three sets of 10 repetitions for each exercise. Balance training consisted of exercises performed under a variety of destabilizing environments (i.e. posterior, anterior and retropulsion exercises) in both eyes-open and eyes-closed condition. These exercises were designed to challenge the vertical position of the body and increase the limits of stability in order to improve equilibrium when the body was destabilized. After training the patients who received strength and balance training demonstrated significant improvements in both balance and strength evaluated by the EquiTest, whereas the control group showed no improvement in any outcome measure. These results are consistent with those reported by Hirsch et al. (Hirsch et al., 2003). They investigated whether balance training combined with lower limb strength training is more effective than balance exercises alone in improving balance in patients with PD. For this purpose, fifteen patients were randomized in two groups. Both groups underwent 10-week balance training under altered visual and somatosensory conditions (3 times a week). Additionally, one group performed a high intensity lower limb resistance training combined with the balance training. The authors showed that both groups improved in balance performance evaluated by means of the Sensory Orientation Test (SOT), but the rate of improvement was higher for the patients who underwent the combined strengthening and balance training Furthermore, muscle strength increased marginally in the balance group while it increased substantially in the combined training group. Data suggest that muscle strengthening is a safe procedure in patients with PD. Moreover, it has the potential to improve PI in spite of the degenerative nature of the illness. In regards to the potential mechanisms that could have benefited from the strengthening training, and thus improved PI, several factors can be identified. First, strengthening intervention could facilitate the use of proprioceptive, visual and vestibular cues in order to stabilize the body, increase equilibrium and consequently prevent falls. Additionally, muscle strengthening may have improved the musculoskeletal system, allowing individuals to have more force to counteract sway during moments of threatened stability. In particular, the subjects used increased muscular strength in the hamstring group and in the quadriceps group to benefit equilibrium. Consistent with this finding, Dietz et al. (Dietz et al., 1993) showed that patients with PD regulated their stance mainly by modulation of leg flexor activation.

6.5 Stepping training

Many researches have focused on the study of postural responses in patients with PD, demonstrating that patients often fall because they respond to a sudden loss of balance with abnormally short (hypometric) steps that are inadequate to help them recover equilibrium (Jacobs & Horak, 2006). Recently, King et al. (King et al., 2010) showed that patients with PD have significantly more PI and falls than age-matched controls, when stepping is required for postural correction in response to lateral disequilibrium. Although they normally choose the same type of postural stepping strategies as the age-matched control subjects, consisting of lateral stepping instead of the cross-over strategy, they have longer latencies of postural responses to external perturbation (King et al., 2010) than age-matched controls. This longer latency turns into a delay in the postural response execution, which may not allow the patient to execute a prompt postural reaction, thus resulting in a fall. It is likely that patients with PD were not able to quickly shift their weight adequately, thus preventing them from taking a fast large step. Furthermore, this deficit did not significantly improve with levodopa antiparkinsonian medication, probably due to the involvement of nondopaminergic pathways (King et al., 2010). These findings support the need to develop specific rehabilitation programs aimed at improving the planning and the execution of postural stepping strategies. It is worth noting here that studies have shown that a specific training for stepping practice could improve lateral postural reactions in both younger and older healthy subjects (Hanke & Tiberio, 2006; Rogers et al., 2001). Jöbges et al. (Jöbges et al., 2004) addressed this issue in patients with PD. The authors enrolled fourteen patients with PD and PI (H&Y stage: 2,5-4) in a case-control study design where each patient's baseline data were compared to his/her post-treatment data. Before training, after training, and 2 weeks and 2 months later, patients were evaluated by means of multiple specific tests containing both clinical and instrumental procedure to evaluate the different effects of PI. Clinical procedures also included the assessment of the quality of life questionnaire (PDQ-39). Instrumental procedures consisted of the analysis of the compensatory steps performed by the patient after the destabilization occurred. Length and initiation of the compensatory steps were recorded by using an ultrasound device (CMS 50; Zebris, Isny, Germany). Gait analyses were performed in order to measure step length, cadence and double support (Win Gait 2.14; Zebris), while posturographical testing was performed using a balance platform to record vertical and horizontal shear forces and to allow calculations of the centre of gravity over time. The training was directed at maintaining stability after the pushes, using large compensatory steps. Thus, the training consisted of repetitive pulls to the patient's back and pushes to her/his right and left side applied by the physiotherapist. The strength of the pulls and pushes was adapted to the degree of the patient's individual PI and in the case of satisfactory compensatory steps, a positive feedback was given, and the intensity of the pulls and pushes was continuously increased. Otherwise, the intensity of pulls and pushes was reduced. Patients were trained for 20 minutes twice daily for two weeks in an outpatient setting. Within these 20 minute training sessions, approximately 180 to 230 pulls and pushes were applied. After training, the length of compensatory steps increased and the step initiation shortened. Gait analysis showed that the cadence and the step length increased, gait velocity improved, and the period of double support shortened. The "mobility" subscore of a quality of life questionnaire (PDQ-39) also improved. All these changes were significant and they were maintained for two months without additional training. In light of this study, a repetitive training of compensatory steps could be beneficial for improving PI also in patients with PD. These effects occurred not only during static tasks but also during gait. Therefore, these findings could have important effects in the rehabilitation of PI in patients with PD. As the authors stated, further studies with larger populations are needed to infer from these findings to the general population with PD and PI prior to this training being included as a standard treatment.

6.6 Treadmill training

Gait abnormalities are one of the most common disabling conditions in PD, consisting of several deficits such as difficulties in gait initiation, turning and balance difficulties. Protas et al. (Protas et al., 2005) showed that in eighteen patients (stage H&Y 2-3) with PD, gait training consisting of walking on the treadmill with body weight support could not only improve gait and dynamic balance, but also reduce the frequency of falls. Cakit at al. (Cakit at al., 2007) replicated these effects in a sample of fifty-four patients randomized to receive experimental training or usual care. Patients who underwent experimental training participated in an eight-week exercise programme using incremental speed-dependent treadmill training. All patients were evaluated before and after the training program by means of a comprehensive battery of tests including balance, gait and fear of falling evaluation. After treatment, the patients in the experimental group showed improvements not only in the outcome measures dealing with gait, but also in the Berg Balance Scale and in the Fall Efficacy Scale. No significant improvements were measured in the control group. Although no follow-up evaluation session was performed in order to evaluate if these important effects may be maintained over time, this treatment method can be applied to patients. Not only is the goal to increase walking speed, and hence give individuals a greater behavioural repertoire in everyday life, but also to reduce the risk of falling and resultant morbidity in the elderly general population and in patients with PD.

6.7 Programs aimed at reducing falls

Exercises programs individually prescribed at home have been shown to be effective in reducing fall frequency among the elderly population. Ashburn et al. (Ashburn et al., 2007) evaluated the effectiveness of a personalized home programme of exercises and strategies for repeat fallers with PD. Participants (n=142) were randomized in the experimental or control group. The experimental group underwent a personalized 6-week home-based exercise and strategy program comprising muscle strengthening, range of movement, balance training and walking. Balance training consisted of static, dynamic and functional exercises, which were chosen at the appropriate level for each individual and if possible progressed by increasing practice repetition. Participants were requested to complete the exercises daily and were given instructions with illustrations for each exercise. The control group underwent usual care, that, for the vast majority, was comprised of contact with a local PD nurse. Findings from the trial showed a consistent trend of reduced rates of falls and injurious falls among participants in the exercise program, even though these differences were not significant. Similar findings were reported in the randomized control trial performed by Allen et al. (Allen et al., 2010). Patients allocated to the exercise group attended a monthly exercise class run by one or two therapists and performed the remaining exercise sessions at home (three times a week) over a 6-month period. Exercises included both strengthening and balance exercises. After treatment, the exercise group showed a greater, but not significant, improvement than the control group in the fall risk score. In contrast, there were statistically significant improvements in the exercise group compared with the control group in FoG Questionnaire, and time sit-to stand. However, no significant trends were found in the exercise group for measures of walking, strength, fear of falling and standing balance. Larger scale studies are warranted to explore this issue (Ashburn et al., 2007; Allen et al., 2010; Canning et al., 2009) because to date no adequately powered studies have investigated exercises interventions aimed at reducing falls in patients with PD. Furthermore, the real cost effectiveness of exercise programs, from the health provider's perspective, has not been established. Hence, recently a study protocol focusing on these important issues has been proposed (Canning et al., 2009). Programs aimed at reducing falls has also been proposed by Brichetto et al. (Brichetto et al., 2006), who performed a pilot study aimed at investigating the effectiveness of a rehabilitation protocol in patients with PD and FoG. Twelve outpatients (H&Y stage 2-3) were selected because of their subjective compliant and occurrence at clinical examination of FoG during the "on" phase of medication. Patients underwent treatment which included different exercises to improve balance, postural control and walking over a period of 6 weeks (three sessions every week). Before, after and 4 weeks after the end of the rehabilitation treatment, patients were examined by means of the UPDRs (motor section), FoG Questionnaire, Parkinson Disease QoL Questionnaire and gait analysis. After treatment, results showed a significant reduction in score on both the FoG Questionnaire and the Parkinson Disease QoL Questionnaire, while no significant changes were found at follow-up. Although this study was based on a small sample, it suggests that the potential short-term efficacy of a rehabilitative approach aimed at FoG in PD may be due to the effects of exercises mainly focused at improving stability and gait (Brichetto et al., 2006).

6.8 Gait rehabilitation in Parkinson's disease

Walking impairments, a hallmark of PD, are characterized by a slow, short stepped, shuffling, forward-stooped gait with asymmetrical arm swing (Morris, 2000, 2006; Morris & Iansek, 1996). To date, many physiotherapy approaches in PD consist mainly of mixed exercises, aimed at the overall remediation of many disturbances that may be associated to PD, including gait. In recent years, many studies have shown that using several sensory cueing strategies may be a valuable approach in order to improve gait performance in patients with PD. Cueing is defined as using external temporal or spatial stimuli to facilitate movement (gait) initiation and continuation. Recent reviews on cueing suggest that it can have an immediate and powerful effect on gait performance in people with PD, indicating improvements in walking speed, step length and step frequency. The influence of cueing has mainly been studied in single-session experiments in laboratory settings (Lim et al., 2005). Results have shown a short-term correction of gait and gait initiation, and suggest that carry-over to uncued performance and its generalisation to activities of daily living (ADL) is limited. Using cues in a therapeutic setting is more complex, as the "modality" of cue delivery (visual, auditory or somatosensory) and the cue "parameter" selected for movement correction (frequency or size of step) have to be adapted to the needs of the patient. Furthermore, improved mobility with cues may have an adverse effect by distracting attention and increasing the risk of falling (Lim et al., 2005). Gait facilitation in patients with PD by means of cueing has been reported since 1942 (Von Wilzenben, 1942). The first detailed analysis of external cueing effect on gait was performed by Martin in 1967 (Martin et al., 1967). To define the word cue is quite problematic. According to Cools et al.

(1993), cues are "contextual or spatial stimuli which are associated with behaviour to be executed, through past experience". Conversely, Horstink distinguishes between cues and stimuli, stating that "cues give information on how an action should be carried out and are hence more specific than simple stimuli" (Horstink et al., 1993). Based on these observations and given that Parkinsonian symptoms particularly affect complex and sequential movements, we decided to define external rhythmical cueing as "applying rhythmical temporal or spatial stimuli associated with the initiation and ongoing facilitation of motor activity".

6.8.1 Putative mechanisms of action

The basal ganglia are the focal point of impairment in PD. They have been shown to be involved in the execution of automatic and repetitive movement (Cunnington et al., 1995; Georgiou et al., 1993). To enhance basal ganglia function, some studies provided external rhythmic auditory cues in order to supplement the deficient internal rhythm. Other studies used visual cues to set the proper stride length, thus providing external information to help augment the defective motor set. To reroute the movement through a non-automatic pathway, attentional cues have been used to focus attention on walking, thus shifting away from the automatic basal ganglia pathway. Alternatively, visual cues may be employed to activate the visual motor pathway instead of the automatic motor pathway.

6.8.2 Auditory cueing

Rhythmic auditory cueing has been gaining popularity over the last years. There is strong evidence that rhythmical auditory cueing enhances gait speed in patients with PD (Lim et al., 2005). Moreover, limited evidence was available for improving stride length and cadence with the use of auditory stimulation (Lim et al., 2005). These improvements have been described to remain evident in the immediate short term even after the cues were removed (Lim et al., 2005). In terms of actual gait training, patients who trained daily while listening to music with an overlaid rhythmic auditory stimulation beat showed more significant and more lasting improvements in gait than patients who did the same exercise program without rhythmic auditory cueing (McIntosh et al., 1997). It has been suggested that perhaps rhythmic auditory stimulation provides an external rhythm that is able to compensate for the defective internal rhythm of the basal ganglia. The finding that the improvements remained even when the cues were removed suggests that rhythmic auditory stimulation may also provide a sort of rhythmic training mechanism. Picelli et al. (Picelli et al., 2010) recently performed a preliminary investigation about the three-dimensional motion analysis of the effects of auditory cueing on gait pattern in patients with PD who underwent auditory cueing respectively at 90, 100 and 110% of their mean cadence at preferred pace. The authors reported that in the presence of auditory cues, walking speed and stride length showed an increase that became more significant matching the higher cueing frequencies. Moreover, the analysis of kinetic gait parameters showed a significant variation of maximal values within the pull-off phase of the hip joint power when subjects were asked to match the rhythm of their stepping to the higher cueing frequency, suggesting that subjects improved their gait by adopting a motor strategy based on a more effective activation of hip flexors and not increasing the more destabilizing ankle extensors function.

6.8.3 Visual cueing

Placement of visual cue floor markers is an approach that can be very effective in regulating stride length. Floor markers were reported to be effective in improving the gait of patients with PD as early as 1967 (Azulay et al., 1999). In some cases, the patient is instructed to walk over each marker to achieve the desirable stride length for each step. In alternative, the patient may be given no specific instructions regarding the floor markers. Interestingly, only certain visual stimuli are apparently effective in improving gait in patients with PD. Transverse lines are effective, whereas zigzag or parallel lines are not. In addition, the lines must be separated by an appropriate width and have a colour that contrasts with the floor in order to achieve the best results. Limited evidence was found for improving speed and stride length when patients with PD were provided with floor markers to externally cue their stepping patterns (Lim et al., 2005). However, a retained positive carryover effect even after the cues were removed has been reported (Rubinstein et al., 2002). Visual cues have also been suggested to be helpful in alleviating freezing episodes (Rubinstein et al., 2002). For example, carrying an inverted walking stick, so that the handle acts as a horizontal cue at foot level, was able to decrease the number of freezing episodes in certain patients. It is not clear exactly how visual cues improve gait in PD. One possibility is that visual cues help to fill in for the motor set deficiency by providing visual data on appropriate stride length (Morris et al., 1996). When patients are told to step over each marker, they are forced to take properly sized steps, normalizing their stride length. Another theory is that visual cues help because they focus attention on gait (Morris et al., 1996). Once the patient is concentrating on walking, it is no longer an automatic task that is being processed through the defective basal ganglia.

6.8.4 Attentional cueing

To evaluate attentional cueing strategies, the effects of different verbal instructional sets on gait have been studied in PD (Rubinstein et al., 2002). Interestingly, while different instructions were able to improve gait speed, the effects were not equivalent. The greatest increase in speed was seen when patients were told to walk fast. However, the resulting gait was abnormal, with an elevated cadence and small stride length. In contrast, walking while focusing on arm swinging or large steps improved the overall velocity to a lesser degree, but resulted in an almost normal gait pattern.

6.8.5 Combined sensory cueing training

In 2007, Nieuwboer et al. (Nieuwboer et al., 2007) performed a single blind, randomized clinical trial with a crossover design (the RESCUE trial) on 153 patients with PD who underwent a 3-week cueing training program (consisting of their preferred modality among auditory, visual and somatosensory) carried out at home by one therapist and a 3-week no training period. The authors observed improvements after intervention on postural stability and gait performance also reporting a reduction in FoG (Nieuwboer et al., 2007). The findings of the RESCUE trial were extended by Rochester et al. (Rochester et al., 2010), who observed that gait training with external rhythmical cues increased single and dual-task cued walking speed and step length.

6.8.6 Physiotherapy combined with sensory cueing

A number of studies have evaluated the effects of physiotherapy combined with sensory cues. In particular, programs that utilized visual and auditory cues as triggers to facilitate initiation and speed of movement or rhythmic and auditory cues to assist in continuous movement have been compared with a control group that did not receive any exercise training. Authors found that the experimental group showed significant improvement in gait immediately after the program, whereas the control group did not (Rubinstein et al., 2002). Other studies compared the effects of a conventional physiotherapy protocol to those of the same physiotherapy protocol enhanced by sensory cueing, reporting that patients who underwent walking training with rhythmic auditory stimulation had significant improvements in gait parameters, whereas the other patients who performed conventional training did not (Rubinstein et al., 2002). Moreover, sensory-enhanced physiotherapy programs have been found not only to improve patients' skills immediately after training, but also at follow-up assessment.

7. References

Abbruzzese, G., & Berardelli, A. (2003). Sensorimotor integration in movement disorders. *Movement Disorders,* Vol. 18, No. 3, pp. 231-40, ISSN 1531-8257.

Adkin, AL., Frank JS., & Jog MS. (2003). Fear of falling and postural control in Parkinson's disease. *Movement Disorders,* Vol. 18, No. 5, pp. 496-502, ISSN 1531-8257.

Ahlborg, L., Andersson, C., & Julin, P. (2006). Whole-body vibration training compared with resistance training: effect on spasticity, muscle strength and motor performance in adults with cerebral palsy. *Journal of Rehabilitation Medicine,* Vol. 38, No. 5, pp. 302-8, ISSN 1651-2081.

Allen, NE., Canning, CG., Sherrington, C., Lord, SR., Latt, MD., Close, JC., O'Rourke, SD., Murray, SM., & Fung, VS. (2010). The effects of an exercise program on fall risk factors in people with Parkinson's disease: a randomized controlled trial. *Movement Disorders,* Vol. 25, No. 9, pp. 1217-25, ISSN 1531-8257.

Amblard, B., Crémieux, J., Marchand, AR., & Carblanc, A. (1985). Lateral orientation and stabilization of human stance: static versus dynamic visual cues. *Experimental brain research,* Vol. 61, No. 1, pp. 21-37, ISSN 1432-1106.

Ashburn, A., Stack, E., Pickering, RM., & Ward, CD. (2001). Predicting fallers in a community-based sample of people with Parkinson's disease. *Gerontology,* Vol. 47, No. 5, pp. 277-81, ISSN 1423-0003.

Ashburn, A., Fazakarley, L., Ballinger, C., Pickering, R., McLellan, LD., & Fitton, C. (2007). A randomised controlled trial of a home based exercise programme to reduce the risk of falling among people with Parkinson's disease. *Journal of Neurology, Neurosurgery & Psychiatry,* Vol. 78, No. 7, pp. 678-84, ISSN 1468-330X.

Azher, SN., & Jankovic, J. (2005). Camptocormia: pathogenesis, classification, and response to therapy. *Neurology,* Vol. 65, No. 3, pp. 355-9, ISSN 1526-632X.

Azulay, J., Mesure, S., Amblanrd, B., Blin, O., Sangla, I., & Pouget, J. (1999). Visual control of locomotion in Parkinson's disease. *Brain,* Vol. 122, No. 1, pp. 111-120,

Balash, Y., Peretz, C., Leibovich, G., Herman, T., Hausdorff, JM., & Giladi, N. (2005). Falls in outpatients with Parkinson's disease: frequency, impact and identifying factors. *Journal of Neurology,* Vol. 252, No. 11, pp. 1310-5, ISSN 1432-1459.

Baldissera, F., Cavallari, P., & Leocani, L. (1998). Cyclic modulation of the H-reflex in a wrist flexor during rhythmic flexion–extension movements of the ipsilateral foot. *Experimental Brain Research,* Vol. 118, No. 3, pp. 427-430, ISSN 1432-1106.

Baltadjieva, R., Giladi, N., Gruendlinger, L., Peretz, C., & Hausdorff, JM. (2006). Marked alterations in the gait timing and rhythmicity of patients with de novo Parkinson's disease. *The European Journal of Neuroscience,* Vol. 24, No. 6, pp. 1815-20, ISSN 1460-9568.

Beckley, DJ., Bloem, BR., & Remler, MP. (1993). Impaired scaling of long latency postural reflexes in patients with Parkinson's disease. *Electroencephalography and Clinical Neurophysiology,* Vol. 89, No. 1, pp. 22-28, ISSN 0013-4694.

Benatru, I., Vaugoyeau, M., & Azulay, JP. (2008). Postural disorders in Parkinson's disease. *Clinical Neurophysiology,* Vol. 38, No. 6, pp. 459-65, ISSN 1769-7131.

Bloem, BR., Beckley, DJ., van Dijk, JG., Zwinderman, AH., Remler, MP., Langston, JW., & Roos, RA. (1994). Medium latency stretch reflexes in young-onset Parkinson's disease and MPTP-induced parkinsonism. *Journal of the Neurological Sciences,* Vol. 123, No. 1-2, pp. 52-8, ISSN 1878-5883.

Bloem, BR., Beckley, DJ., van Dijk, JG., Zwinderman, AH., Remler, MP., & Roos, RA. (1996). Influence of dopaminergic medication on automatic postural responses and balance impairment in Parkinson's disease. *Movement Disorders,* Vol. 11, No. 5, pp. 509-521, ISSN 1531-8257.

Bloem, BR., Allum, JHJ., Carpenter, MG., & Honegger, F. (2000a). Is lower leg proprioception essential for triggering human automatic postural responses? *Experimental Brain Research,* Vol. 130, No. 3, pp. 375–391, ISSN 1435-1106.

Bloem, BR., Lammers, GJ., Overeem, S., Grimbergen, YA., & Tetrud, J. (2000b). Outcome assessment of retropulsion tests in Parkinson's disease. *Movement Disorders,* Vol. 15, No. 3, pp. S179, ISSN 1531-8257.

Bloem, BR., Grimbergen, YA., Cramer, M., Willemsen, M., & Zwinderman, AH. (2001). Prospective assessment of falls in Parkinson's disease. *Journal of Neurology,* Vol. 248, No. 11, pp. 950-8, ISSN 1432-1459.

Bloem, BR., Allum, JHJ., Carpenter, MG., Verschuuren, JJGM., & Honegger, F. (2002). Triggering of balance corrections and compensatory strategies in a patient with total leg proprioceptive loss. *Experimental brain research,* Vol. 142, No. 1, pp. 91–107.

Bloem, BR., & Bhatia, KP. (2004). Gait and balance in basal ganglia disorders, In: *Clinical disorders of balance, posture and gait,* Bronstein, AM., Brandt, T., Nutt, JG., Woollacott, MH., (2 ed.), pp. 173–206, Arnold, ISBN 0340806575, London.

Bloem, BR., Grimbergen, YA., van Dijk, JG., & Munneke, M.. (2006). The "posture second" strategy: a review of wrong priorities in Parkinson's disease. *Journal of Neurological Sciences,* Vol. 248, No. 1-2, pp. 196-204, ISSN 1878-5883.

Boonstra, TA., van der Kooij, H., Munneke, M., & Bloem, BR. (2008). Gait disorders and balance disturbances in Parkinson's disease: clinical update and pathophysiology. *Current Opinion in Neurology,* Vol. 21, No. 4, pp. 461-71, ISSN 1473-6551.

Bouisset, S., & Zattara, M. (1987). Biomechanical study of the programming of anticipatory postural adjustments associated with voluntary movement. *Journal of Biomechanics,* Vol. 20, No. 8, pp. 735-42. ISSN 1873-2380.

Brichetto, G., Pelosin, E., Marchese, R. & Abbruzzese, G. (2006). Evaluation of physical therapy in parkinsonian patients with freezing of gait: a pilot study. *Clinical Rehabilitation,* Vol. 20, No. 1, pp. 31-5, ISSN 1477-0873 .

Bronstein, AM., Hood, JD., Gresty, MA., & Panagi, C. (1990). Visual control of balance in cerebellar and Parkinsonian syndromes. *Brain,* Vol. 113, Pt. 3, pp. 767-779, ISSN 1460-2156.

Bronte-Stewart, HM., Minn, AY., Rodrigue, K., Buckley, EL., & Nashner, LM. (2002). Postural instability in idiopathic Parkinson's disease: the role of medication and unilateral pallidotomy. *Brain,* Vol. 125, Pt. 9, pp. 2100-2114, ISSN 1460-2156.

Brusse, KJ., Zimdars, S., Zalewski, KR., & Steffen, TM. (2005). Testing functional performance in people with Parkinson disease. *Physical Therapy,* Vol. 85, No. 2, pp. 134-41, ISSN 1538-6724.

Bruyere, O., Wuidart, MA., Di Palma, E., Gourlay, M., Ethgen, O., Richy, F., & Reginster, JY. (2005). Controlled whole body vibration to decrease fall risk and improve health-related quality of life of nursing home residents. *Archives of Physical Medicine and Rehabilitation,* Vol. 86, No. 2, pp. 303-7, ISSN 1532-821X.

Caap-Ahlgren, M., & Dehlin, O. (2001). Insomnia and depressive symptoms in patients with Parkinson's disease. Relationship to health-related quality of life. An interview study of patients living at home. *Archives of Gerontology and Geriatrics,* Vol. 32, No. 1, pp. 23-33, ISSN 1872-6976.

Cacciatore, TW., Gurfinkel, VS., Horak, FB., Cordo, PJ., & Ames, KE. (2010). Increased dynamic regulation of postural tone through Alexander Technique training. *Human movement science,* Vol. 30, No. 1, pp. 74-89, ISSN1872-7646.

Cakit, BD., Saracoglu, M., Genc, H., Erdem, HR., & Inan, L. (2007). The effects of incremental speed-dependent treadmill training on postural instability and fear of falling in Parkinson's disease. *Clinical Rehabilitation,* Vol. 21, No. 8, pp. 698-705, ISSN 1477-0873.

Canning, CG., Sherrington, C., Lord, SR., Fung, VS., Close, JC., Latt, MD., Howard, K., Allen, NE., O'Rourke, SD., & Murray, SM. (2009). Exercise therapy for prevention of falls in people with Parkinson's disease: a protocol for a randomised controlled trial and economic evaluation. *BMC Neurology,* Vol. 22, No. 9, p. 4, ISSN 1471-2377.

Carpenter, MG., Allum, JH., Honegger, F., Adkin, AL., & Bloem, BR. (2004). Postural abnormalities to multidirectional stance perturbations in Parkinson's disease. *J. Neurol. Neurosurg. Psychiatry,* Vol. 75, pp. 1245–1254.

Carpenter, MG., & Bloem, BR. (2011). Postural control in Parkinson patients: a proprioceptive problem? *Experimental Neurology,* Vol. 227, No. 1, pp. 26-30, ISSN 1090-2430.

Cazalets, JR., & Bertrand, S. (2000). Coupling between lumbar and sacral motor networks in the neonatal rat spinal cord. *The European Journal of Neuroscience,* Vol. 12, No. 8, pp. 2993-3002, ISSN 1460-9568.

Chapuis, S., Ouchchane, L., Metz, O., Gerbaud, L., & Durif, F. (2005) Impact of the motor complications of Parkinson's disease on the quality of life. *Movement Disorders,* Vol. 20, No. 2, pp. 224-30, ISSN 1531-8257.

Chaudhry, H., Bukiet, B., Ji, Z., & Findley, T. (2011). Measurement of balance in computer posturography: Comparison of methods--A brief review. *The Journal of Bodywork and Movement Therapies*, Vol. 15, No. 1, pp. 82-91, ISSN 1532-9283.

Clark, RD., Lord, SR., & Webster, IW. (1993). Clinical parameters associated with falls in an elderly population. *Gerontology*, Vol. 39, No. 2, pp. 117-23, ISSN 1423-0003.

Cohen, H., Heaton, LG., Congdon, SL., & Jenkins, HA. (1996). Changes in sensory organization test scores with age. *Age and Ageing*, Vol. 25, No. 1, pp. 39-44, ISSN 1468-2834.

Commissaris, DA., Toussaint, HM., & Hirschfeld, H. (2001). Anticipatory postural adjustments in a bimanual, whole-body lifting task seem not only aimed at minimising anterior-posterior centre of mass displacements. *Gait Posture*, Vol. 14, No. 1, pp. 44-55, ISSN 1879-2219.

Cools, AR., Berger, HJC., Buytenhuis, EL., Horstink, MWIM., & Van Spaendonck, KPM. (1993). Manifestations of switching disorders in animal and man with dopamine deficits in A10 and/or A9 circuitries, *Proceedings of the European Congress on Mental Dysfunction in Parkinson's Disease*, pp. 49-67, ISBN 3-905-277-19-0, Amsterdam, The Netherlands, October 20-23.

Coughlin, L., & Templeton, J. (1980). Hip fractures in patients with Parkinson's disease. *Clinical Orthopaedics and Related Research*, Vol. 148, pp. 192-5, ISSN 1528-1132.

Crenna, P., Carpinella, I., Rabuffetti, M., Calabrese, E., Mazzoleni, P., Nemni, R., & Ferrarin, M. (2007). The association between impaired turning and normal straight in Parkinson's disease. *Gait & Posture*, Vol. 26, No. 2, pp. 172-8, ISSN 1879-2219.

Cunnington, R., Iansek, R., Bradshaw, J., & Phillips, J. (1995). Movement-related potentials in Parkinson's disease: presence and predictability of temporal and spatial cues. *Brain*, Vol. 118, No. 4, pp. 935-950, ISSN 1460-2156.

Davis, RB. (1997). Reflections on clinical gait analysis. *Journal of Electromyography and Kinesiology*, Vol. 7, No. 4, pp. 251-257, ISSN 1873-5711.

de Noordhout, AM., Rapisarda, G., Bogacz, D., Gèrard, P., De Pasqua, V., Pennisi, G., & Delwaide, PJ. (1999). Corticomotoneuronal synaptic connections in normal man: an electrophysiological study. *Brain*, Vol. 122, No. 7, pp. 1327-40, ISSN 1460-2156.

Deane, KHO., Jones, D., Ellis-Hill, C., Clarke, CE., Playford, ED., & Ben-Shlomo, Y. (2001a). Physiotherapy for Parkinson's disease: a comparison of techniques. In: *The Cochrane Library*, No. 4, Available from: Update Software, Oxford, ISSN 1469-493X.

Deane, KHO, Jones D, Playford, ED., Ben-Shlomo, Y., & Clarke, CE. (2001b). Physiotherapy versus placebo or no intervention in Parkinson's disease. In: *The Cochrane Library*, No. 4, 2001. Available from: Update Software, Oxford, ISSN 1469-493X.

Debaere, P., Swinnen, SP., Béatse, E., Sunaert, S., Van Hecke, P., & Duysens, J. (2001). Brain areas involved in interlimb coordination: a distributed network. *Neuroimage*, Vol. 14, No. 5, pp. 947-958, ISSN 1095-9572.

Di Fabio, RP., & Badke, MB. (1990). Relationship of sensory organization to balance function in patients with hemiplegia. *Physical Therapy*, Vol. 70, No. 9, pp. 542-8, ISSN 1538-6724.

Diamond, A., & Jankovic, J. (2005). The effect of deep brain stimulation on quality of life in movement disorders. *Journal of Neurology, Neurosurgery and Psychiatry*, Vol. 76, No. 9, pp. 1188-93, ISSN 1468-330X.

Dietz, V. (1993). Reflex behaviour and programming in Parkinson's disease. *Advances in Neurology*, Vol. 60, pp. 375-80, ISSN 0091-3952.

Dietz, V. (2002). Do human bipeds use quadrupedal coordination? *Trends in Neurosciences*, Vol. 25, No. 9, pp. 462-467, ISSN 1878-108X.

Dietz, V., & Michel, J. (2008). Locomotion in Parkinson's disease: neuronal coupling of upper and lower limbs. *Brain*, Vol. 131, No. 12, pp. 3421-3431, ISSN 1460-2156.

Dietz, V., & Michel, J. (2009). Human bipeds use quadrupedal coordination during locomotion. *Annals of the New York Academy of Sciences*, Vol. 1164, No. 1, pp. 97-103, ISSN 1749-6632.

Duncan, PW., Weiner, DK., Chandler, J., & Studenski, S. (1990). Functional reach: a new clinical measure of balance. *Journal of Gerontology*, Vol. 45, No. 6, pp. M192-7, ISSN 0022-1422.

Ebersbach, G,. Edler, D., Kaufhold, O., & Wissel, J. (2008). Whole body vibration versus conventional physiotherapy to improve balance and gait in Parkinson's disease. *Archives of Physical Medicine and Rehabilitation*, Vol. 89, No. 3, pp. 399-403, ISSN 1532-821X.

Faherty, CJ., Raviie Shepherd, K., Herasimtschuk, A., & Smeyne, RJ. (2005). Environmental enrichment in adulthood eliminates neuronal death in experimental Parkinsonism. *Brain research. Molecular brain research*, Vol. 134, No. 1, pp. 170-9, ISSN 0169-328X.

Falvo, MJ., & Earhart, GM. (2009). Six-minute walk distance in persons with Parkinson disease: a hierarchical regression model. *Archives of Physical Medicine Rehabilitation*, Vol. 90, No. 6, pp. 1004-8, ISSN 1532-821X.

Foster, M. (1892). *A text book of physiology. The central nervous system*, Vol. III (6th ed.), Macmillan, London.

Fox, CM., Ramig, LO., Ciucci, MR., Sapir, S., McFarland, DH., & Farley, BG. (2006). The science and practice of LSVT/LOUD: neural plasticity-principled approach to treating individuals with Parkinson disease and other neurological disorders. *Seminars in Speech and Language*, Vol. 27. No. 4, pp. 283-99, ISSN 1098-9056.

Fung, J., Henry SM., & Horak FB. (1995). Is the force constraint strategy used by humans to maintain stance and equilibrium? *Proceedings of the Neuroscience Meeting Planner of Society for Neuroscience, Society for Neuroscience Abstract*, No. 21, p. 683, San Diego, California, November 11-16.

Gambarin, M., Antonini, A., Moretto, G., Bovi, P., Romito, S., Fiaschi, A., & Tinazzi, M. (2006). Pisa syndrome without neuroleptic exposure in a patient with Parkinson's disease: case report. *Movement Disorders*, Vol. 21, No. 2., pp. 270-3, ISSN 1531-8257.

Gauthier, L., Dalziel, S., & Gauthier, S. (1987). The benefits of group occupational therapy for patients with Parkinson's disease. *The American Journal of Occupational Therapy: official publication of the American Occupational Therapy Association*, Vol. 41, pp. 360–365, ISSN 0272-9490.

Georgiou, N., Iansek, R., Bradshaw, J., Phiullips, J., Mattingley, J., & Bradshaw, J. (1993). An evaluation of the role of internal cues in the pathogenesis of parkinsonian hyperkinesias. *Brain*, Vol. 116, No. 6, pp. 1575-1587, ISSN 1460-2156.

Giladi, N., McMahon, D., Przedborski, S., Flaster, E., Guillory, S., Kostic, V., & Fahn S. (1992). Motor blocks in Parkinson's disease. *Neurology*, Vol. 42, No. 2, pp. 333-9, ISSN 1526-632X.

Giladi, N., Shabtai, H., Simon, ES., Biran, S., Tal, J., & Korczyn, AD. (2000). Construction of freezing of gait questionnaire for patients with Parkinsonism. *Parkinsonism and Related Disorders*, Vol. 6, No. 3, pp. 165-170, ISSN 1873-5126.

Goldie, PA., Matyas, TA., Spencer, KI., & McGinley, RB. (1990). Postural control in standing following stroke: test-retest reliability of some quantitative clinical tests. *Physical Therapy*, Vol. 70, No. 4, pp. 234-43, ISSN 1538-6724.

Goodwin, VA., Richards, SH., Taylor, RS., Taylor, AH., & Campbell, JL. (2008). The effectiveness of exercise interventions for people with Parkinson's disease: a systematic review and meta-analysis. *Movement Disorders*, Vol. 23, No. 5, pp. 631-40. ISSN 1531-8257.

Grasso, R., Prevost, P., Ivanenko, YP., & Berthoz, A. (1998). Eye–head coordination for the steering of locomotion in humans: an anticipatory synergy. *Neuroscience Letters*, Vol. 253, No. 2, pp. 115–8, ISSN 1872-7972.

Greenspan, SL., Myers, ER., Kiel, DP., Parker, RA., Hayes, WC., & Resnick, NM. (1998). Fall direction, bone mineral density, and function: risk factors for hip fracture in frail nursing home elderly. *American Journal Medicine*, Vol. 104, No. 6, pp. 539-45, ISSN 1555-7162.

Grillner, S. (1981). Control of locomotion in bipeds, tetrapods, and fish. In: *Handbook of Physiology. The Nervous System. Motor Control*, JM. Brookhart, VB. Mountcastle, (Eds.), pp. 1179–1236, American Physiology Society, ISBN 978-068-3011-05-0, Washington DC, USA.

Grimbergen, YA., Munneke, M., & Bloem, BR. (2004). Falls in Parkinson's disease. *Current Opinion in Neurology*, Vol. 17, No. 4, pp. 405-15, ISSN 1473-6551.

Haas, CT., Turbanski, S., Kessler, K., & Schmidtbleicher, D. (2006). The effects of random whole-body-vibration on motor symptoms in Parkinson's disease. *NeuroRehabilitation*, Vol. 21, No. 1, pp. 29-36, ISSN 1878-6448.

Hanke, TA., & Tiberio, D. (2006). Lateral rhythmic unipedal stepping in younger, middle-aged, and older adults. *Journal of Geriatric Physical Therapy*, Vol. 29, No. 1, pp. 22-7, ISSN 1539-8412.

Hase, K., & Stein, RB. (1999). Turning strategies during human walking. *Journal of Neurophysiology*, Vol. 81, No. 6, pp. 2914–22, ISSN 1522-1598.

Hausdorff, JM., Schaafsma, JD., Balash, Y., Bartels, AL., Gurevich, T., & Giladi, N. (2003). Impaired regulation of stride variability in Parkinson's disease subjects with freezing of gait. *Experimental Brain Research*, Vol. 149, No. 2, pp. 187-94, ISSN 1432-1106.

Hausdorff, JM. (2009). Gait dynamics in Parkinson's disease: common and distinct behaviour among stride length, gait variability, and fractal-like scaling. *Chaos*, Vol. 19, No. 2, pp. 026113, ISSN 1089-7682.

Hely, MA., Morris, JG., Traficante, R., Reid, WG., O'Sullivan, DJ., & Williamson, PM. (1999). The sydney multicentre study of Parkinson's disease: progression and mortality at 10 years. *Journal of Neurology, Neurosurgery & Psychiatry*, Vol. 67, No. 3, pp. 300-7, ISSN 1468-330X.

Hely, MA., Reid, WG., Adena, MA., Halliday, GM., & Morris, JG. (2008). The Sydney multicenter study of Parkinson's disease: the inevitability of dementia at 20 years. *Movement Disorders*, Vol. 23, No. 6, pp. 837-44, ISSN 1531-8257.

Herlofson, K., & Larsen, JP. (2003). The influence of fatigue on health-related quality of life in patients with Parkinson's disease. *Acta Neurologica Scandinavica*, Vol. 107, No. 1, pp. 1-6, ISSN 1600-0404.

Hess, JA., Woollacott, M., & Shivitz, N. (2006). Ankle force and rate of force production increase following high intensity strength training infrail older adults. *Aging Clinical and Experimental Research*, Vol. 18, No. 2, pp. 107-15, ISSN 1594-0667.

Hill, K., Bernhardt, J., McGann, A., Maltese, D., & Berkovits, D. (1996). A new test of dynamic standing balance for stroke patients: Reliability, validity and comparison with healthy elderly. *Physiotherapy Canada*, Vol. 48, No. 4, pp. 257-262.

Hirsch, MA., Toole, T., Maitland, CG., & Rider, RA. (2003). The effects of balance training and high-intensity resistance training on persons with idiopathic Parkinson's disease. *Archives of Physical Medicine and Rehabilitation*, Vol. 84, No. 8, pp. 1109-17, ISSN 1532-821X.

Hollands, MA., Patla, AE., & Vickers, JN. (2002).''Look where you're going!'': gaze behaviour associated with maintaining and changing the direction of locomotion. *Experimental Brain & Research*, Vol. 143, No. 2, pp. 221–30, ISSN 1432-1106.

Horak, FB., & Nashner, LM. (1986). Central programming of postural movements: adaptation to altered support-surface configurations. *Journal of Neurophysiology*, Vol. 55, No. 6, pp. 1369-81, ISSN 1522-1598.

Horak, FB., Nutt, JG., & Nashner LM. (1992). Postural inflexibility in parkinsonian subjects. *Journal of Neurological Sciences*, Vol. 111, No. 1, pp. 46-58, ISSN 1878-5883.

Horak, FB., Frank, J., & Nutt, J. (1996). Effects of dopamine on postural control in parkinsonian subjects: scaling, set, and tone. *Journal of Neurophysiology*, Vol. 75, No. 6, pp. 2380-96, ISSN 1522-1598.

Horak, FB., Dimitrova, D., & Nutt, JG. (2005). Direction-specific postural instability in subjects with Parkinson's disease. *Experimental Neurology*, Vol. 193, No. 2, pp. 504-21, ISSN 1090-2430.

Horstink, MWIM., De Swart, BJM., Wolters, EC., & Berger, HJC. (1993). Paradoxical behaviour in Parkinson's disease, *Proceedings of the European Congress on Mental Dysfunction in Parkinson's Disease*, pp. 81-93, ISBN 3-905-277-19-0, Amsterdam, The Netherlands, October 20-23.

Huxham, F., Baker, R., Morris, ME., & Iansek, R. (2008). Head and trunk rotation during walking turns in Parkinson's disease. *Movement Disorders*, Vol. 23, No. 10, pp. 1391-7, ISSN 1531-8257.

Idjadi, JA., Aharonoff, GB., Su, H., Richmond, J., Egol, KA., Zuckerman, JD., & Koval, KJ. (2005). Hip fracture outcomes in patients with Parkinson's disease. *American Journal of Orthopaedic (Belle Mead NJ)*, Vol. 34, No. 7, pp. 341-6, ISSN 1934-3418.

Imai, T., Moore, ST., Raphan, T., & Cohen, B. (2001). Interaction of the body, head, and eyes during walking and turning. *Experimental Brain & Research,* Vol. 136, No. 1, pp. 1–18, ISSN 1432-1106.

Jacobs, JV., & Horak, FB. (2006). Abnormal proprioceptive-motor integration contributes to hypometric postural responses of subjects with Parkinson's disease. *Neuroscience,* Vol. 141, No. 2, pp. 999-1009, ISSN 1873-7544.

Jacobs, JV., & Horak, FB. (2007). Cortical control of postural responses. *Journal of Neural Transmission,* Vol. 114, No. 10, pp. 1339–1348, ISSN 1435-1463.

Jankovic, J. (2008). Parkinson's disease: clinical features and diagnosis. *Journal of Neurology, Neurosurgery & Psychiatry,* Vol. 79, No. 4, pp. 368-76, ISSN 1468-330X.

Jöbges, M., Heuschkel, G., Pretzel, C., Illhardt, C., Renner, C., & Hummelsheim, H. (2004). Repetitive training of compensatory steps: a therapeutic approach for postural instability in Parkinson's disease. *Journal of Neurology, Neurosurgery & Psychiatry,* Vol. 75, No. 12, pp. 1682-7, ISSN 1468-330X.

Kegelmeyer, DA., Kloos, AD., Thomas, KM., & Kostyk, SK. (2007). Reliability and validity of the Tinetti Mobility Test for individuals with Parkinson disease. *Physical Therapy,* Vol. 87, No. 10, pp. 1369-78, ISSN 1538-6724.

Kerr, GK., Worringham, CJ., Cole, MH., Lacherez, PF., Wood, JM., & Silburn, PA. (2010). Predictors of future falls in Parkinson disease. *Neurology,* Vol. 75, No. 2, pp. 116-24, ISSN 1526-632X.

Keus, SH., Bloem, BR., van Hilten, JJ., Ashburn, A., & Munneke, M. (2007). Effectiveness of physiotherapy in Parkinson's disease: the feasibility of a randomised controlled trial. *Parkinsonism and Related Disorders,* Vol. 13, No. 2, pp. 115-21, ISSN 1873-5126.

Khudados, E., Cody, FW., & O'Boyle, DJ. (1999). Proprioceptive regulation of voluntary ankle movements, demonstrated using muscle vibration, is impaired by Parkinson's disease. *Journal of Neurology, Neurosurgery & Psychiatry,* Vol. 67, No. 4, pp. 504-10, ISSN 1468-330X.

King, LA., & Horak, FB. (2008). Lateral stepping for postural correction in Parkinson's disease. *Archives of Physical Medicine and Rehabilitation,* Vol. 89, No. 3, pp. 492-9, ISSN 1532-821X.

King, LA., St George, RJ., Carlson-Kuhta, P., Nutt, JG., & Horak, FB. (2010). Preparation for compensatory forward stepping in Parkinson's disease. *Archives of Physical Medicine and Rehabilitation,* Vol. 91, No. 9, pp. 1332-8, ISSN 1532-821X.

Kitamura, J., Nakagawa, H., Iinuma, K., Kobayashi, M., Okauchi, A., Oonaka, K., & Kondo, T. (1993). Visual influence on center of contact pressure in advanced Parkinson's disease. *Archives of Physical Medicine and Rehabilitation,* Vol. 74, No. 10, pp. 1107–1112, ISSN 1532-821X.

Koller, W., & Kase, S. (1986). Muscle strength testing in Parkinson's disease. *European Neurology,* Vol. 25, No. 2, pp. 130-3, ISSN 1421-9913.

Konczak, J., Corcos, DM., Horak, F., Poizner, H., Shapiro, M., Tuite, P., Volkmann, J., & Maschke, M. (2009). Proprioception and motor control in Parkinson's disease. *Journal of Motor Behaviour,* Vol. 41, No. 6, pp. 543-52, ISSN 0022-2895.

Kuo, AD. (2005). An optimal state estimation model of sensory integration in human postural balance. *Journal of Neural Engineering,* Vol. 2, No. 3, pp. S235-49, ISSN 1741-2552.

Latt, MD., Lord, SR., Morris, JG., & Fung, VS. (2009). Clinical and for elucidating falls risk in Parkinson's disease. *Movement Disorders,* Vol. 24, No. 9, pp. 1280-9, ISSN 1531-8257.

Lee, RG., Tonolli, I., Viallet, F., Aurenty, R., & Massion, J. (1995). Preparatory postural adjustments in Parkinsonian patients with postural instability. *Canadian Journal of Neurological Sciences,* Vol. 22, No. 2, pp. 126-135, ISSN 0317-1671.

Leonard, JA., Brown, RH., & Stapley, PJ. (2009). Reaching to multiple targets when standing: the spatial organization of feedforward postural adjustments. *Journal of neurophysiology,* Vol. 101, No. 4. pp. 2120-33, ISSN 1522-1598.

Lim, I., van Wegen, E., de Goede, C., Deutekom, M., Nieuwboer, A., Willems, A., Jones, D., Rochester, L., & Kwakkel, G. (2005). Effects of external rhythmical cueing on gait in patients with Parkinson's disease: a systematic review. *Clinical Rehabilitation,* Vol. 19, No. 7, pp. 695-713, ISSN 1477-0873.

Maier, MA., Illert, M., Kirkwood, PA., Nielsen, J., & Lemon, RN. (1998). Does a C3-C4 propriospinal system transmit corticospinal excitation in the primate? An investigation in the macaque monkey. *J Physiol,* Vol. 511, No. 1, pp. 191-212.

Marchese, R., Bove, M., & Abbruzzese, G. (2003). Effect of cognitive and motor tasks on postural stability in Parkinson's disease: a posturographic study. *Movement Disorders,* Vol. 18, No. 6, pp. 652-8, ISSN 1531-8257.

Marshall, J.F., & Ungerstedt, U. (1997). Striatal efferent fibers play a role in maintaining rotational behavior in the rat. *Science,* Vol. 198, No. 4312, pp. 62-4, ISSN 0193-4511.

Martin, JP. (1967). *The basal ganglia and posture.* Pitman Publishing, *ISBN* 914-154-5429-0, London, UK.

Martínez-Martín, P. (1998). An introduction to the concept of "quality of life in Parkinson's disease". *Journal of Neurology,* Vol. 245, No. 1, pp. S2-6, ISSN 1432-1459.

Masani, K., Sin, VW., Vette, AH., Thrasher, AT., Kawashima, N., Morris, A., et al. (2009). Postural reactions of the trunk muscles to multi-directional perturbations in sitting. *Clinical Biomechanics,* Vol. 24, No. 2, pp. 176–182, ISSN 1879-1271.

Maschke, M., Tuite, PJ., Pickett, K., Wachter, T., & Konczak, J. (2005). The effect of subthalamic nucleus stimulation on kinaesthesia in Parkinson's disease. *Journal of Neurology, Neurosurgery & Psychiatry,* Vol. 76, No. 4, pp. 569-71, ISSN 1468-330X.

McIntosh, GC., Brown, SH., Rice, RR., & Thaut, MH. (1997). Rhythmic auditory-motor facilitation of gait patterns in patients with Parkinson's disease. *Journal of Neurology, Neurosurgery, and Psychiatry,* Vol. 62, No. 1, pp. 22-26, ISSN 1468-330X.

Melton, LJ. 3rd, Leibson, CL., Achenbach, SJ., Bower, JH., Maraganore, DM., Oberg, AL., & Rocca, WA. (2006). Fracture risk after the diagnosis of Parkinson's disease: Influence of concomitant dementia. *Movement Disorders,* Vol. 21, No. 9, pp. 1361-7, ISSN 1531-8257.

Moore, G., Robertson, D., Kuasar, SA., & Taylar, G. (2000). Postural awareness and falls in Parkinson's disease. *Proceedings of the conference "Multidisciplinary care in Parkinson's disease and parkinsonism, from science to practice",* London, 20 July 2000, p. 14.

Moore, O., Peretz, C., & Giladi, N. (2007). Freezing of gait affects quality of life of peoples with Parkinson's disease beyond its relationships with mobility and gait. *Movement disorders,* Vol. 22, No. 15, pp. 2192-5, ISSN 1531-8257.

Morris, ME., Iansek, R., Matyas, TA., & Summers, JJ. (1994). Ability to modulate walking cadence remains intact in Parkinson's disease. *Journal of Neurology, Neurosurgery, and Psychiatry*, Vol. 57, No. 12, pp. 1532-1534, ISSN 1468-330X.

Morris, ME., Iansek, R., Matyas, TA., & Summers, JJ. (1996). Stride length regulation in Parkinson's disease. Normalization strategies and underlying mechanisms. *Brain,* Vol. 119, No. 2, pp. 551-568, ISSN 1460-2156.

Morris, ME. (2000). Movement disorders in people with Parkinson disease: a model for physical therapy. *Physical Therapy*, Vol. 80, No. 6, pp. 578-597, ISSN 1538-6724.

Morris, S., Morris, ME., & Iansek, R. (2001). Reliability of measurements obtained with the Timed "Up & Go" test in people with Parkinson disease. *Physical Therapy*, Vol. 81, No. 2, pp. 810-8, ISSN 1538-6724.

Morris, ME. (2006). Locomotor training in people with Parkinson disease. *Physical Therapy,* Vol. 86, No. 10, pp. 1426-1435, ISSN 1538-6724.

Morris, ME., Iansek, R., & Galna, B. (2008). Gait festination and freezing in Parkinson's disease: pathogenesis and rehabilitation. *Movement Disorders,* Vol. 23, No. 2, pp. S451-460, ISSN 1531-8257.

Nakajima, K., Maier, MA., Kirkwood, PA., & Lemon, RN. (2000). Striking differences in transmission of corticospinal excitation to upper limb motoneurones in two primate species. *Journal of Neurophysiology*, Vol. 84, No. 2, pp. 698-709, ISSN 1522-1598.

Nardone, A., & Schieppati, M. (2010) The role of instrumental assessment of balance in clinical decision making. *European Journal of Physical Rehabilitation and Medicine,* Vol. 46, No. 2, pp. 221-37, ISSN 1973-9095.

Nashner, LM. (1977). Fixed patterns of rapid postural responses among leg muscles during stance. *Experimental Brain Research*, Vol. 24, No. 301, pp. 13-24, ISSN 1432-1106.

Nelson, AJ., Zwick, D., Brody, S., Doran, C., Pulver, L., Rooz, G., Sadownick, M., Nelson, R., & Rothman, J. (2002). The validity of the GaitRite and the Functional Ambulation Performance scoring system in the analysis of Parkinson gait. *NeuroRehabilitation,* Vol. 17, No. 3, pp. 255-62, ISSN 1878-6448.

Nicolas, G., Marchand-Pauvert, V., Burke, D., & Pierrot-Deseilligny, E. (2001). Corticospinal excitation of presumed cervical propriospinal neurones and its reversal to inhibition in humans. *Journal de Physiologie,* Vol. 533, No. 3, pp. 903-919, ISSN 0021-7948.

Nieuwboer, A., Kwakkel, G., Rochester, L., Jones, D., van Wegen, E., Willems, AM., Chavret, F., Hetherington, V., Baker, K., & Lim, I. (2007). Cueing training in the home improves gait-related mobility in Parkinson's disease: the RESCUE trial. *Journal of Neurology, Neurosurgery, and Psychiatry*, Vol. 78, No. 2, pp. 134-137, ISSN 1468-330X.

Obeso, JA. Marin, C., Rodriguez-Oroz, C., Blesa, J., Benitez-Temiño, B., Mena-Segovia, J., Rodríguez, M., & Olanow, CW. (2008). The basal ganglia in Parkinson's disease: current concepts and unexplained observations. *Annals of Neurology*, Vol. 64, No. 2, pp. S30-46, ISSN 1531-8249.

Orendurff, MS., Segal, AD., Berge, JS., Flick, KC., Spanier, D., & Klute, GK. (2006). The kinematics and kinetics of turning: limb asymmetries associated with walking a circular path. *Gait & Posture,* Vol. 23, No. 1, pp. 106-11, ISSN 1879-2219.

Orr, R. (2010). Contribution of muscle weakness to postural instability in the elderly. A systematic review. *European Journal of Physical Rehabilitation and Medicine,* Vol. 46, No. 2, pp. 183-220, ISSN 1973-9095.

Pastor, MA., Day, BL., & Marsden, CD. (1993). Vestibular induced postural responses in Parkinson's disease. *Brain,* Vol. 116, No. 5, pp. 1177-90, ISSN 1460-2156.

Patla, AE., Prentice, SD., Robinson, C., & Neufeld, J. (1991). Visual control of locomotion: strategies for changing direction and for going over obstacles. *Journal of Experimental Psychology: Human Perception and Performance,* Vol. 17, No. 3, pp. 603–34, ISSN 1939-1277.

Peto, V., Jenkinson, C., Fitzpatrick, R., & Greenhall, R. (1995). The development and validation of a short measure of functioning and well being for individuals with Parkinson's disease. *Quality of life research : an international journal of quality of life aspects of treatment, care and rehabilitation,* Vol. 4, No. 3, pp. 41-8, ISSN 1573-2649.

Picelli, A., Camin, M., Tinazzi, M., Vangelista, A., Cosentino, A., Fiaschi, A., & Smania, N. (2010). Three-dimensional motion analysis of the effects of auditory cueing on gait pattern in patients with Parkinson's disease: a preliminary investigation. *Neurological Sciences*, Vol. 31, No. 4, pp. 423-430, ISSN 1590-3478.

Pickering, RM., Grimbergen, YA., Rigney, U., Ashburn, A., Mazibrada, G., Wood, B., Gray, P., Kerr, G., & Bloem, BR. (2007). A meta-analysis of six prospective studies of falling in Parkinson's disease. *Movement Disorders*, Vol. 22, No. 13, pp. 1892-900, ISSN 1531-8257.

Plotnik, M., Giladi, N., & Hausdorff, JM. (2007). A new measure for quantifying the bilateral Coordination of human gait: effects of aging and Parkinson's disease. *Experimental Brain Research,* Vol. 181, No. 4, pp. 561–570, ISSN 1432-1106.

Proctor, F., Riklan, M., Cooper, IS., & Teuber, HL. (1964). Judgment of visual and postural vertical by parkinsonian patients. *Neurology*, Vol. 14, pp. 287–293, ISSN 1526-632X.

Protas, EJ., Mitchell, K., Williams, A., Qureshy, H., Caroline, K., & Lai, EC. (2005). Gait and step training to reduce falls in Parkinson's disease. *NeuroRehabilitation*, Vol. 20, No. 3, pp. 183-90, ISSN 1878-6448.

Qutubuddin, AA., Pegg, PO., Cifu, DX., Brown, R., McNamee, S., & Carne, W. (2005). Validating the Berg Balance Scale for patients with Parkinson's disease: a key to rehabilitation evaluation. *Archives of Physical Medicine and Rehabilitation,* Vol. 86, No. 4, pp. 789-92, ISSN 1532-821X.

Qutubuddin, AA., Cifu, DX., Armistead-Jehle, P., Carne, W., McGuirk, TE., & Baron, MS. (2007). A comparison of computerized dynamic posturography therapy to standard balance physical therapy in individuals with Parkinson's disease: a pilot study. *NeuroRehabilitation*, Vol. 22, No. 4, pp. 261-5, ISSN 1878-6448.

Rochester, L., Baker, K., Hetherington, V., Jones, D., Willems, AM., Kwakkel, G., Van Wegen, E., & Lim, I., Nieuwboer, A. (2010). Evidence for motor learning in Parkinson's disease: acquisition, automaticity and retention of cued gait performance after training with external rhythmical cues. *Brain Research*, Vol. 10, No. 1319, pp. 103-111, ISSN 1872-6240.

Rogers, MW., Kukulka, CG., Brunt, D., Cain, TD., & Hanke, TA. (2001). The influence of stimulus cue on the initiation of stepping in young and older adults. *Archives of Physical Medicine and Rehabilitation*, Vol. 82, No. 5, pp. 619-24, ISSN 1532-821X.

Rubinstein, TC., Giladi, N., & Hausdorff, JM. (2002). The power of cueing to circumvent dopamine deficits: a review of physical therapy treatment of gait disturbances in Parkinson's disease. *Movement Disorders*, Vol. 17, No. 6, pp. 1148-1160, ISSN 1531-8257.

Schaafsma, JD., Giladi, N., Balash, Y., Bartels, AL., Gurevich, T., & Hausdorff, JM. (2003). Gait dynamics in Parkinson's disease: relationship to Parkinsonian features, falls and response to levodopa. *Journal of Neurological Sciences*, Vol. 212, No. 1-2, pp. 47-53, ISSN 1878-5883.

Schieppati, M., & Nardone, A. (1991). Free and supported stance in Parkinson's disease: the effect of posture and "postural set" on leg muscle responses to perturbation, and its relation to the severity of the disease. *Brain*, Vol. 114, pp. 1227-1244, ISSN 1460-2156.

Schuhfried, O., Mittermaier, C., Jovanovic, T., Pieber, K., & Paternostro-Sluga, T. (2005). Effects of whole-body vibration in patients with multiple sclerosis: a pilot study. *Clinical Rehabilitation*, Vol. 19, No. 8, pp. 834-42, ISSN 1477-0873.

Smania, N., Picelli, A., Romano, M., & Negrini, S. (2008). Neurophysiological basis of rehabilitation of adolescent idiopathic scoliosis. *Disability and rehabilitation*, Vol. 30, No. 10, pp. 763-71. ISSN 1464-5165.

Smania, N., Corato, E., Tinazzi, M., Stanzani, C., Fiaschi, A., Girardi, P., & Gandolfi, M. (2010). Effect of balance training on postural instability in patients with idiopathic Parkinson's disease. *Neurorehabilitation and Neural Repair*, Vol. 24, No. 9, pp. 826-34, ISSN 1552-6844.

Smiley-Oyen, AL., Cheng, HY., Latt, LD., & Redfern, MS. (2002). Adaptation of vibration-induced postural sway in individuals with Parkinson's disease. *Gait & Posture*, Vol. 16, No. 2, pp. 188-97, ISSN 1879-2219.

Smithson, F., Morris, ME., & Iansek, R. (1998). Performance on clinical tests of balance in Parkinson's disease. *Physical Therapy*, Vol. 78, No. 6, pp. 577-92, ISSN 1538-6724.

Snijders, AH., van de Warrenburg, BP., Giladi, N., & Bloem, BR. (2007). Neurological gait disorders in elderly people: clinical approach and classification. *Lancet Neurology*, Vol. 6, No. 1, pp. 63-74, ISSN 1474-4465.

Snijders, AH., Nijkrake, MJ., Bakker, M., Munneke, M., Wind C., & Bloem BR. (2008). Clinimetrics of freezing of gait. *Movement Disorders*, Suppl. 2, pp. S468-74, ISSN 1538-6724.

Stack, E., Jupp, K., & Ashburn, A. (2004). Developing methods to evaluate how people with Parkinson's Disease turn 180 degrees: an activity frequently associated with falls. *Disability and Rehabilitation*, Vol. 22, No. 26, pp. 478-84. ISSN 1464-5165.

Steinberg, M., Cartwright, C., Peel, N., & Williams, G. (2000). A sustainable programme to prevent falls and near falls in community dwelling older people: results of a randomised trial. *The Journal of Epidemiology and Community Health*, Vol. 54, No. 3, pp. 227-32, ISSN 1470-2738.

Stolze, H., Klebe, S., Baecker, C., Zechlin, C., Friege, L., Pohle, S., & Deuschl, G. (2005). Prevalence of gait disorders in hospitalized neurological patients. *Movement Disorders,* Vol. 20, No. 1, pp. 89-94, ISSN 1531-8257.

Swinn, L., Schrag, A., Viswanathan, R., Bloem, B.R., Lees, A., & Quinn, N. (2003). Sweating dysfunction in Parkinson's disease. *Movement Disorders*, Vol. 8, No. 12, pp. 1459-63, ISSN 1531-8257.

Temlett, JA., & Thompson, PD. (2006). Reasons for admission to hospital for Parkinson's disease. *Internal Medicine Journal*, Vol. 36, No. 8, pp. 524-6, ISSN 1445-5994.

Thomas, AA., Rogers, JM., Amick, MM., & Friedman, JH. (2010). Falls and the falls efficacy scale in Parkinson's disease. *Journal of Neurology*, Vol. 257, No. 7, pp. 1124-8, ISSN 1432-1459.

Ting, LH, & Macpherson, JM. (2004). Ratio of shear to load ground-reaction force may underlie the directional tuning of the automatic postural response to rotation and translation. *Journal of Neurophysiology*, Vol. 92, No. 2, pp. 808-23, ISSN 1522-1598.

Toole, T., Hirsch, MA., Forkink, A., Lehman, DA., & Maitland, CG. (2000). The effects of a balance and strength training program on equilibrium in Parkinsonism: A preliminary study. *NeuroRehabilitation*, Vol. 14, No. 3, pp. 165-174, ISSN 1878-6448.

Van Nes, IJ., Latour, H., Schils, F., Meijer, R., van Kuijk, A., & Geurts, AC. (2006). Long-term effects of 6-week whole-body vibration on balance recovery and activities of daily living in the postacute phase of stroke: a randomized, controlled trial. *Stroke,* Vol. 37, No. 9, pp. 2331-5, ISSN 1524-4628.

Vaugoyeau, M., Viallet, F., Aurenty, R., Assaiante, C., Mesure, S, & Massion J. (2006). Axial rotation in Parkinson's disease. *Journal of Neurology, Neurosurgery, and Psychiatry*, Vol. 77, No. 7, pp. 815-21, ISSN 1468-330X.

Vaugoyeau, M., Viel, S., Assaiante, C., Amblard, B., & Azulay, J.P. (2007). Impaired vertical postural control and proprioceptive integration deficits in Parkinson's disease. *Neuroscience*, Vol. 146, No. 2, pp. 852-63, ISSN 1873-7544.

Vaugoyeau, M., Viel, S., Amblard, B., Azulay, JP., & Assaiante, C. (2008). Proprioceptive contribution of postural control as assessed from very slow oscillations of the support in healthy humans. *Gait & posture,* Vol. 27, No. 2, pp. 294-302, ISSN 1879-2219.

Vaugoyeau, M., & Azulay, JP. (2010). Role of sensory information in the control of postural orientation in Parkinson's disease. *Journal of the Neurological Sciences*, Vol. 289, No. 1-2, pp. 66-8, ISSN 1878-5883.

Vestergaard, P., Rejnmark, L., & Mosekilde, L. (2007). Fracture risk associated with parkinsonism and anti-Parkinson drugs. *Calcified tissue international,* Vol. 81, No. 3, pp. 153-61, ISSN 1432-0827.

Visser, JE., Voermans, NC., Oude Nijhuis, LB., van der Eijk, M., Nijk, R., Munneke, M., & Bloem, BR. (2007). Quantification of trunk rotations during turning and walking in Parkinson's disease. *Clinical Neurophysiology*, Vol. 118, No. 7, pp. 1602-6, ISSN 1769-7131.

Visser, JE., Allum, JH., Carpenter, MG., Esselink, RA., Limousin-Dowsey, P., Honegger, F., Borm, GF., & Bloem, BR. (2008). Effect of subthalamic nucleus deep brain stimulation on axial motor control and protective arm responses in Parkinson's disease. *Neuroscience,* Vol. 157, No. 4, pp. 798-812, ISSN 1873-7544.

Von Wilzenben, HD. (1942). *Methods in the treatment of post encephalic Parkinson's*. Grune and Stratten, ISBN 951-42-8070-9, New York, USA.

Wannier, T., Bastiaanse, C., Colombo, G., & Dietz, V. (2001). Arm to leg coordination in humans during walking, creeping and swimming activities. *Experimental Brain Research,* Vol. 141, No. 3, pp. 375–379, ISSN 1432-1106.

Wood, BH., Bilclough, JA., Bowron, A., & Walker, RW. (2002). Incidence and prediction of falls in Parkinson's disease: a prospective multidisciplinary study. *Journal of Neurology, Neurosurgery & Psychiatry,* Vol. 72, No. 6, pp. 721-5, ISSN 1468-330X.

Wright, WG., Gurfinkel, VS., Nutt, J., Horak, FB., & Cordo, PJ. (2007). Axial hypertonicity in Parkinson's disease: direct measurements of trunk and hip torque. *Experimental Neurology,* Vol. 208, No. 1, pp. 38-46, ISSN 1090-2430.

Young, LR. (1981). Visual and vestibular influences in human self-motion perception. In: *The Vestibular System: Function and Morphology,* Gualatieratti, T. (Ed.), pp. 393–424, Springer, New York.

Zehr, EP., & Kido, A. (2001). Neural control of rhythmic, cyclical human arm movement: task dependency, nerve specificity and phase modulation of cutaneous reflexes. *The Journal of Physiology,* Vol. 15, No. 537, pp. 1033-45, ISSN 1469-7793.

10

How to Stay Active with Parkinson's Disease

Abu A. Qutubuddin
Virginia Commonwealth University, Richmond, Virginia, U.S.A.

1. Introduction

The key management of Parkinson's disease (PD) other than medications is rehabilitation. Three main areas - flexibility, strength, and cardio respiratory endurance must be considered for rehabilitation with these patients. The following are the basics of the rehabilitation:

1. Physical therapy (PT),
2. Occupational therapy (OT),
3. Recreational therapy (RT) and
4. Speech and language therapy (SLP).

One should be working with these disciplines closely to overcome any limitations and eventually to attain their functional goals. We all know flexibility can be restricted by rigidity or tightness in any of the structures surrounding the joints, by pathology of the joints like arthritis, or by pain.

Older adults lose cardio respiratory endurance or stamina primarily due to decreased physical activities with age. People with PD go through the same age-related changes in range of motion (ROM), strength, flexibility, power, and endurance as does the general geriatric population. However, PD patients have a greater risk of secondary musculoskeletal impairments because of their primary disease process. ROM can be affected by the decreased amplitude and bradykinesia (slowness of movements), rigidity, and impaired proprioception commonly seen in PD patients. Activities can be further reduced secondary to the increased difficulty with movements.

The focus of this chapter is to offer guidelines and examples of various types of exercise. Our goal is to achieve rehabilitation and long-term maintenance of desired activity through educating the PD population and their caregivers. However, knowledge alone is insufficient. Participation and adherence to the program is vital and up to the individual with Parkinson's.

To optimize gains, patients should exercise when they are ON STATE with medications because it reduces the rigidity and bradykinesia. Exercise should not cause any pain. If pain occurs, any exercise should be discontinued or modified.

The ultimate goal or purpose of exercise is to help the PD patients to lead a better quality of life.

We need to understand that before starting any exercise one should consult his/her doctor. Generally, a combination of medications and exercise well tailored to your individual situation and needs will provide an improved state of activity and functioning.

Flexibility and balance are important first considerations in start an exercise program. By improving flexibility, ROM and pain free movement will be improved. By improving balance, safety and life enjoyment will be maximized. If the exercise prescription is right, they will feel comfort rather than pain and discomfort.

Strength is the next exercise priority. It requires weight lifting with different kinds of weight for muscle strength.

The next goal is to increase stamina with different types of movements so that the cardio respiratory condition of the PD patients can be improved.

Dexterity is another important, but often overlooked, factor in assisting the PD patients. Due to tremor, rigidity and inflexibility these patients have difficulties buttoning dresses, holding and turn pages, and writing or signing their checks. To improve these we do have several rehabilitative activities that often are helpful in assisting these patients with their daily tasks that allow for independence and dignity.

2. Rehabilitation

What is Rehabilitation: It is a process of active change by which a person who has become disabled acquires the knowledge and skills needed for optimum physical, psychological and social function.

2.1 Neurological rehabilitation of PD

The patient with PD needs multiple ways to keep themselves active and mobile. Though we know that rehabilitation is the KEY to success, there is presently a lack of well-designed research studies looking at specific rehabilitation techniques. While there are reviews examining studies involving various physical therapy techniques in Parkinson's disease, they have found insufficient evidence to support or refute the efficacy of any form of physical therapy over another form.

The aim of rehabilitation with persons with PD will vary between individuals and between client groups. In general the aim is to provide individuals and their families with the knowledge, skills and support necessary to maintain their autonomy, minimize disability and maximize their level of participation. This includes prevention of complications and secondary disabilities.

Before explaining the different exercise modules, we need to emphasize speech and voice problems that occur with PD progression. Many patients have trouble with speech clarity, volume and swallowing. As we all know if we want to communicate with others we need our voice to be heard loud and clear. So, PD patients need to keep up with their voice exercises to prevent low voice volume (hypophonia) and word slurring (dsyarthria). A simple way to maintain our voice/speech is daily practice preferably twice a day. A simple exercise is to scream at the top of the voice the vowel sounds "A E I O U" for 2-5 minutes. The other simple way to keep your voice loud and clear is to sing along with your favorite song. In my practice most of my patients are benefiting from these two simple, cheap, and easy exercises to keep their speech or to improve their voice. This also helps to improve the swallowing process. There are no real well designed research studies comparing rehabilitation for voice, speech or swallowing. This is purely from my experience.

Before prescribing any exercise program, one has to take into consideration the patient's underlying physical condition and other disease processes. As we know, PD patients appear to exercise with decreased metabolic and mechanical efficiency. To overcome this disadvantage they might be amenable to treatment with aerobic conditioning. Prescribing conditioning exercise to PD patients is only useful in the setting of an optimized medication regimen. This is why it has been agreed to start exercise when the patient is on "ON STATE". That means they should wait at least 30-45 minutes after the dose when most of the patients medication kicks in.

3. Flexibility

For a well-rounded routine exercise, stretching is an important component. Some basic guidelines and practical examples for an effective stretching program are discussed below.

3.1 General considerations

To be effective and to maximize flexibility, patients should and need to be educated about the three components of stretching and how they affect their flexibility. First, they must achieve their current available full range of movement to maintain their flexibility. Compensatory strategies might be required for PD patients. Second, optimal frequency of stretching must be addressed. And finally, holding time for stretching should be determined.

3.2 Achieving maximum range of motion

Slow movements, referred to as bradykinesia in the PD population, can contribute to losing potential flexibility of all the joints of the body. Centrally impaired proprioceptive integration can also contribute hypo metric movements (Jacobs & Horak, 2006).

Cueing strategies may be used to overcome and encourage a larger excursion of movement to obtain full range of motion. This has been shown in gait improvements.

Cueing can also help in an exercise program as well. Attention strategies may be sufficient for obtaining full range in patients with mild PD patents. But to achieve the same results with moderate to severe PD, patients, may need more that just attention strategy. Those patients may do better with verbal, visual, or tactile cues from professionals and caregivers to accomplish optimal flexibility.

To optimize trunk rotation, a person first stands with the back to the wall. Then he or she is asked to touch the wall on the left side by reaching across with his or her right hand. The movement is then reversed. Touching the wall ensures that maximum range has been achieved (Fig.1). Types of cueing needed should be assessed on an individual basis. The patient should be encouraged to obtain full range. Available range will not maximize or be maintained if full range of motion is not utilized "if you don't use it, you lose it".

3.3 Frequency

The American College of Sports Medicine (ACSM) guidelines recommend that adults should stretch a minimum of 2-3 days per week and ideally 5-7 days a week focusing on the areas of reduced range of motion (ROM). There are no specific guidelines for patients with PD. In my experience it is a good practice to do stretching 5-10 minutes at least twice a day, first after getting up from bed in the morning and then before retiring at night. This is in addition to the regular exercise. Holding for the stretching 45-60 seconds with 4-6 repetitions has been shown to be optimal.

3.4 Range of motion exercises

ROM exercises depend on the exercise goals. It is also important to consider the effectiveness, tolerance, and adherence to exercise. It is very important to consider the diagnosis of osteoporosis among the PD patients as many of them have sedentary life styles. Precautions should be observed prescribing ROM exercises to minimize complications.

3.5 Cervical retraction

This type of exercise improves balance and swallowing. This can be done sitting on a chair or lying in bed. While sitting on a chair push the back and head against the wall. The wall will serve as a tactile cue. If it is difficult a pillow can be placed between the head and the wall.

3.6 Cervical rotation

Practicing this exercise helps walking, driving and even sitting with friends in a meeting or restaurants. We need our neck to be flexible in all directions so that when we are walking we can scan our walking path and when driving we can move the neck when needed without much intervention due to tightness. Cervical rotation should be done with the neck in an optimal neutral position without much forward flexion. Having said this, it is advisable to do the cervical retraction exercise before the cervical rotation.

3.7 Shoulder flexion

This can cause loss of balance and falling backwards when trying to reach up.
Ex: if someone has limited shoulder flexion it will restrict reaching for a high shelf. Commonly, people substitute with extending and rotating the trunk. This is not a suitable position for people who already have postural instability as seen in some patients. Sitting with the back fully supported in a chair can help isolate the motion in the shoulder. Folding hands together in front of the chest and above the shoulder can reduce the irritation to the rotator cuff muscles. Patients can then focus on excursion rather than just arm position. As with any exercise it should not cause any pain, it should be performed to comfort. Pre-existing problems of shoulder should require individualized attention.

3.8 Trunk

Tightness or stiffness of the trunk is pretty common and often leads to discomfort or pain. Patients with PD can have this type of stiffness which is partly due to bradykinesia.

3.9 Trunk flexion

PD patients have common problems with the low back due to paravertebral muscle tightness. This can aggravate the symptoms of spinal stenosis. Forward trunk bending while sitting in a chair helps relief of symptoms than just sitting. While keeping the hand on the knees and forward flexion of the trunk helps stretch the back muscles. Patients can easily perform this exercise as needed for pain control.

3.10 Trunk extension

Typically there is limited extension in thoracic and lumbar spine so tolerance to these exercises varies widely. Younger people have fewer co-morbidities that restrict trunk extension. Trunk extension exercises can range from prone press-up to a gentle supine position. This can be performed by longitudinal stretch with reaching arms and legs. Extension can aggravate symptoms of spinal stenosis so the patient may need to rely on a gentle approach.

3.11 Trunk rotation

This exercise can be performed in a supine, sitting, or standing position. This type of exercise should be avoided by people who have osteoporosis. Golf players understand the relevance of trunk rotation exercises. The patient can use tactile cues by attempting to touch the elbow to the opposite knee. Patients who are less flexible may attempt to touch the forearm to the opposite knee. Visual cues can facilitate the motion in which the patient attempts to look at a target behind.

4. Lower extremity

Limitations in range of motion in the lower extremities can affect ones balance, gait, activities of daily living (ADLs), and transfers.

4.1 Hip extension

Sedentary people exhibit an increased forward-flexed posture due to hip flexors tightness. They also walk with reduced stride length. Hip flexors tightness can also contribute to low back strain and aggravates the symptoms of spinal stenosis. Hip flexors stretching vary widely.

One method of stretching the quadriceps (hip flexors) is to lie supine with one leg hanging off a bed while holding the opposite knee to the chest. Pulling the knee to the chest prevents arching of the back. If it is difficult just lie flat in the bed, resting one leg on the bed and try to pull the other knee close to the chest. It might be difficult the first couple of times, but eventually it is possible to do. This way the hip flexors are stretched, not the back. People who cannot tolerate the hip flexors stretching can do active hip extension while standing. They also can perform this exercise by forward lunge.

4.2 Hip abduction

Activities like getting in and out of the bathtub and maintaining hygiene need relaxed adductors muscles of the hip. If the adductors are tight it causes limitations in hip abduction, i.e. difficulty moving the hips and thigh outwards. It also sometimes causes narrowing the base of support which may interfere with ambulation. Another way this can be achieved is by standing behind a chair holding the backrest of the chair. Squat halfway keeping the heels together and the front of the feet spread outside. This will help release the tone of the adductors.

4.3 Hip flexion

It is difficult to don and doff shoes and socks when hip flexion is restricted. Restricted hip flexion can cause lack of forward trunk leaning. One common reason people do not lean forward because of fear of falling. This can reduce ability to stand up from a sitting position. This can be improved by sitting in a chair straight then forward flex the trunk and try to touch the feet with the hands. If there is back pain then keep the hands on the knees.

4.4 Hamstring tightness

This interferes with bed mobility. Presence of rigidity in PD patients and if there is hamstring tightness, this will create bed mobility difficult. It is easier to stretch the hamstring muscles in a sitting position. The patient sits on the edge of a chair with one knee straight and heel on the ground. Then the patient slides both the hands down the extended leg until they feel the stretch in back of the leg while keeping the spine in a neutral position. This can be done safely at home as one of the regular home exercises. Another easy way to stretch the hamstrings is while sitting in a chair with the back supported in a neutral position just extend the knees actively.

4.5 Ankle dorsiflexion or calf tightness

Reduced dorsiflexion of the ankle can be the cause of falls. Falls are common in PD patents. An easy way to stretch the calf tightness is to stand with the forefeet on the edge of a wooden/cement block with the heels resting on the ground. Stretch can be modified by adjusting forward lean. This can also be done easily by standing on the forefeet without any block, holding the edge of a table, sink or kitchen counter, provided they are securely placed. Then do the repetitions by standing on the forefeet with 10 to 20 reps.

Other training for the PD patient includes resistance exercises like strength training, training for power, and also to increase cardio respiratory endurance.

The above exercises can be done with the help of trained therapist to start with if necessary. The important aspect to keeping our body in shape is to adhere to the exercise program. Exercise is a lifelong commitment, not just for the short time. There is no short cut in keeping our body fit for the activities of daily living.

5. References

[1] Parkinson's Disease Diagnosis and Clinical Management, Second Edition by Stewart A. Factor/William J. Weiner

[2] Movement Disorders Neurologic Principles and Practice by Ray L. Watts and William C. Koller.

[3] Neurological Rehabilitation of Parkinson's Disease, Queen Square Neurological Rehabilitation Series, Edited by Diane Playford.

[4] Health Professionals' Guide to Physical Management of Parkinson's Disease by Miriam P. Boelen.

[5] Exercise & Physical Activity, Your Everyday Guide from The National Institute on Aging.

11

Invasive and Non-Invasive Stimulation in Parkinson's Disease

Caspar Stephani
Department of Clinical Neurophysiology, University Medical Center Göttingen, Göttingen Germany

1. Introduction

The ability of the brain to process information relies on its control of the conduction of electric currents. Brain diseases invariably affect this capability. One of the therapeutic approaches to a variety of neurological disorders therefore includes the application of electric currents and fields to the brain. A successful example of this strategy is the introduction of deep brain stimulation which has become a cornerstone of the therapy of advanced Parkinson's disease (PD), dystonia and essential tremor. Several studies have proven its effectiveness and often patients respond immediately to this therapy. Invasiveness and complexity of this treatment restrict its indication. On the other hand, there are techniques for the non-invasive modulation of cortical excitability namely transcranial magnetic stimulation (TMS) as well as transcranial direct current stimulation (tDCS). These techniques have been investigated in several studies including patients with PD. However results so far are heterogeneous and limit their therapeutic value. In the following chapter the basic principles of as well as therapeutic experiences with invasive and non-invasive electrical stimulation techniques and their applications in patients with PD will be discussed.

2. Electrical stimulation in Parkinson's disease

2.1 Invasive electrical stimulation in Parkinson's disease

In the modern era of medicine the modification of cerebral function by electrical stimulation for therapeutic purposes was considerably influenced by the introduction of stereotactic methods into neurosurgery in the middle of the 20th century (Hariz et al., 2010). The stereotactic induction of lesions in the medial nucleus of the thalamus (medial thalamotomy) was reported in a first series with psychiatric patients "in order to reduce the emotional reactivity by a procedure much less drastic than frontal lobotomy" (Spiegel et al., 1947). The frontal lobotomy which was a psychosurgical treatment for psychoses at that time was associated with significant irreversible cerebral destruction. Therefore, applying thermocoagulation with a wire or cannula inserted stereotactically through the intact dura to induce a defined lesion within a distinct cerebral structure in patients with psychiatric disorders revealed a significant therapeutic advancement. Simultaneously, the potential of this technique for the treatment of movement disorders or pain syndromes was suggested (Spiegel et al., 1947). Indeed, the first pallidotomies performed at that time had morbidity rates of 45% and a mortality rate of 15% (Gildenberg P.L., 2003). Stereotactically implanted intracranial electrodes offered the opportunity not only to induce a structural lesion by thermocoagulation but also to identify the basal ganglia electrographically by its distinct pattern of recordable neuronal activity. A related approach without the use of stereotactic instruments but with a similar technique was named chemopallidectomy and consisted in the instillation of absolute alcohol in the globus pallidus with an intracranial cannula. Reduction of rigidity or tremor in several geriatric parkinsonian patients who were considered to old for the alternative and complex anterior choroidal artery occlusion provided evidence for the potential of surgically targeting the basal ganglia for the treatment of movement disorders (Cooper I.S., 1955). Intracranial intraoperative electrical stimulation of the inserted electrodes was conducted early on in order to thereby identify potential targets for the induction of a lesion. Stimulation was performed with low (~ <30 Hz) and high (~ >30 Hz) frequencies in different centers at that time and a significant therapeutic effect of high frequency stimulation at 100 Hz with intracranial stimulation has been described in the early phase of this new therapy (Gildenberg P.L., 2003). Still, even though electrodes were left in place intracranially up to several days electrical stimulation was applied for diagnostic and not for therapeutic purposes. With the introduction of levo-dopa for the treatment of PD its surgical therapy became infrequent. In the following years intracranial electrical stimulation was tested as experimental procedure for a variety of disorders e.g. as a treatment for refractory pain or with cerebellar implants for the treatment of epilepsy (Gol A., 1967; Shealy et al., 1967; Cooper et al., 1976). Devices for chronic subdural electrical stimulation were developed within the same time. The idea of chronically implanted subdural electrodes on the visual cortex working as "prosthesis" for the blind by inducing meaningful visual perceptions in blind patients by electrocortical stimulation was realized in a few patients (Brindley G.S. and Lewin W.S., 1968). Still, this method was not implemented in larger groups of patients for a variety of reasons. Also, early promising results of therapeutic deep brain stimulation in epilepsy or pain could not be reproduced by following studies leading to a subsequent decline of deep brain stimulation in epilepsy. In succession torticollis spasmodicus appears to be the first disorder of the motor system that has been treated with chronic electrical stimulation of the spinal cord (Gildenberg P.L., 1977). Then, in the 1980s the group of Benabid and colleagues rediscovered the beneficial therapeutic effect of intracranial electrical stimulation. Their report of the suppression of parkinsonian and non-parkinsonian tremor when stimulating the nucleus ventralis intermedius of the thalamus (VIM) intraoperatively before VIM thalamotomy as well as the first description of permanent implantation of deep brain stimulators into the VIM in four patients pioneered the surgical treatment of PD by deep brain stimulation as applied today (Benabid et al. 1987).

2.1.1 The object of invasive electrical stimulation in Parkinson's disease

The important role of the basal ganglia for movement control has probably been recognized in the 17th century (Lanska D.J., 2010). Modern concepts of function of the basal ganglia have lead to and benefit from the introduction of neurosurgical approaches in the therapy of movement disorders like PD. The basal ganglia include the striatum (putamen and caudate nucleus), the globus pallidus internus (GPi), the globus pallidus externus (GPe), the subthalamic nucleus (STN), the subtantia nigra pars reticularis (SNr) and the substantia nigra pars compacta (SNc). The basal ganglia receive their main external input from the primary motor cortex (M1), premotor areas including the supplementary sensorimotor area (SSMA) and the cingulate motor area in the anterior cingulum. Additionally, the ventrolateral and the ventral anterior nuclei of the thalamus project to the basal ganglia. The striatum is the first relay and therefore the main gate for a majority of the afferents to the basal ganglia. Also the STN receives primary afferents from the aforementioned cortical areas (Table 1). Importantly, the projections to the basal ganglia are highly organized by means of their functional and topographic origin into three main groups of afferents (Parent A., 1990). First, afferents from M1 and premotor areas including the SSMA preferentially project to the postcommissural putamen; second, afferents from prefrontal cortex project to the precommissural putamen and the caudate nucleus; third, those afferents originating in limbic areas including the anterior cingulum and the orbitofrontal cortex project primarily to the ventral striatum. Additionally, afferents from the primary motor regions are organized somatotopically including distal limb projections (Bauswein et al., 1989). This organizational principle of afferents has been recognized in the striatum as well as in the STN whose dorsolateral part receives information from M1, while its ventrolateral part receives projections from the caudal cingulate motor area. The SSMA and the pre-SSMA as well as the rostral part of the cingulate motor area project to the dorsomedial part of the STN, while other premotor areas connect to its ventromedial part (Hartmann-von Monakow et al., 1978; Takada et al., 2001). Electrophysiological studies in non-human primates revealed that corticostriatal neurons differ in their neurophysiological properties from corticospinal neurons. The former show slower conduction velocities, lower discharge rates and a different response pattern to somatosensory input. Indeed, both systems appear to be supplied by completely different populations of cortical neurons (Turner and DeLong, 2000). Another important source of input to the striatum are mesencephalic nuclei with the dopamiergic projections of the SNc being the most significant. The SNc is itself influenced by feedback projections from the STN, the SNr and external afferent sources like the prefrontal and orbitofrontal cortex, the raphe nuclei, the superior colliculi. Functionally, a tonic firing pattern that can be modified by reward-learning has been recognized as a characteristic electrophysiological pattern of dopaminergic neurons of the SNc (Hollerman & Schultz, 1998, Wichmann and DeLong, 2007).

On a cellular level afferents to the striatum terminate almost exclusively on medium spiny neurons that represent 90-95% of all striatal neurons. The information processing within these GABAergic neurons is further modulated by intrinsic cholinergic and peptidergic interneurons (Wichmann and DeLong, 2007). The large majority of target-neurons in the STN is glutamatergic unlike all other nuclei of the basal ganglia and only few neurons in the human STN were found to be GABAergic (Levesque and Parent, 2005). The information is further processed via two different systems: the direct and indirect pathway. The former projects directly to the output nuclei of the basal ganglia, the GPi and the SNr. The indirect pathway is polysynaptic and its information is modulated in the GPe and STN from where it then projects to GPi and SNr as well. Medium spiny neurons forming the direct pathway preferentially exhibit dopamine D1-receptors and express substance P. Indirect pathway medium spiny neurons on the contrary do express predominantly D2-receptors and enkephalin (Gerfen et al., 1990). Therefore, both major classes of dopamine receptors - the D1-like family whose activation increases and the D2-like family whose activation decreases the concentration of the second messenger cyclic adenosine monophosphate (cAMP) - are represented in the striatofugal system. The dopaminergic projections from the SNc balance direct and indirect striatal projections within the basal ganglia, the net effect of which promotes an inhibitory influence on the output of the basal ganglia to the thalamus leading to increased thalamocortical activity in case of the direct pathway and to an opposite effect in case of the indirect pathway (Wichman and DeLong, 2007). Loss of function of the neurons of the SNc in Parkinson's disease causes a functional imbalance of the output of the basal ganglia.

The output of the basal ganglia that arises mainly from the GPi and SNr is primarily directed towards the ventral anterior nucleus and the ventrolateral nucleus of the thalamus. From this nucleus the information is further transmitted to motor-, premotor- and prefrontal cortex (Hoover and Strick, 1993). As mentioned previously the relative topographic segregation between the three main functional input systems of the basal ganglia is maintained through the different stages of information processing including its output projections (Shink et al., 1996). Other neurons of the SNr project to the superior colliculus or the reticular formation.

While the aforementioned subcortical network maintains normal motor function in the healthy state its dysfunction in Parkinson's disease is correlate of the clinical symptoms like tremor, hypokinesia, rigidity. The depletion of dopamine in the striatum due to degeneration of the SNc is decisive in this pathophysiology and both the dysinhibition of the direct pathway as well as the increased inhibitory activity of the striatopallidal fibers of the indirect pathway finally lead to a reduced activity of thalamocortical projections to the various motor areas. Aside from the pure imbalance of inhibitory and excitatory mechanisms in PD recent research has recognized alterations in frequency and synchronization of basal ganglia circuits (Hammond et al., 2007). Some evidence suggests that increased synchronization of oscillations in the beta-frequency range between basal ganglia and cortical projection areas impair movement control and are a correlate of PD. This synchronization indeed can be suppressed by dopaminergic therapy. Further research on this subject is required.

Anatomical structure	Main transmitter
Striatum	GABA
STN	Glutamate
GPi	GABA
GPe	GABA
SNc	Dopamine
SNr	GABA

Table 1. This table lists the predominant neurotransmitters of substructures of the basal ganglia. STN = subthalamic nucleus, GPi = globus pallidus internus, GPe = globus pallidus externus, SNc = substantia nigra pars compacta, SNr = substantia nigra pars reticulata. GABA = gamma-amino-butyric acid.

2.1.2 The medium of invasive electrical stimulation in Parkinson's disease

Currently, the hardware implanted for deep brain stimulation includes the stimulation device or internal pulse generator, the stimulating electrode(s) and a connector between these elements. The battery driven stimulator is usually implanted subcutaneously in the subclavicular area. This device is connected to two or less often one deep brain electrode(s) by a stimulator cable that is tunneled through cervical, retroauricular and cranial subcutaneous tissue. The deep brain electrodes have four electrode contacts at their tip counting from the most central electrode contact that is labeled as contact zero. The diameter of the lead body is 1.27 mm. The length of the electrode contact varies between 1.5 and 3 mm whereas the electrode spacing varies between 0.5 and 4 mm depending on the model of the lead. This system is controlled by an external telemetric programmer that allows to modify current intensity, pulse width, frequency of stimulation, polarity of the stimulus and electrode configuration. A typical type of deep brain stimulator offers a range of 0 - 25.5 mA in the current mode or 0 - 10.5 V in the voltage mode regarding adjustment of the stimulation intensity. The frequency of stimulation can be modified within a range of 2-250 Hz and the pulse width can be altered between 60 and 450 µs according to the manufacturer of deep brain stimulation devices (Medtronic; Minnesota, U.S.A.). However, the parameters stimulation frequency as well as pulse width are infrequently subject to changes and the fine tuning of the stimulator is commonly done by changing the stimulus intensity. Stimulation frequency is most often set at around 130 Hz providing a good ratio between efficiency and energy consumption (Volkmann et al., 2006). This is based on studies which demonstrated a high efficiency of electrical stimulation within a range of stimulation frequencies between 30 and 250 Hz when stimulation intensity is left constant (Mihailovic and Delgado, 1956). Similarly the range in which the pulse width can be varied closely reflects the most efficient and safest interval for neuronal excitation which is between 100 and 500 µs (Mihailovic and Delgado, 1956). In general and due to different time constants a shorter pulse width is more likely to excite axons or axon hillocks at least in the case of single pulse stimulation (Ranck, 1975; Nowak and Bullier, 1998). And commonly the pulse width of a deep brain stimulator is set at 60 µs (Perlmutter and Mink, 2006). In contrast to these parameters, the configuration and polarity of the electrodes are typically modified in the course of the treatment. A monopolar montage with a single "active" cathodal electrode contact on the deep brain electrode referenced to the "inactive" anodal pulse generator or a bipolar montage between two of the four electrode contacts with one serving as cathode and one as anode can be chosen. The monopolar configuration with an inactive reference is often preferred since it improves the ability to relate a therapeutic effect to a specific electrode contact. Nonetheless, monopolar as well as bipolar stimulation should both be regarded as being relatively focal. The preference of the cathodal polarity for monopolar stimulation results from its higher efficiency in stimulating neurons compared to anodal pulses regarding intracerebral application of electrical stimulation. Indeed, threshold currents for the induction of action potentials in pyramidal tract cells can differ up to more than factor ten between cathodal and anodal current (Stoney et al., 1968). Neuroanatomically electrical stimulation preferentially activates structures parallel to the electrical field (Ranck, 1975). Knowledge of this factor may help to interpret the effects of DBS. DBS in PD is continuous and therefore energy consuming. Optimal parameters of DBS account for this factor increasing the interval for exchange of the battery. In fact, modern devices are advertised with having a longevity of 9 years (Medtronic; Minnesota, U.S.A.). However, patients need to be aware of the potential necessity of a second surgical intervention for battery changes. Also the existence of intracranial metallic material as well as the stimulation device impose vigilance on the possible hazards and restrict use of magnetic resonance imaging (MRI), transcranial magnetic stimulation (TMS), diathermia or other external electromagnetic sources in patients with DBS.

2.1.3 The mechanism of action of invasive stimulation in Parkinson's disease

The choice of the target to be stimulated in order to reduce symptoms of PD has been decisively influenced by previous experiences with lesional surgery for the therapy of PD. In fact Benabid et al. (2009) stated that "DBS mimics the effects of ablation in all targets used to date." However, dependence on active stimulation of the electrode contacts clearly indicates a dynamic neurophysiologic mechanism of action of DBS which has not been fully elucidated so far (Perlmutter and Mink, 2006). The similarities between the effects of a lesion and stimulation of particular neuroanatomical targets supported the theory that high-frequency deep brain stimulation of the STN and other targets acts in general inhibitory on the neuron and hence on the functional output of the stimulated structure i.e. of the STN. In accordance with that hypothesis a study using single neuron patch-clamp-technique in prepared slices of the STN of Wistar rats has shown that electrical high-frequency stimulation (stimulation frequency = 100-250 Hz, pulse width = 100 μs, duration of stimulation = 60 seconds) is able to block single-spiking or bursting activity of STN-neurons for about six minutes after stimulation an effect that can be evoked repeatedly (Beurrier et al., 2001). This effect did neither depend on Ca2+ mediated transmitter release nor was it the consequence of membrane hyperpolarization. In another study using in-vivo records of patients undergoing surgery for advanced PD single pulses with an intensity of 50 μA induced short-lasting inhibition of tonically firing neurons of the GPi within a radius of up to more than 600 μm. In this study however, a transmitter-dependent mechanism was proposed (Dostrovsky et al., 2000). Moreover, it was demonstrated in a Positron-emission-tomography (PET)-study that the regional cerebral blood flow (rCBF) of the SSMA, the cingulate motor cortex and the dorsolateral prefrontal cortex (DLPFC) during active stimulation of the STN is significantly increased compared to inactive stimulation. These findings resembled the results of studies which compared changes of rCBF before and after pallidotomy (Grafton et al., 1995; Limousin et al., 1997). Also, it was shown by PET that the pathophysiological hypoactivity of the SSMA as found in PD is reversed by active DBS of the STN as well as pallidotomy (Ceballos-Bauman A.O., 2003). Nevertheless, the view of a predominant inhibitory action of DBS has been challenged for several reasons (Vitek J.L., 2002). Importantly, other studies focused on the effects that DBS of the STN exerts on related nuclei of the basal ganglia. Supporting increased excitatory action of the STN elevated levels of glutamate were found in SNr and GP of normal rats after DBS of the STN with intracerebral microdialysis (Windels et al., 2003). This effect depended strongly on the frequency of stimulation with a maximum increase of glutamate in the GP and SNr at 130 Hz, weaker increases at either 60 or 350 Hz and no effect at 10 Hz being concordant with the well-known frequency dependence of the clinical effect of DBS of the STN in humans. Studies that demonstrated an increased activity of neurons in the SNr after DBS of the STN are in line with these results. Nonetheless, effects were depending on stimulation intensity and while high intensities of high-frequency DBS induced the aforementioned increase in neuronal activity, low-stimulation intensity reversed this effect (Maurice et al., 2003). In light of the evidence suggesting blocking of activity of STN neurons it is likely that the excitation measured in related nuclei is due to activation of efferent fibers from the STN rather than the neurons themselves. Experimental evidence suggest that the threshold for activation by intracranial electrical stimulation is lowest at axons and their initial segments and in fact much higher at the neuronal cell body (Nowak and Bullier, 1998). Another effect of intracerebral brain stimulation may be relevant for the efficacy of this treatment which is the "anodal surround" effect. With increasing intensity of cathodal DBS the depolarizing outward current induced by the stimulation around the electrode is compensated by an increasing hyperpolarizing inward current which is highest in relative proximity to the current source hence resembling the effect of anodal stimulation. Therefore, conduction of action potentials of an excited axon may be blocked completely in orhodromic and antidromic direction. With greater distance from the electrode contact the anodal-like effect decreases and action potentials will not be interrupted (Ranck, 1975). Consequently, action potentials of those elements centered closest around the stimulating electrode contact may not leave this zone around the contact further supporting a theory of central inhibition and peripheral excitation. An influence of DBS on oscillations and firing patterns in the basal ganglia has been proposed as relevant correlate of its therapeutic efficiency more recently (Welter et al., 2004).

2.1.4 The indication for invasive electrical stimulation in Parkinson's disease

Despite its invasive nature, the perioperative risk and the highly specialized therapy DBS offers some advantages over the classical pharmacological treatment of PD that hold true regardless of the stage of the disease. DBS acts continuously reducing fluctuation of symptoms that often are due to variable serum levels of antiparkinsonian drugs. Therefore, if implantation succeeded DBS has a good therapeutic predictability. Also, psychiatric side-effects like hallucinations due to levo-dopa administration or use of dopaminergic drugs are less common with DBS. However, the therapeutic value of DBS depends to a significant extent on the correct identification of appropriate patients for this therapy. Since other parkinsonian syndromes do not respond sufficiently to DBS the diagnosis of an idiopathic Parkinson syndrome (IPS) or PD must be firm. Criteria for the adequacy of the diagnosis of PD have to be checked before indicating a surgical approach in the treatment of PD. An asymmetric onset of the disease and early and satisfying response to levo-dopa are typical and crucial features of PD. Also tremor is typical of PD whereas it is infrequent in other parkinsonian syndromes. On the other hand early existence of significant postural instability, autonomic dysfunction or cognitive decline point to an atypical Parkinson syndrome. In any case the presurgical evaluation must include the performance of a levo-dopa-test (Charles et al., 2002). A single high-dose application of levo-dopa e.g. 250 mg 12 hours after discontinuation of antiparkinsonian treatment is sufficient. The motor symptoms of PD then should be evaluated in the state off medication and in the best on-state or 1 hour after application of the single test-dose of l-dopa. Part III of the Unified Parkinson's disease rating scale (UPDRS) is the preferred tool to asses the outcome of this test and an improvement of 30% in this part of the UPDRS is regarded as significant and typical of PD. However, some centers demand an even better presurgical response to this test (Welter et al., 2002). Since dementia should preclude surgery for DBS a neuropsychological testing is part of the presurgical evaluation. As a screening tool for surgery the mini-mental state examination (MMSE) is useful and a result of less than 24 points would omit further testing. However, it has to be taken into considerations that often candidate patients are not unfamiliar with this test and results may incorporate training effects. Age is negatively correlated with a favourable outcome of the procedure. Often an age of 75 is regarded as upper limit for performing an implantation of deep brain electrodes. Still, this guideline is not exclusive. A recent cranial MRI is essential for the presurgical evaluation and should rule out leukoencephalopathy, atrophy or other functionally relevant abnormalities. Also a preexisting psychiatric disorders will preclude a patient from surgery for DBS. Therefore patients will need to be assessed by a psychiatrist presurgically. A multidisciplinary setting is required for taking the decision for implantation of a deep brain stimulator. Today, DBS is a treatment choice for advanced PD that is not manageable by pharmacotherapy e.g. due to motor fluctuations, dyskinesias or psychiatric side effects of medication. Currently, a multicentre randomized, open-label clinical trial is investigating a potential role of STN-DBS compared to best medical treatment on quality of life for earlier stages of the disease (NCT00354133).

2.1.5 The outcome of invasive electrical stimulation in Parkinson's disease

According to the manufacturer of the medical devices for deep brain stimulation (DBS), the healthcare company Medtronic (Minnesota, U.S.A.), more than 80.000 patients have received deep brain stimulators since 1995 as of March 2011. DBS first was approved for the therapy of essential tremor in Europe in 1995 and in the U.S.A. in 1997. In 1998 it was licensed for therapy of advanced Parkinson's disease in Europe, Canada and Australia while the approval of the food and drug administration (FDA) in the U.S.A. followed in 2002. An approval for the treatment of dystonia in the U.S.A. came in 2003. Additionally, DBS can now be applied for severe obsessive compulsive disorders (OCD) and focal epilepsy refractory to pharmaceutical treatment in Europe.

Three structures are currently targeted for invasive therapy of PD: the nucleus ventralis intermedius of the thalamus (VIM), the globus pallidus internus (GPi) and the nucleus subthalamicus (STN). The effectiveness of electrical deep brain stimulation of these intracerebral structures for the therapy of PD has each been proven by several clinical outcome studies. Among the aforementioned target structures the VIM was the first which was investigated for therapy of PD (Benabid et al., 1987). Today it is the target least often chosen for DBS in PD. However, it remains a particularly effective therapy for resting or postural tremor in PD, both of which are less well controlled by the alternative strategies of DBS of the GPi or STN. Conversely, improvement of akinesia and rigidity is less satisfying with DBS of the VIM compared to DBS of STN or GPi. Hence, DBS of the VIM is a valuable therapeutic choice in patients with tremor dominant forms of PD and is effective in about 90% of these patients (Tarsy et al., 2008). Also, the results of a prospective randomized study indicate that DBS of the VIM is superior to thalamotomy regarding clinical outcome with significantly higher effectiveness concerning activities of daily living and upper extremity mobility as well as a more favorable benefit risk ratio (Schuurman et al., 2000). The second most frequently targeted structure for DBS for PD is the GPi. The motor score of the UPDRS improves by 30-40% on average with results ranging from 10-70% after uni- or bilateral DBS of the GPi as measured 3 to 12 months after surgery in most studies (Weaver et al., 2008). In two studies the clinical benefit of bilateral DBS of the GPi remained relatively stable in a long-term perspective after two and three to four years compared to short-term results after six and twelve months respectively indicating a long-term benefit of this treatment (Ghika et al., 1998; Rodriguez-Oroz et al., 2005). This improvement in motor function is reflected by patients self-reporting a significant increase of daily time in an on-state from 26 to 69% following bilateral electrode implantation in the GPi (Rodriguez-Oroz et al., 2005). The main target of DBS for PD today is the STN. A reduction of the motor part of the UPDRS of 50% on average can be expected after implantation of depth electrodes into the STN. Also, STN DBS is effective regarding bradykinesia, rigidity as well as tremor. Additionally, dyskinesias and motor fluctuations are likely to be reduced significantly. On the other hand, postural stability more often does not improve satisfactorily following DBS of the STN and may even worsen in some cases. Regarding non-motor consequences of this therapy it has been suggested that a decline in cognitive abilities may be related to DBS of the STN. However, from current data it is not clear to which extent this finding is the consequence of the natural course of the disease. A decisive advantage of STN DBS is the potential postsurgical reduction in the levo-dopa dosis which may in a subgroup of patients even lead to a temporary cessation of pharmacotherapy (Merello, 2008). In general, the procedure results in a better quality of life for patients on average. One study compared DBS of the STN in addition to medication against best pharmacotherapy alone in patients with advanced PD. Significant superiority of the former treatment was demonstrated in both the UPDRS as well as in a PD quality of life scale after six month in patients under 75 years of age (Deuschl et al., 2006). Even though DBS does not exceed the overall effectiveness of levo-dopa therapy off states are less frequent with DBS. Comparison between DBS of the STN and the GPi based on the literature suggests that both procedures are equally effective regarding motor outcome and self-reported function (Follett et al., 2010). Due to different parameters of stimulation battery life of stimulators of the GPi may be shorter compared to devices implanted for stimulation of the STN. Also, patients undergoing STN DBS require a lower dose of dopaminergic treatment compared to patients after GPi DBS. In contrast, neuropsychological complications may be less frequent with stimulation of the GPi (Weaver et al., 2008; Follett et al., 2010). Aside from the potential benefits of any type of DBS patients need to be made aware of the perioperative risks including implantation site infection or intracranial hemorrhage and long-term risks like breakage of material, dislocation of the electrodes or an immunological reaction. Finally it must be clarified to the patient that the procedure occasionally may fail to improve the symptoms of PD.

2.2 Non-invasive stimulation in Parkinson's disease

There is good evidence from basic research that application of rTMS and tDCS can have a lasting impact on cortical plasticity and several studies suggest that these techniques may offer a new therapeutic approach to a variety of neurological disorders. Still, compared to DBS the therapeutic effects of transcranial stimulation in Parkinson's disease so far appear to be rather small and variable. This may in part be due to a heterogeneity of study protocols regarding several parameters of stimulation. Representing innovative mechanisms exploration of the therapeutic potential of these techniques deserves further attention.

2.2.1 Technical aspects of non-invasive electrical stimulation

Transcranial magnetic stimulation: Current flow in an iron coil will induce a magnetic field perpendicular to the electric current flow. The magnetic field again induces an electric field perpendicular to itself. In consequence, this electric field is parallel and in opposite direction to the inducing current flow. When applied on the scalp above the cortex brief currents of an electric coil are able to produce direct excitation of neurons. While single pulse transcranial magnetic stimulation (TMS) is used to induce a neuronal action potential which then may produce a motor evoked potential the single pulses of repetitive TMS (rTMS) usually do not reach the threshold for inducing action potentials. Several parameters that can be determined with single pulse TMS reflect different aspects of cortical excitability: 1) the resting motor threshold (RMT) or active motor threshold (AMT) probably reflect membrane properties, 2) the silent period (SP) which is a quiescent phase in the electromyogram (EMG) is partially of cortical origin and is related to the function of GABA-B receptors. 3) short intracortical inhibition (SICI) and short intracortical facilitation (SICF) occur when a subthreshold stimulus precedes a suprathreshold stimulus by less than 5 ms or 8-30 ms respectively. SICI likely depends on GABAergic function while mechanisms of the SICF are less clear and probably involve function of GABA receptors as well as N-methyl-D-aspartate (NMDA)-receptors (Hallett, 2007; Ziemann, 2004).

On the other hand, rTMS has the potential to alter the cortical excitability depending on duration and mode of stimulation (Hallett, 2007). rTMS frequencies of around 1 Hz induce an inhibitory effect on cortical excitability (Chen et al., 1997) and rates of more than 5 Hz generate facilitation (Pascual-Leone et al., 1994; Hallett, 2007). Huang et al. (2005) developed a different high-frequency transcranial magnetic stimulation (TMS) - called Theta-burst stimulation (TBS) - with excitability modulating after effects of up to 60 minutes in healthy volunteers. Here the repetition rate of the rTMS is irregular with three pulses with an inter-pulse interval of 20 ms (50 Hz) repeated every 200 ms (5 Hz) applied either continuously for 40 seconds as continuous TBS (cTBS) or for two seconds repeated 20 times every 10 seconds then named intermittent TBS (iTBS). cTBS produces a short-lasting inhibitory effect on cortical excitability and iTBS induces a short-lasting cortical facilitation. This induction of cortical plasticity or metaplasticity resembles the effects of repetitive electrical stimuli of single neurons which lead to either long-term potentiation (LTP) or long-term depression (LTD). Hence, the effects of rTMS are often referred to as LTP-like facilitation and LTD-like inhibition, respectively. Therapeutic applications of rTMS is based on these facilitatory or inhibitory effects that outlast the stimulation procedure itself and are aimed to modulate excitability of the cortex at least transiently.

Several substances were found to alter the effects of TMS on cortical excitability or rTMS on cortical plasticity. Based on a review by Ziemann (2004) carbamazapine, phenytoin and lamotrigine which all are blocking sodium-channels reduce the motor threshold. Lorazepam and diazepam increase the SICI while they reduce the SICF. The NMDA-receptor antagonists dextrometorphan and memantine also reduce the ICF while SICI is enhanced. This pattern is also observed in a dose-dependent manner for ethanol. And D2-agonists like bromocriptine or cabergoline as well as the combined D1-/D2-agonist pergolid are enhancers of the SICI as well while an opposite effect is observed for the dopamine-antagonist haloperidol. Therefore dopamine receptor agonists or antagonists have been termed "inverse modulators of motor cortex excitability" (Ziemann et al., 1997). LTP-like cortical plasticity as studied mainly with paired associative stimulation (PAS) is increased during treatment with D2-agonist cabergoline as well as methylphenidate and decreased under treatment with NMDA-receptor antagonist dextrometorphan as well as haloperidol, lamotrigine, lorazepam and biperiden (Ziemann et al., 2006).

Aside from medical drugs the duration of stimulation may decisively affect the result of rTMS. Whereas 40 seconds of continuous TBS decreases cortical excitability, halving the same stimulation to 20 seconds induces facilitatory effects (Gentner et al., 2008). A similar reversal of the impact of a stimulation has been reported by others (Gamboa et al., 2010). An additional influence on the effect of cortical stimulation may results from the state of pre-activation of target muscles during a stimulation. As an example, effects of iTBS can be abolished when the muscle of interest is contracted with approximately 10% of maximal power (Huang et al., 2008). It is important to note that in PD rigidity may be more often present at rest in contrast to situations in most studies which are performed with healthy individuals. Pre-activation of a muscle e.g. due to rigidity or tremor in these patients may shift intracortical homeostasis, which then may influence MEP-amplitudes and neuronal recruitment.

Transcranial direct current stimulation: In 1980 it was demonstrated that a high-voltage shock applied transcranially over the primary motor cortex is able to produce a motor-evoked potential (Merton and Morton, 1980). Despite being non-invasive the application of this transcranial electric stimulation (TES) is painful which limits its applicability. A well-tolerated technique of transcranial electric stimulation has been introduced into research on neuroplasticity in the recent past (Nitsche and Paulus, 2000). Here instead of directly inducing action potentials a weak direct current is applied on the scalp and is able to gradually modulate cortical excitability in humans. An "active" electrode placed on the scalp above a cortical target region to be stimulated – e.g. above the primary motor cortex – and a distant reference electrode that is usually placed supraorbitally and contralaterally to the active electrode are both connected to a battery-driven stimulator forming an electric circuit. In healthy young individuals the cerebral cortex beneath a cathodal electrode can be hyperpolarized whereas the cortex beneath an anodal electrode can be depolarized as shown by decrease or increase of the amplitude of motor evoked potentials (MEPs). This effect can last up to 60 minutes after stimulation and even longer under circumstances (Nitsche et al., 2007). More recently, Terney et al. (2008) similarly showed that alternating current stimulation with random amplitude and frequency variation - transcranial random noise stimulation (tRNS) – is able to produce a significant increase in regional motor-cortical excitability in healthy subjects for up to 60 minutes after the end of stimulation. Studies have demonstrated a relevance of different neuronal transmitter systems for the mediation of this effect. For example, the NMDA-receptor antagonist dextrometorphan is able to completely abolish the effect of either anodal or cathodal tDCS (Liebetanz et al., 2002). It has been shown that the decreased cortical excitability following cathodal tDCS can be prolonged by administration of pergolide, a combined D1/D2 agonist, and can be diminished by sulpiride, a D2-antagonist. Additionally, co-administration of pergolide and sulpiride abolishes effects of cathodal as well as anodal tDCS with a tendency of reversing effects of anodal stimulation (Nitsche et al., 2006). Confirmatory, it has been reported more recently that the facilitating effect of anodal tDCS in healthy volunteers can be reversed under the influence of l-dopa and may lead to a significant decrease in cortical excitability (Kuo et al., 2008). Indeed, a complex U-shaped or inversely U-shaped dose-dependent effect of D2-receptor stimulation on MEP-amplitudes in healthy individuals after cathodal or anodal tDCS respectively has been proposed (Monte-Silva et al., 2009). These results highlight especially the role of dopamine in cortical plasticity affecting strategies on the application of this technique in patients with Parkinson's disease.

2.2.2 Neurophysiology of non-invasive electrical stimulation in Parkinson's disease

Transcranial magnetic stimulation: Some of the basic parameters measured by single pulse or paired pulse TMS are affected by PD and medication for the disease. Typically, there is no change in motor threshold in patients with PD compared to healthy individuals. The silent period as well as the SICI are decreased and can be normalized by application of parkinsonian medication in patients with PD (Priori et al., 1994; Lefaucheur et al., 2004; Hallett, 2007). Most studies do not report a significant effect of PD on ICF (Cantello et al., 2002). However, results regarding the effect on this parameter are heterogeneous (Bareš et al., 2003).

The effects of rTMS on neurophysiologic parameters in patients with PD can significantly differ from those in healthy persons. Gilio et al. (2002) already described a lack of MEP-changes after 5-Hz rTMS in patients with PD in contrast to healthy subjects. Moreover, they found that voluntary contraction of the target-muscle during 5 Hz rTMS did abolish changes in cortical excitability. Accordingly, a recent study showed that iTBS does not induce cortical plasticity in patients with PD under dopaminergic medication (Stephani et al., 2011). Despite findings of Ueki et al. (2006) who reported a restored cortical plasticity in patients with PD after administration of dopaminergic drugs in response to interventional paired associative stimulation (iPAS) this may not be the case in response to iTBS. And in a placebo-controlled, double-blind, randomized trial on iTBS in patients with PD there was no improvement of the UPDRS after 8 sessions of stimulation over the motor cortex and dorsolateral prefrontal cortex (Benninger et al., 2011; table 2). Comparably, no change in cortical excitability after application of an inhibitory continuous TBS (cTBS) protocol could be found in a recent report (Eggers et al., 2010).

Transcranial direct current stimulation: Within the few studies published on tDCS in patients with PD there is only one that also reports on the effects of stimulation on a neurophysiological parameter (Fregni et al., 2006). This study demonstrated a 70%-increase of the MEP-amplitude at a single time-point directly after 20 minutes of anodal tDCS over the primary motor cortex with an intensity of 1 mA. The same protocol with cathodal stimulation over the primary motor cortex induced a significant decrease of the MEP-amplitude of around 20%. These results are analogue to those of healthy persons and interestingly, antiparkinsonian drugs in these patients were held for approximately 12 hours prior to the experiment. In a recent study a new technique of transcranial alternating current stimulation (tACS) termed transcranial random noise stimulation (tRNS) was applied. This technique uses randomly alternating currents of ± 500 μA. Patients with PD showed a decrease in cortical excitability in contrast to results on healthy subjects whose cortical excitability increased after 10 minutes of tRNS (Stephani et al., 2011; Terney et al., 2008). Continued dopaminergic therapy may have contributed to this paradoxic effect.

2.2.3 Therapeutic use of non-invasive electrical stimulation in Parkinson's disease

Both, rTMS and tDCS offer the possibility of non-invasively altering cortical excitability and inducing cortical plasticity in humans (Pascual-Leone et al., 1994, Nitsche and Paulus, 2000). However, they share the disadvantage of not being able to directly modulate subcortical structures like the basal ganglia due to a restricted operating distance. Hence, their therapeutic potential depends on disease processes that directly or indirectly affect cortical function. A pathological decrease or increase in excitability of cortical areas like the supplementary motor area (SMA), the dorsolateral prefrontal cortex (DLPFC) and the primary motor cortex (M1) has been demonstrated in various stages of Parkinson's disease thus providing potential targets for therapeutic applications of non-invasive stimulation in PD (Lefaucheur, 2005).

Transcranial magnetic stimulation: Based on these concepts rTMS has been applied in patients with PD in several studies with a variety of different stimulation protocols (Table 2 and Table 3). A meta-analysis of studies that reported on effects of rTMS on the UPDRS between 1985 and 2007 included 10 sufficient prospective trials with control groups on different sham conditions. Whereas in 6 trials high-frequency rTMS was used 3 trials applied low-frequency rTMS and in one trial both techniques were used. A significant effect size of 0.58 was only found for high-frequency rTMS whereas meta-analysis of low-frequency rTMS revealed no therapeutic effect (Elahi et al., 2008). In the one study that tested 10 Hz as well as 0.5 Hz real rTMS in patients with Parkinson's disease both were shown to improve motor performance 20 minutes after their application. However, their effects on parameters of excitability were reversed compared to healthy individuals indicating an altered motor cortex excitability in these patients (Lefaucheur et al., 2004).

Improvement in the UPDRS has been reported after low and high-frequency rTMS of varying duration and location by others (Wu et al., 2008). However, the largest study of rTMS in PD so far had 85 participants that were assigned to three different groups. Applying very low frequency rTMS (0.2 Hz) there was no improvement of UPDRS III (Okabe et al., 2003). In an early study Siebner et al. (2000) e.g. detected a significantly improved mobility of the arm one hour after 5 Hz rTMS over the contralateral M1 area of the hand. Favouring the effectiveness of high-frequency rTMS, Strafella et al. (2001) could show that 10 Hz rTMS for one second every 10 seconds for 15 times which then was repeated three times every ten minutes over the prefrontal cortex conditions a dopamine release in the striatum. Still, in a series with 22 patients who each underwent single sessions of 0.5 Hz rTMS, 10 Hz rTMS, iTBS, cTBS and sham stimulation no significant effect of either stimulation was found on the UPDRS III while training effects may have masked any possible therapeutic effect of the TMS (Rothkegel et al, 2009). In accordance with this result, the most recent studies evaluating the clinical effectiveness of cTBS or iTBS both of which are powerful techniques for the modulation of cortical plasticity in healthy individuals did fail to demonstrate a significant therapeutic benefit further suggesting a lack of change in cortical excitability in patients with PD (Eggers et al., 2010; Benninger et al., 2011).

Authors	Year	Verum	Sham	No. Of ses.	Coil	Hz	Sec	dd	RMT	n	Method	Results
Shimamoto et al.	2001	Bilateral frontal cortex	Acoustic sham	8 (once a week)	Round	0.2	300	On	100 ±10%	9	1(150s left+150s right)	Mild but significant improvement of UPDRS III after 2 months. No improvement after 1 month. Significant effect on activities of daily living.
Ikeguchi et al.	2003	F3 (clockwise) or F4 (counterclockwise)	Occipital stimulation between inion and auditory meatus (clockwise on the left, counterclockwise on the right)	6 in 2 weeks	Round	0.2	600	On	70% of max. output	12	1(150s left+300s Pause(?) +150s right)	Mild but significant decrease of UPDRS III in up to 7 days after rTMS
Okabe et al.	2003	Motor cortex	Sham condition + occipital lobe	8 (once a week)	Round	0.2	500	On	110% AMT	85	1(250s clockwise-250s anticlockwise)	No sigificant effect on UPDRS
Lefaucheur et al.	2004	M1(hand)	Sham coil	1	F8	0.5	1200	Off	80%	12	continuous	Significant decrease in UPDRS equal to 28-32% of the l-dopa effect
Arias et al.	2010	Vertex	Two coils (inactive coils beneath an active coil	10	Round	1	100	On	90%	9	1(50s clockwise-5min pause-50s anticlockwise)	No significant effects on any signs compared to placebo stimulation
Eggers et al.	2010	M1(hand)	Same coil placed 90° in angulation over M1	1	F8	50/5	40	Off	80% AMT	8	1(40s)	No significant effect on UPDRS III nor measures of cortical excitability

Table 2. Studies on the therapeutic use of low-frequency rTMS in patients with PD. Study-results reported here mainly refer to the UPDRS while other measures of motor excitability are mainly neglected. M1 = primary motor cortex, no. of ses. = number of sessions, F8 = figure of eight, Hz = Hertz, dd = dopaminergic drugs during stimulation, RMT = resting motor threshold, AMT = active motor threshold, DLPFC = dorsolateral prefrontal cortex, mA = milli Ampere, UPDRS = unified Parkinson's disease rating scale.

Authors	Year	Verum	Sham	No. Of ses.	Coil	Hz	Sec	dd	RMT	n	Method	Results
Siebner et al.	2000	M1(hand)	Midfrontal	1	F8	5	600	Off	90%	10	15(30 s stimulation + 10 s pause)	Significant decrease in UPDRS III 1 h after stimulation
Khedr et al.	2003	Lower limbs+M1(hand l+r)	Same condition, elevated+angled away from head	10 (consecutive days)	F8	5	400	Off	120%	36	200 s over lower limbs + 100s each over left and right hand	Significant decrease in UPDRS 1h after 1th, 5th, 10th stimulation and after one month
Lefaucheur et al.	2004	M1(hand)	Sham coil	1	F8	10	1200	Off	80%	12	20(10s stimulation+50s pause)	Significant decrease in UPDRS equal to 28-32% of the l-dopa effect
Lomarev et al.	2006	M1(hand) + DLPFC each left and right	Verum coil turned around 180°	8 (within 4 weeks)	Solid core coil	25	1200	On	100%	8+8	4(12s) each on left+right M1, left+right DLPFC	No significant effect on UPDRS; Significant improvement in other motor tests.
Del Olmo et al.	2007	DLPFC	Verum coil 7 cm rostrally to the vertex	10	F8	10	1800	On	90%	8+5	3(15(1s stimulation +10s pause)) separated by 10 min.	No significant change in UPDRS after stimulation. Significant improvement of other motor tests.
Benninger et al.	2011	M1(hand) + DLPFC each left and right	Sham coil	8	Solid core	50/5	190	On	80% AMT	13+13	20(2s TBS+8s pause)	No significant effect on UPDRS III; significant effect on mood

Table 3. Studies on the therapeutic use of high-frequency rTMS in patients with PD. Study-results reported here mainly refer to the UPDRS while other measures of motor excitability are mainly neglected.M1 = primary motor cortex, no. of ses. = number of sessions, F8 = figure of eight, Hz = Hertz, dd = dopaminergic drugs during stimulation, RMT = resting motor threshold, AMT = active motor threshold, TBS = theta burst stimulation, DLPFC = dorsolateral prefrontal cortex, mA = milli Ampere, UPDRS = unified Parkinson's disease rating scale.

Transcranial direct current stimulation:

There are few studies in which the therapeutic efficiency of tDCS in PD was investigated (Table 4). An improvement of motor function in patients with PD measured by the UPDRS after 20 minutes anodal but not cathodal tDCS over the M1 region has been reported (Fregni et al., 2006). Boggio et al. (2006) demonstrated that patients with PD performed better in a memory and alertness test during a left prefrontal tDCS than during sham-stimulation. In another study the technique of rTMS was combined with tDCS in order to improve bradykinesia in PD (Grüner et al., 2010). In this study low frequency rTMS over the primary motor cortex contralateral to the more effected upper extremity was preceded by either sham, cathodal or anodal tDCS. Whereas the results in different tests of movement control (frequency of finger and hand tapping, horizontal pointing movements) improved significantly after performing rTMS preceded by either sham or anodal tDCS the beneficial effect of 1 Hz rTMS on bradykinesia was reduced when preconditioning was performed with cathodal tDCS. Patients were tested while they were on dopaminergic drugs in this study as well. In the most recent study 25 participants with PD received 20 minutes of 2 mA anodal tDCS over the (pre)motor or prefrontal cortex on 8 days within 2.5 weeks each while on parkinsonian medication. A significant clinical improvement of the mobility of the upper extremity in the on- and off-state one day after the last stimulation was the main result in this study. But neither the velocity of gait nor the overall UPDRS score differed between sham and verum stimulation (Benninger et al., 2010). Also, there was a significant placebo effect in most conditions. However, size and montage of the electrodes used in this study differed from previous attempts possibly confounding the comparability of these results to earlier approaches and studies in healthy individuals. Finally, techniques of transcranial electrical stimulation may be able to improve symptoms of PD even though current data indicate that the effect size may be moderate. Development of new stimulation protocols may improve understanding of pathophysiological concepts of PD and increase therapeutic efficacy (Pogosyan et al., 2009; Moliadze et al., 2010).

Authors	Year	Location	Conditions	mA	Min	dd	n	Object	Results
Fregni et al.	2006	M1 DLPFC	Anodal/cathodal	1	20	Off	8/9	Motor performance	Significant improvement of UPDRS III (about 22% reduction) only after anodal stimulation of M1
Boggio et al.	2006	LDLPFC M1	Anodal/Sham Anodal/Sham	1 vs. 2	20	Off	9	Working memory	Significant improvement of working memory only with 2mA anodal stimulation of the LDLPFC
Grüner et al.	2010	M1	Anodal/Cathodal/ Sham	1	10	On	15	Motor performance	Significant improvement of motor performance (hand tapping and horizontal pointing frequency) after 1 Hz rTMS preconditioned by anodal or sham tDCS
Benninger et al.	2010	M1/M2 + Prefront. cortex	Anodal/Sham	2	20	On	25	Gait + hand and arm movements	Improvement of upper extremity bradykinesia 1 day after anodal stimulation

Table 4. Summary of the therapeutic studies of transcranial direct current stimulation (tDCS) in Parkinson's disease. M1 = primary motor cortex, M2 = premotor cortex, LDLPFC = left dorsolateral prefrontal cortex, mA = milli Ampere, UPDRS = unified Parkinson's disease rating scale.

3. Conclusion

Electrical or magnetic stimulation techniques amend the therapeutic tools for the treatment of PD. Among them, deep brain stimulation is the only approved treatment. It's positive effect on tremor and bradykinesia is significant and immediate in patients with advanced PD. In contrast, rTMS and tDCS are experimental techniques and their therapeutic effects, if present, are comparably small. Still, these techniques are relatively new and future protocols may improve their efficacy.

4. Acknowledgment

This work has been supported by the grant ZN 2187 of the Niedersachsen-Israel Research Cooperation Program, and by the DFG, grant NI 683/6-1.

5. References

Arias, P., Vivas, J., Grieve, K.L., et al. (2010). Controlled trial on the effect of 10 days low-frequency repetitive transcranial magnetic stimulation (rTMS) on motor signs in Parkinson's Disease. *Movement Disorders*, Vol. 25, pp. 1830-1838.

Bareš, M., Kaňovský, P., Klajblová, H., et al. (2003). Intracortical inhibition and facilitation are impaired in patients with early Parkinson's disease: a paired TMS study. *European Journal of Neurology*, Vol. 10, pp. 385-389.

Bauswein, E., Fromm, C. & Preuss, A. (1989). Corticostriatal cells in comparison with pyramidal tract neurons : contrasting properties in the behaving monkey. Brain *Research*, Vol. 493, pp. 198-203.

Benabid A.L., Pollak, P., Louveau, A., et al. (1987). Combined (thalamotomy and stimulation) stereotactic surgery of the VIM thalamic nucleus for bilateral Parkinson disease. *Applied Neurophysiology*, Vol. 50, pp. 344-346.

Benabid, A.L., Chabardes, S., Mitrofanis, J., et al. (2009). Deep brain stimulation of the subthalamic nucleus for the treatment of Parkinson's disease. *The Lancet Neurology*, Vol. 8, pp. 67-81.

Benninger, D.H., Lomarev, M., Lopez, G., et al. (2010). Transcranial direct current stimulation for the treatment of Parkinson's disease. *Journal of Neurology Neurosurgery and Psychiatry*, Vol. 81, pp. 1105-1111.

Benninger, D.H., Berman, B.D., Houdayer, E., et al. (2011). Intermittent theta-burst transcranial magnetic stimulation for treatment of Parkinson's disease. *Neurology*, Vol. 76, pp. 601-609.

Beurrier, C., Bioulac, B., Audin, J., et al. (2001). High-frequency stimulation produces a transient blockade of voltage-gated currents in subthalamic neurons. *Journal of Neurophysiology*, Vol. 85, pp. 1351-1356.

Boggio, P.S., Ferrucci, R., Rigonatti, S.P., et al. (2006). Effects of transcranial direct current stimulation on working memory in patients with Parkinson's disease. *Journal of the Neurological Sciences*, Vol. 249, pp. 31-38.

Brindley, G.S. & Lewin, W.S. (1968). The sensations produced by electrical stimulation of the visual cortex. *Journal of Physiology*, Vol. 196, pp. 479-493.

Cantello, R., Tartelli, R. & Civardi, C. (2002). Transcranial magnetic stimulation and Parkinson's disease. *Brain Research Reviews*, Vol. 38, pp. 309-327.

Ceballos-Baumann, A.O. (2003). Functional imaging in Parkinson's disease: activation studies with PET, fMRI and SPECT. *Journal of Neurology*, Vol. 250, Suppl. 1, pp. 15-23.

Charles, P.D., van Blercom, N., Krack, P., et al. (2002). Predictors of effective bilateral subthalamic nucleus stimulation for PD. *Neurology*, Vol. 59, pp. 932-934.

Chen, R., Classen, J., Gerloff, C., et al. (1997). Depression of motor cortex excitability by low-frequency transcranial magnetic stimulation. *Neurology*, Vol. 48, pp. 1398–1403.

Cooper, I.S. (1955). Chemopallidectomy : an investigative technique in geriatric parkinsonians. *Science*, Vol. 121, pp. 217-218.

Cooper, I.S., Amin, I., Riklan, M., et al. (1976). Chronic cerebellar stimulation in epilepsy. Clinical and anatomical studies. *Archives of Neurology*, Vol. 33, No. 8, pp. 559–570.

Del Olmo, M.F., Bello, O. & Cudeiro, J. (2007). Transcranial magnetic stimulation over dorsolateral prefrontal cortex in Parkinson's disease. *Clinical Neurophysiology*, Vol. 118, pp. 131-139.

Deuschl, G., Schade-Brittinger, C., Krack, P., et al. (2006). A randomized trial of deep-brain stimulation for Parkinson's disease. *New England Journal of Medicine*, Vol. 355, pp. 896-908.

Dostrovsky, J.O., Levy, R., Wu, J.P., et al. (2000). Microstimulation-induced inhibition of neuronal firing in human globus pallidus. *Journal of Neurophysiology*, Vol. 84, pp. 570-574.

Eggers, C., Fink, G.R. & Nowak, D.A. (2010). Theta burst stimulation over the primary motor cortex does not induce cortical plasticity in Parkinson's disease. *Journal of Neurology*, Vol. 257, No. 10, pp. 1669-1674.

Elahi, B., Elahi, B. & Chen, R. (2008). Effect of transcranial magnetic stimulation on Parkinson motor function-systematic review of controlled clinical trials. *Movement Disorders*, Vol. 24, No.3, pp. 357-363.

Follett, K.A., Weaver, F.M., Stern, M., et al. (2010). Pallidal versus subthalamic deep-brain stimulation for Parkinson's disease. *New England Journal of Medicine*, Vol. 362, pp. 2077-2091.

Fregni, F., Boggio, P.S., Santos, M.C., et al. (2006). Noninvasive cortical stimulation with transcranial direct current stimulation in Parkinson's disease. *Movement Disorders*, Vol. 21, No. 10, pp. 1693-1702.

Gamboa, O.L., Antal, A., Moliadze, V. et al. (2010). Simply longer is not better: reversal of theta burst after-effect with prolonged stimulation. *Experimental Brain Research*, Vol. 204, pp. 181-187.

Gentner, R., Wankerl, K., Reinsberger, C., et al. (2008). Depression of human corticospinal excitability induced by magnetic Theta-burst stimulation: evidence of rapid polarity-reversing metaplasticity. *Cerebral Cortex*, Vol. 18, pp. 2046-2053.

Gerfen, C.R., Engber, T.M., Mahan, L.C., et al. (1990). D1 and D2 dopamine receptor-regulated gene expression of striatonigral and striatopallidal neurons. *Science*, Vol. 250, pp. 1429-1432.

Gildenberg, P.L. (1977). Treatment of spasmodic torticollis with dorsal column stimulation. *Acta Neurochirurgica Supplement (Wien)*, Vol. 24, pp. 65–66.

Gildenberg, P.L. (2003). History repeats itself. *Stereotactic and Functional Neurosurgery*, Vol. 80, No. 1-4, pp. 61-75.

Gilio, F., Currà, A., Inghilleri, M., et al. (2002). Repetitive magnetic stimulation of cortical motor areas in Parkinson's disease: implications for the pathophysiology of cortical function. *Movement Disorders*, Vol. 17, pp. 467-473.

Ghika, J., Villemure, J., Fankhauser, H., et al. (1998). Efficiency and safety of bilateral contemporaneous pallidal stimulation (deep brain stimulation) in levodopa-responsive patients with Parkinson's disease with severe motor fluctuations: a 2 year follow-up. *Journal of Neurosurgery*, Vol. 89, pp. 713-718.

Gol, A. (1967). Relief of pain by electrical stimulation of the septal area. *Journal of the Neurological Science*, Vol. 5, pp. 115–120.

Grafton, S.T., Waters, C. & Sutton, J. (1995). Pallidotomy increases activity of motor association cortex in Parkinson's disease: a positron emission tomographic study. *Annals of Neurology*, Vol. 37, pp. 776-783.

Grüner, U., Eggers, C., Ameli, M., et al. (2010). 1 Hz rTMS preconditioned by tDCS over the primary motor cortex in Parkinson's disease : effects on bradykinesia of arm and hand. Journal of Neural Transmission, Vo. 117, pp. 207-216.

Hallett, M. (2007). Transcranial magnetic stimulation : a primer. *Neuron*, Vol. 55, pp. 187-199.

Hammond, C., Bergman, H. & Brown, P. (2007). Pathological synchronization in Parkinson's disease: networks, models and treatments. *Trends in Neuroscience*, Vol. 30, No. 7, pp. 357-264.

Hariz, M.I., Blomstedt, P. & Zrinzo, L. (2010). Deep brain stimulation between 1947 and 1987: the untold story. *Neurosurgery Focus*, Vol. 29, No. 2 :E1, pp. 1-10.

Hartmann-von Monakow, K., Akert, K. & Künzle, H. (1978). Projections of the precentral motor cortex and other cortical areas of the frontal lobe to the subthalamic nucleus in the monkey. *Experimental Brain Research*, Vol. 33, pp. 395-403.

Hollerman, J.R. & Schultz, W. (1998). Dopamine neurons report an error in the temporal prediction of reward during learning. *Nature Neuroscience*, Vol. 1, pp. 304-309.

Hoover, J.E. & Strick, P.L. (1993). Multiple output channels in the basal ganglia. *Science*, Vol. 259, pp. 819-821.

Huang, Y.-Z., Edwards, M.J., Rounis, E., et al. (2005). Theta burst stimulation of the human motor cortex. *Neuron*, Vol. 45, pp. 201-206.

Huang, Y.-Z., Rothwell, J.C., Edwards, M.J., et al. (2008). Effect of physiological activity on an NMDA-dependent form of cortical plasticity in human. *Cerebral Cortex*, Vol. 18, pp. 563-570.

Ikeguchi, M., Touge, T., Nishiyama, Y., et al. (2003). Effects of successive repetitive transcranial magnetic stimulation on motor performances and brain perfusion in idiopathic Parkinson's disease. *Journal of the Neurological Sciences*, Vol. 209, pp. 41-46.

Khedr, E.M., Farweez, H.M. & Islam, I. (2003). Therapeutic effect of repetitive transcranial magnetic stimulation on motor function in Parkinson's disease patients. *European Journal of Neurology*, Vol. 10, pp. 567-572.

Kuo, M.-F., Paulus, W. & Nitsche, M.A. (2008). Boosting focally-induced brain plasticity by dopamine. *Cerebral Cortex*, Vol. 18, pp. 648-651.

Lanska, D.J. (2010). The history of movement disorders, In: *Handbook of Clinical Neurology, Vol. 95 History of Neurology*, S. Finger, F. Boller, K.L. Tyler, (Eds.), pp. 501-546, Elsevier, ISBN 978-0-444-52009-8, Amsterdam, The Netherlands.

Lefaucheur, J.-P. (2005). Motor cortex dysfunction revealed by cortical excitability studies in Parkinson's disease: influence of antiparkinsonian treatment and cortical stimulation. *Clinical Neurophysiology*, Vol. 116, pp. 244-253.

Lefaucheur, J.-P. Drouot, X., Von Raison, F., et al. (2004). Improvement of motor performance and modulation of cortical excitability by repetitive transcranial magnetic stimulation of the motor cortex in Parkinson's disease. *Clinical Neurophysiology*, Vol.115, No., pp. 2530-2541.

Levesque, J.C. & Parent, A. (2005). GABAergic interneurons in human subthalamic nucleus. *Movement Disorders*, Vol. 20, pp. 574-584.

Liebetanz, D., Nitsche, M.A., Tergau, F., et al. (2002). Pharmacological approach to the mechanisms of transcranial DC-stimulation-induced after-effects of human motor cortex excitability. *Brain*, Vol. 125, pp. 2238-2247.

Limousin, P., Greene, J., Pollak, P., et al. (1997). Changes in cerebral activity pattern due to subthalamic nucleus or internal pallidum stimulation in Parkinson's disease. *Annals of Neurology*, Vol. 42, pp. 283-291.

Lomarev, M.P., Kanchana, S., Bara-Jimenez, W., et al. (2006). Placebo-controlled study of rTMS for the treatment of Parkinson's disease. *Movement Disorders*, Vol. 21, No. 3, pp. 325-331.

Maurice, N., Theirry, A.-M., Glowinski, J., et al. (2003). Spontaneous and evoked activity of substantia nigra pars reticulata neurons during High-frequency stimulation of the subthalamic nucleus. *The Journal of Neuroscience*, Vol. 2003, No. 30, pp. 9929-9936.

Merello, M. (2008). Deep brain stimulation of the subthalamic nucleus for the treatment of Parkinson's disease. In: *Deep brain stimulation in neurological and psychiatric disorders*, Tarsy, D., Vitek, J.L., Starr, P.A. & Okun, M.S. (Eds.), pp. 253-276, Humana Press, Totowa, The United States of America.

Merton, P.A. & Morton, H.B. (1980). Stimulation of the cerebral cortex in the intact human subject. *Nature*, Vol. 285., p. 227.

Mihailovic, L. & Delgado, J.M.R. (1956). Electrical stimulation of monkey brain with various frequencies and pulse durations. *Journal of Neurophysiology*, Vol. 19, No. 1, pp. 21-36.

Moliadze, V., Antal, A. & Paulus, W. (2010). Boosting brain excitability by transcranial high frequency stimulation in the ripple range. *Journal of Physiology*, Vol. 588, pp. 4891-4904.

Monte-Silva, K., Kuo, M-F., Thirugnanasambandam, N., et al. (2009). Dose-dependent inverted U-shaped effect of dopamine (D2-like) receptor activation on focal and nonfocal plasticity in humans. *The Journal of Neuroscience*, Vol. 29, pp. 6124-6131.

Nitsche, M.A. & Paulus, W. (2000). Excitability changes induced in the human motor cortex by weak transcranial direct current stimulation. *Journal of Physiology*, Vol. 527, No., pp. 633-639.

Nitsche, M.A., Lampe, C., Antal, A., et al. (2006). Dopaminergic modulation of long-lasting direct current-induced cortical excitability changes in the human motor cortex. *European Journal of Neuroscience*, Vol. 23, pp. 1651-1657.

Nitsche, M.A., Roth, A., Kuo, M.-F., et al. (2007). Timing-dependent modulation of associative plasticity by general network excitability in the human motor cortex. *The Journal of Neuroscience*, Vol. 27, No. 14, pp. 3807-3812.

Nowak, L.G. & Bullier, J. (1998). Axons, but not cell bodies are activated by electrical stimulation in cortical gray matter. I. Evidence from chronaxie measurements. *Experimental Brain Research*, Vol. 118, pp. 477-488.

Okabe, S., Ugawa, Y., Kanazawa, I., et al. (2003). 0.2-Hz repetitive transcranial magnetic stimulation has no add-on effects as compared to a realistic sham stimulation in Parkinson's disease. *Movement Disorders*, Vol. 18, No. 4, pp. 382-388.

Parent, A. (1990). Extrinsic connections of the basal ganglia. *Trends in Neuroscience*, Vol. 13, No. 7, pp. 254-258.

Pascual-Leone, A., Valls-Solé, J., Wassermann, E.M., et al. (1994). Responses to rapid-rate transcranial magnetic stimulation of the human cortex. *Brain*, Vol. 117, pp. 847-858.

Perlmutter, J.S. & Mink, J. (2006). Deep brain stimulation. *Annual Reviews of Neuroscience*, Vol. 29, No., pp. 229-257.

Pogosyan, A., Gaynor, L.D., Eusebio, A., et al. (2009). Boosting cortical activity at beta-band frequencies slows movement in humans. *Current Biology*, Vol. 19, No. 19, pp. 1637-1641.

Priori, A., Berardelli, A., Inghilleri. M., et al. (1994). Motor cortical inhibition and the dopaminergic system. Pharmacological changes in the silent period after transcranial brain stimulation in normal subjects, patients with Parkinson's disease and drug-induced parkinsonism. *Brain*, Vol. 117, pp. 317–323.

Ranck, J.B. (1975). Which elements are excited in electrical stimulation of mammalian central nervous system: A review. *Brain Research*, Vol. 98, pp. 417-440.

Rodriguez-Oroz, M.C., Obeso, J.A., Lang, A.E., et al. (2005). Bilateral deep brain stimulation in Parkinson's disease: a multicentre study with 4 years follow-up. *Brain*, Vol. 128, pp. 2240-2249.

Rothkegel, H., Sommer, M., Rammsayer, T., et al. (2009). Training effects outweigh effects of single-session conventional rTMS and theta burst stimulation in PD patients. *Neurorehabilitation and Neural Repair*, Vol. 23, pp. 373-381.

Schuurman, P.R., Bosch, D.A., Bossuyt, P.M.N., et al. (2000). A comparison of continuous thalamic stimulation and thalamotomy for suppression of severe tremor. *New England Journal of Medicine*, Vol. 342, pp. 461-468.

Shealy, C.N., Mortimer, J.T. & Reswick, J.B. (1967). Electrical inhibition of pain by stimulation of the dorsal columns. Preliminary clinical report. *Anesthesia and Analgesia (Cleveland)*, Vol. 46, pp. 489–491.

Shimamoto, H., Takasaki, K., Shigemori, M., et al. (2001). Therapeutic effect and mechanism of repetitive transcranial magnetic stimulation in Parkinson's disease. *Journal of Neurology*, Vol. 248, Suppl. 3, III/48-III/52.

Shink, E., Bevan, M.D., Bolam, J.P., et al. (1996). The subthalamic nucleus and the external pallidum: two tightly interconnected structures that control the output o the basal ganglia in the monkey. *Neuroscience*, Vol. 73, No. 2, pp. 335-357.

Siebner, H.R., Rossmeier, C., Mentschel, C., et al. (2000). Short-term motor improvement after sub-threshold 5-Hz repetitive transcranial magnetic stimulation of the primary motor hand area in Parkinson's disease. *Journal of the Neurological Sciences*, Vol. 178, pp. 91-94.

Spiegel, E.A., Wycis, H.T., Marks, M., et al. (1947). Stereotaxic apparatus for operations on the human brain. *Science*, Vol. 106, pp. 349-350.

Stephani, C., Nitsche, M.A., Sommer, M., et al. (2011). Impairment of motor cortex plasticity in Parkinson's disease, as revealed by theta-burst transcranial magnetic stimulation and transcranial random noise stimulation. *Parkinsonism and Related Disorders*, Vol. 17, pp. 297-298.

Stoney, S.D., Thompson, W.D. & Asanuma, H. (1968). Excitation of pyramidal tract cells by intracortical microstimulation: effective extent of stimulating current. *Journal of Neurophysiology*, Vol. 31, pp. 659-669.

Strafella, A.P., Paus, T., Barrett, J., et al. (2001). Repetitive transcranial magnetic stimulation of the human prefrontal cortex induces dopamine release in the caudate nucleus. *The Journal of Neuroscience*, Vol. 21RC157, No., pp. 1-4.

Takada, M., Tokuno, H., Hamada, I., et al. (2001). Organization of inputs from cingulate motor areas to basal ganglia in macaque monkey. *European Journal of Neuroscience*, Vol. 14, pp. 1633-1650.

Tarsy, D., Papavassiliou, E., Lyons, K.E., et al. (2008). Thalamic deep brain stimulation for Parkinson's disease tremor. In: *Deep brain stimulation in neurological and psychiatric disorders*, Tarsy, D., Vitek, J.L., Starr, P.A. & Okun, M.S. (Eds.), pp. 229-242, Humana Press, Totowa, The United States of America.

Terney, D., Chaieb, L., Moliadze, V., et al. (2008). Increasing human brain excitability by transcranial high-frequency random noise stimulation. *The Journal of Neuroscience*, Vol. 28, No. 52, pp. 14147-14155.

Turner, R.S. & DeLong, M.R. (2000). Corticostriatal activity in primary motor cortex of the macaque. *The Journal of Neuroscience*, Vol. 20, No. 18, pp. 7096-7108.

Ueki, Y., Mima, T., Kotb, M.A., et al. (2006). Altered plasticity of the human motor cortex in Parkinson's disease. *Annals of Neurology*, Vol. 59, pp. 60-71.

Vitek, J.L. (2002). Mechanisms of deep brain stimulation: excitation or inhibition. *Movement Disorders*, Vol. 17, Suppl. 3, pp. S69-S72.

Volkmann, J., Moro, E. & Pahwa, R. (2006). Basic algorithms for the programming of deep brain stimulation in Parkinson's disease. *Movement Disorders*, Vol. 21, Suppl. 14, pp. S284-S289.

Weaver, F., Follett, K. & Stern, M. (2008). Globus pallidus deep brain stimulation for Parkinson's disease. In: *Deep brain stimulation in neurological and psychiatric disorders*, Tarsy, D., Vitek, J.L., Starr, P.A. & Okun, M.S. (Eds.), pp. 243,-252, Humana Press, Totowa, The United States of America.

Welter, M.L., Houeto, J.L., Tezenas du Montcel, S. et al. (2002). Clinical predictive factors of subthalamic stimulation in Parkinson's disease. *Brain*, Vol. 125, pp. 575-583.

Welter, M.L., Houeto, J.L., Bonnet, A.M., et al. (2004). Effects of high-frequency stimulation on subthalamic neuronal activity in parkinsonian patients. *Archives of Neurology*, Vol. 61, pp. 89-96.

Windels, F., Bruet, N., Poupard, A., et al. (2003). Influence of the frequency parameter on extracellular glutamate and gamma-aminobutyric acid in substantia nigra and globus pallidus during electrical stimulation of subthalamic nucleus in rats. *Journal of Neuroscience Research*, Vol. 72, No. 2, pp. 259-267.

Wichmann, T. & DeLong, M.R. (2007). Anatomy and physiology of the basal ganglia : relevance to Parkinson's disease and related disorders. In: *Handbook of Clinical Neurology, Vol. 83, Parkinson's disease and related disorders Part I*, Koller, W.C. & Melamed, E. (Eds.), pp. 3-18, ISBN 978-0-444-52900-9, Amsterdam, The Netherlands.

Wu, A.D., Fregni, F., Simon, D.K., et al. (2008). Noninvasive brain stimulation for Parkinson's disease and dystonia. *Neurotherapeutics*, Vol. 5, No. 2, pp. 345-361.

Ziemann, U. (2004). TMS and drugs. *Clinical Neurophysiology*, Vol. 115, pp. 1717-1729.

Ziemann, U., Meintzschel, F., Korchounov, A., et al. (2006). Pharmacological modulation of plasticity in the human motor cortex. *Neurorehabilitation and Neural Repair*, Vol. 20, pp. 243-251.

Ziemann, U., Tergau, F., Bruns, D., et al. (1997). Changes in human motor cortex excitability induced by dopaminergic and anti-dopaminergic drugs. *Electroencephalography and Clinical Neurophysiology*, Vol. 105, pp. 430-437.

12

Mechanisms of High Frequency Stimulation of the Subthalamic Nucleus in Parkinson's Disease: From Local to Distal Effects on the Basal Ganglia Network

Marc Savasta, Carole Carcenac and Sabrina Boulet
Grenoble Institute of Neuroscience,
Dynamic and Pathophysiology of Basal Ganglia,
France

1. Introduction

1.1 Parkinson's disease, basal ganglia and the value of the subthalamic nucleus as a treatment target

Parkinson's disease (PD) is the second most common neurodegenerative disorder affecting about 1% of adults over the age of 60 years (Samii et al., 2004). It is caused by a progressive loss of the dopaminergic neurons of the substantia nigra pars compacta (SNc) and of their axons, which project to the striatum (Ehringer & Hornykiewicz, 1960). Degeneration of the nigrostriatal pathway results in the development of the motor symptoms characteristic of the disease, including tremor, rigidity, postural abnormalities and bradykinesia. These cardinal signs of PD reflect striatal dopamine (DA) depletion, leading to the global disorganization of the activity of the basal ganglia (BG), a complex network of subcortical nuclei involved in the control and execution of motor behavior.

According to the classical model of BG organization (Albin et al., 1989; Alexander et al., 1990; DeLong, 1990), the interruption of dopaminergic transmission induces an imbalance between the activity of the two striatal circuits, the so-called 'direct' and 'indirect' pathways (Fig. 1). The activity of the inhibitory striatal neurons projecting directly to the substantia nigra pars reticulata (SNr) and the globus pallidus internalis (GPi), the direct pathway, is decreased. Conversely, the activity of the inhibitory striatal neurons projecting to the globus pallidus externalis (GPe) is increased, disinhibiting the activity of the subthalamic nucleus (STN), which projects excitatory glutamatergic neurons to the SNr and the GPi (indirect pathway). As efferent neurons of the SNr and GPi are GABAergic and are tonically active, this increase in indirect pathway activity results in an increase in the inhibitory output from the BG output structures to the thalamus and the thalamocortical neurons. The resulting reduction of cortical activation accounts for some of the signs of PD, such as akinesia (Albin et al., 1989; Bolam et al., 2000; DeLong, 1990; Obeso et al., 2008; Parent & Hazrati, 1995a, b). Based on this model and the results of others studies demonstrating the key role of the STN in controlling movement (Kita & Kitai, 1987; Kitai & Deniau, 1981; Smith et al., 1998), it has been suggested that the abnormal glutamatergic hyperactivity observed in the STN in the parkinsonian state plays a critical role in the expression of motor symptoms (Bergman et al.,

1994; Blandini et al., 1996, 2000; Carlsson & Carlsson, 1990; Hassani et al., 1996). Thus, it may be possible to restore equilibrium by decreasing STN neuronal output, through procedures such as lesioning or other manipulations (DeLong, 1990).

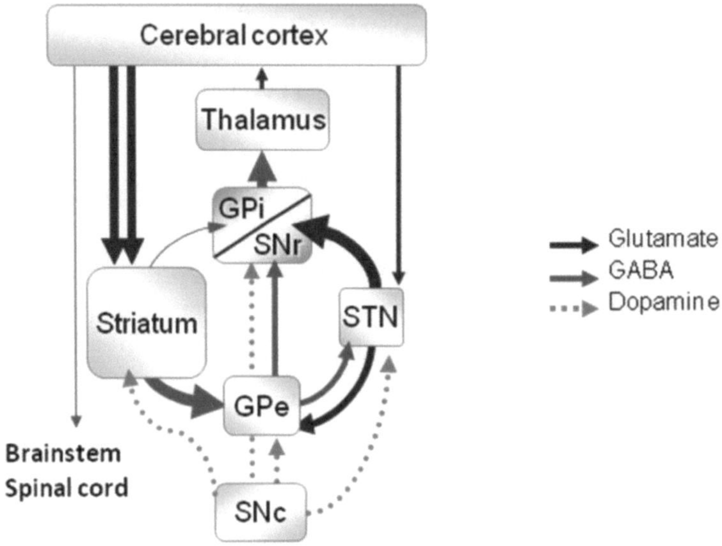

Fig. 1. Functional organization of the basal ganglia and classical pathophysiological model of Parkinson's disease. SNr, substantia nigra pars reticulata; SNc, substantia nigra pars compacta; STN, subthalamic nucleus; GPe, globus pallidus externalis; GPi, globus pallidus internalis.

This hypothesis has been supported by several experimental studies in animal models of PD in which neurotoxic lesions (Aziz et al., 1991; Bergman et al., 1990) and pharmacological blockade of the STN (Levy et al., 2001) or the administration of glutamatergic (NMDA) antagonists (Greenamyre & O'Brien, 1991) are used to reduce motor impairments. These results obtained, together with the observation that the gold standard pharmacological treatment of PD - the daily administration of the DA precursor levodopa (L-DOPA) - induces severe side effects, such as motor fluctuations and dyskinesia after several years of use (Poewe et al., 1986; Rascol, 2000; Starr, 1995), have excited renewed interest in surgical approaches to PD treatment, with the STN as a target of choice. Surgical or accidental lesions of the STN in PD patients improve parkinsonian symptoms, including the tremor in particular, and are associated with a large decrease in the dose of L-DOPA required (Barlas et al., 2001; Gill & Heywood, 1997; Patel et al., 2003). However, such lesions may also result in permanent hemiballismus (for a review, see Guridi & Obeso, 2001). The behavioral effects of high-frequency stimulation (HFS) are usually similar to those of lesions of the structure stimulated. Futhermore, it has been demonstrated in a primate model of PD that STN-HFS improves parkinsonian motor symptoms (Benazzouz et al., 1993). This led to the initiation of clinical trials using STN-HFS for the treatment of PD (Limousin et al., 1995a, b).

Many studies on the efficacy of STN-HFS for the treatment of parkinsonian motor syndrome have since been carried out. STN-HFS has been reported to induce clinical improvement in both PD patients and experimental animal models, resulting in large decrease in L-DOPA requirement, and consequently decreasing L-DOPA-induced dyskinesia (Bejjani et al., 2000;

Benabid et al., 1998, 2000; Krack et al., 1998, 2003; Krause et al., 2001; Moro et al., 1999). STN-HFS is now widely agreed to be a powerful surgical option for the treatment of advanced PD. Nevertheless, despite its remarkable clinical efficacy, the precise mechanisms by which STN-HFS exerts its effects remain a matter of debate.

2. Mechanisms of action of subthalamic nucleus high frequency stimulation: inhibition or excitation?

2.1 The first hypothesis

As the functional effects of STN-HFS resemble those of STN lesion (Benazzouz et al., 1995), it was initially assumed that HFS inhibited STN neurons (Benabid et al., 2002; Dostrovsky & Lozano, 2002) via a depolarization-induced blockade of their activity, resulting in depression of the STN-driven BG output nuclei. This HFS-induced inhibition hypothesis was supported by several lines of experimental evidence, including slice recordings (Beurrier et al., 2001; Magarinos-Ascone et al., 2002), in vivo recordings in rodents (Benazzouz et al., 2000; Tai et al., 2003) and primates (Boraud et al., 1996) and recordings in human patients (Benabid et al., 1998; Filali et al., 2004). However, due to technical problems precluding recording during the stimulation period, most of these electrophysiological data were obtained immediately after STN-HFS was stopped. Furthermore, they concerned very short periods of stimulation (5 seconds to 1 minute).

These technical limitations, together with the work of Benazzouz et al. reporting the activation of 100% of GP cells immediately after STN-HFS cast doubt on the depolarization block hypothesis (Benazzouz et al., 1995). However, the first real challenge to the silencing hypothesis came in the form of neurochemical data obtained in normal anesthetized rats subjected to one hour of subthalamic stimulation applied with therapeutic parameters. These data showed that STN-HFS induced the release of glutamate in the SNr and entopeduncular nucleus (EP, the rat equivalent of GPi), two direct target structures of STN neurons (Windels et al., 2000, 2003). This effect, measured during stimulation, conflicted with the depolarization block hypothesis as it showed that STN neurons and their axons could be activated during HFS. Following technical improvements, these pioneering results were soon supported by electrophysiological recordings. In particular, data acquired in MPTP-treated monkeys showed that STN-HFS, when applied at parameters that decrease akinesia, changes the spontaneous irregular firing of STN target cells (GPe and GPi) to a high-frequency regular pattern of discharge time-locked to the stimulation and resulting in a significant increase in the mean discharge rate of both structures (Hashimoto et al., 2003). Another study in rats suggested that the activity of SNr cells was increased by the application of STN-HFS at a 'high' stimulation intensity (Maurice et al., 2003). However, although the authors described this intensity (300 μA) as 'high' based on a comparison with the other intensities used in their study (20-80 μA), it corresponds to intensities commonly used in rats. Finally, Garcia et al. showed that the application of HFS at clinical parameters drove the STN activity in rat slices in vitro, suppressing all types of spontaneous STN activity and imposing a new pattern of activity on STN neurons (Garcia et al., 2003). All these studies argue against the notion that HFS totally silences STN neurons, thereby reducing the excitatory input of basal ganglia output nuclei. However, these results are consistent with previous work showing that STN neurons are able to fire at much higher frequencies than 130 Hz, following current injections, suggesting that they are unlikely to show a substantial depolarization block in the frequency range generally known to have therapeutic effects (Bevan & Wilson, 1999).

2.2 Sites of action within the brain

Many others neurochemical (Galati et al., 2006; Lee et al., 2007; Stefani et al., 2005; Windels et al., 2005), electrophysiological (Degos et al., 2005; Kita et al., 2005; Li et al., 2010; Shi et al., 2006) and functional imaging (Hilker et al., 2008) studies in both animal models and PD patients have generated apparently conflicting results on the effects of HFS on neuronal activities. Based on these observations, the impact of therapeutic STN-HFS cannot be limited to the simple blockade of STN neurons activity. Instead, it probably involves complex and distinct effects on the cell soma and axons, combining local inhibitory and excitatory effects and resultant distal effects.

2.2.1 Effects at the local level

A number of studies have revealed the complexity of the effects of HFS on STN neuron activity. Three main types of effects have been reported: 1) extinction or strong inhibition of neuronal activity 2) an increased in activity and 3) dual effects combining inhibition and the induction of high frequency bursts (Fig. 2).

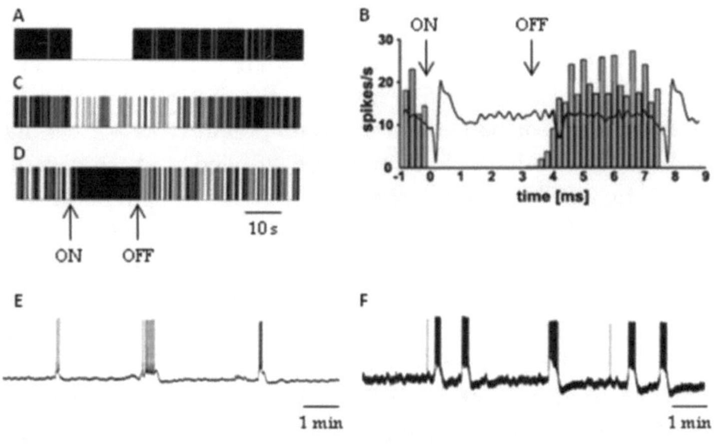

Fig. 2. Electrophysiological effects of STN-HFS at local level. Raster displays (A, C and D) and filter analogue recordings (B) representing a typical example of complete (*A and B*) and partial inhibition (C) or of excitation (D) in STN neurons during HFS of the STN. A, C and D modified from Tai et al. (2003), B modified from Meissner et al. (2005). E and F, control spontaneous bursting activity of STN neurons (E) and bursting activity of STN neurons (F) evoked by 10 minutes duration 185Hz HFS, modified from Garcia et al. (2003).

The inhibition and suppression of STN activity are the effects most frequently induced by stimulation in both animal models of the disease and humans (Fig. 2A, B and C). Indeed, while recording STN discharge during surgery in PD patients, both Welter et al. (2004) and Filali et al. (2004) reported the inhibition of activity in a significant number of STN neurons (50 to 75%), associated with a decrease in the mean firing rate of the cells. However, this decrease did not prevent residual neuronal activity, which persisted in 70% of the recorded neurons and was associated in some cases with a change in the firing pattern (Welter et al., 2004).This change in firing pattern, although not systematically observed, may make an important contribution to the clinical effects of STN-HFS. Indeed, studies recording the activity of STN neurons activity in PD patients during clinically effective deep brain stimulation (DBS) have reported a change in discharge pattern, with about one half of the neurons originally classified as bursting or tonic firing neurons shifting to a random pattern during and after delivery of the stimulus train (Carlson et al., 2010; Walker et al., 2010). Inhibition of neuronal activity was also obtained in in vitro (Beurrier et al., 2001; Magarinos-Ascone et al., 2002) and in vivo studies. In rats, Tai et al. (2003) observed a significant decrease in firing rate or even the inhibition of most neurons during the stimulation, combined with a decrease in CoI mRNA levels. In non human primates, a substantial decrease in overall firing rate was also shown (Meissner et al., 2005). According to the authors, this decrease in mean firing rate can be accounted for by a pause in firing lasting several milliseconds after each pulse and resulting from the resetting of the firing probability of STN neurons to almost zero by the stimulus pulse (Carlson et al., 2010; Meissner et al., 2005). As the firing probability returned to baseline values 7 ms after the onset of the electrical stimulus, the overall decrease in mean firing rate resulted from the repetition of a dynamic process with a frequency of 130 Hz (inter stimulus interval 7.7ms) allowing the neuron to fire with its baseline firing rate only for a very short period. None of these studies addressed the issue of the mechanisms giving rise to this observed inhibition, but they clearly demonstrated that this phenomenon could not be due to a depolarization block of STN neurons as it was initially supposed. Another hypothesis can be put forward to account for this partial or total inhibition of STN neurons activity. STN neurons are glutamatergic, so the observed inhibition may result from the stimulation of extrinsic sources of synaptic inputs. The release of GABA following excitation of the GPe, the main GABAergic afferents in STN, is clearly one possible mechanism (Meissner et al., 2005; Tai et al., 2003) potentially accounting for these findings, including the short duration of inhibition observed after a single stimulus (Filali et al., 2004). Synaptic inhibitory processes of this type have major implications for the therapeutic mechanisms of STN-HFS as, unlike lesions and functional inactivation, they do not completely block the transmission of information through the STN. HFS seems to inhibit the activity of a clear majority of STN neurons, but some neurons in animal models of PD (Tai et al., 2003) and in patients (Walker et al., 2010) responded to stimulation by an increase in activity (Fig. 2D).These apparently conflicting findings are not necessarily inconsistent, as inhibition of the cell body does not preclude simultaneous excitation of the axon or even excitation of the cell body together with the inhibition of spontaneous firing. Indeed, computational modeling has shown that, despite the suppression of somatic neuronal activity during HFS, axonal stimulation may still occur within the STN at relatively high stimulation frequencies (McIntyre et al., 2004). This theoretical model is supported by the results of in vivo and in vitro studies. Using an enzyme-linked glutamate sensor, Lee et al. (2007) showed that HFS increased the extracellular concentration of glutamate in the STN of anesthetized rats, providing support for the notion that HFS can activate afferent axons of the STN. Glutamate within the STN may initially be excitatory. However, the post-synaptic effects of glutamate receptor activation are mediated by various glutamate receptors, including the AMPA and kaïnate ionotropic receptors. These receptors are rapidly desensitized in the presence of glutamate.

The prolonged increase in glutamate concentration induced by STN-HFS may eventually desensitize local AMPA/kaïnate receptors, thereby preventing any further spontaneous activity of STN neurons, despite continued electrical stimulation. However, it does not prevent the direct activation of the neuronal membrane. Consistent with these data and the hypothesized coexistence of simultaneous excitation and inhibition mechanisms within the STN level, Garcia et al. (2003) showed, in an in vitro study, that HFS has a dual effect at therapeutically relevant frequencies (80-185Hz); it entirely abolishes all types of spontaneous activity within the STN and generates a robust pattern of recurrent bursts of spikes, with each spike being time locked to a stimulus pulse, thus reflecting direct activation of the axon and back-firing of the soma (Fig. 2E and F). This HFS driven discharge of STN neurons has not been reported in vivo, but is fully consistent with earlier reports of antidromic activation elicited by HFS in the nuclei anatomically connected to the STN (Li et al., 2010; Maurice et al., 2003). It also provides an additional line of evidence that information transmission via the trans-subthalamic pathway is not completely blocked during STN-HFS.

These observations highlight the multiplicity of effects recorded at local level, which may differ considerably according to the experimental conditions. The electrical field generated by the clinical DBS electrode has been extensively modeled (Butson & McIntyre, 2006; 2008; Miocinovic et al., 2009). Estimation of the current density surrounding a microelectrode tip is more challenging, but currents in the range of 50 to 500 μA are used, yielding a current density one to two orders of magnitude greater than those obtained with a DBS electrode. The particular neural element activated depends on current density (Rattay & Aberham, 1993), so extrapolation from the effects of a microelectrode to DBS electrode stimulation may be erroneous. Furthermore, despite the major contribution of computational models to our understanding of how and where neural elements are affected by stimulation pulses, these models remain of limited value for predicting the full extent of the effects induced by DBS, as they do not take into account the intranuclear organization of connection fibers. Depending on the spatial arrangement of fiber paths and intranuclear connections, neurons located well beyond the limit of the efficient stimulating current may be influenced by fibers activated by the stimulating electrode. Finally, detailed knowledge of the organization of intranuclear fiber paths, the precise location of the electrode and the electric field it generates must be taken into account when trying to understand the mechanisms of action of STN-HFS.

2.2.2 Effects at distal level

By activating axons, STN-HFS may generate widespread and heterogeneous distal effects. Experimental support for this hypothesis is provided by the observation that therapeutic stimulation of the STN in PD patients and animal models of the disease induces a change in the activity of BG structures anatomically connected to the STN, including its main direct target structures, the SNr (Benazzouz et al., 1995; Boulet et al., 2006; Burbaud et al., 1994; Degos et al., 2005; Galati et al., 2006; Maltete et al., 2007; Maurice et al., 2003; Shi et al., 2006; Tai et al., 2003; Windels et al., 2000, 2003) and GPi (Burbaud et al., 1994; Hahn et al., 2008; Hashimoto et al., 2003; Kita et al., 2005; Reese et al., 2008; Shi et al., 2006; Stefani et al., 2005), GPe (Hahn et al., 2008; Hashimoto et al., 2003; Kita et al., 2005; Windels et al., 2000, 2003), striatum (Bruet et al., 2001; Hilker et al., 2003; Lee et al., 2006 ; Meissner et al., 2001, 2002; Strafella et al., 2003), cortex (Butson & McIntyre, 2008; Fraix et al., 2008; Kuriakose et al., 2009) and thalamus (Benazzouz et al., 2000; Dorval et al., 2008).

As already observed for local effects, the effects of STN-HFS on distal structures appear contradictory. The first electrophysiological studies on anesthetized rats focused on the activity of the principal BG output nuclei, the SNr and EP. They reported a decrease of neuronal activity and firing rate in these structures after (Benazzouz et al., 1995, 2000) or during (Burbaud et al., 1994) application of STN-HFS. Others recordings acquired in normal or parkinsonian animals and in humans confirmed and extended these initial findings (Kita et al., 2005; Maltete et al., 2007; Maurice et al., 2003; Tai et al., 2003).This inhibition was initially thought to result from the suppression of STN cell activity (Benazzouz et al., 1995, 2000). However, it is actually more likely to result from the activation of GABAergic inputs as it is blocked by the local iontophoretic application of bicucculine, a $GABA_A$ receptor antagonist (Maurice et al., 2003)and as STN-HFS induces GABA release in the SNr (Boulet et al., 2006; Tai et al., 2003; Windels et al., 2000, 2003) (Fig. 3A). Lesions of the GP completely abolished this increase in GABA concentration in the SNr, then suggesting that GP GABAergic neurons constitute a major source of GABA in the SNr and that the activation of the GABAergic pallido-nigral pathway by HFS-STN contributes to the effects of this treatment (Windels et al., 2005) (Fig. 3B).This activation may occur in different ways, given the connections of the GP (Kita, 2007): a synaptic activation of the pallido-nigral neurons via the glutamatergic subthalamo-pallidal projections, an axon reflex resulting from antidromic activation of the pallidal neurons projecting to both the STN and the SNr and/or a direct stimulation of the pallido-nigral axons in the STN.

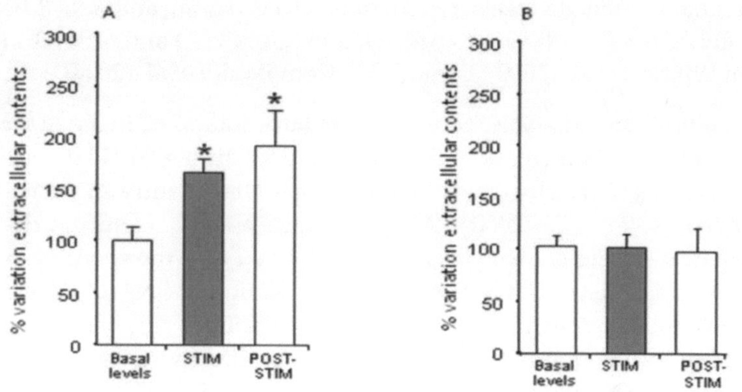

Fig. 3. Extracellular GABA levels determined before, during and after 1 hour STN-HFS in the ipsilateral SNr of 6-OHDA (A) or ibotenic acid GP plus SNc lesioned rats (B). Modified from Windels et al. (2005).

However, as shown by electrophysiological studies in rodents (Maurice et al., 2003; Tai et al., 2003), primates (Hashimoto et al., 2003; Kita et al., 2005) and PD patients (Hahn et al., 2008) and by functional MRI (Jech et al., 2006) and PET (Hershey et al., 2003; Perlmutter et al., 2002) studies in humans, STN-HFS can also increase the activity and the mean firing rate of basal ganglia output nuclei and the GPe. These excitatory effects, probably resulting from activation of the subthalamo-nigral and subthalamo-pallidal pathway, are not surprising as those axons are primarily glutamatergic (Kita & Kitai, 1987). The significant increase in extracellular glutamate concentration in the GP (Fig. 4A) and SNr (Fig. 4B) observed during prolonged STN HFS in microdialysis studies (Boulet et al., 2006; Tai et al., 2003; Windels et al., 2000, 2003) and the latencies of the excitatory responses evoked in nigral cells by STN-HFS (Maurice et al., 2003) are consistent with this hypothesis. Nevertheless, the effect of STN-HFS on the excitatory influence of the trans-subthalamic pathway on SNr cells appears to be dependent on the stimulation intensity used. Indeed, increasing HFS intensity facilitates excitatory responses, as low-intensity HFS induces principally an inhibition in SNr cells and an increase in extracellular GABA concentration, whereas higher HFS induces excitation and an increase in extracellular glutamate concentration (Boulet et al., 2006; Maurice et al., 2003; Tai et al., 2003).

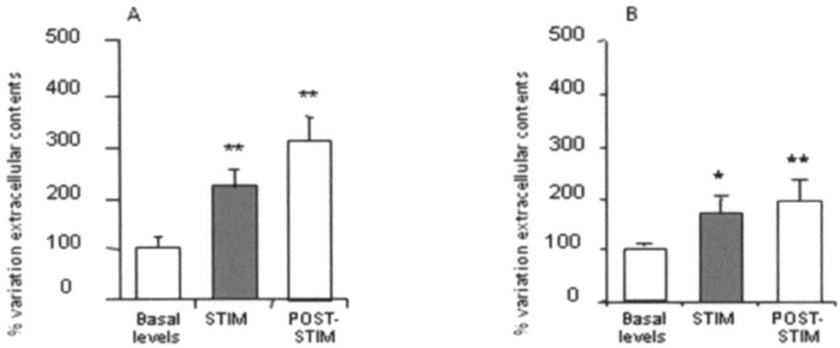

Fig. 4. Extracellular Glutamate levels determined before, during and after 1 hour STN-HFS in the GP (A) and SNr (B) ipsilateral to STN-HFS in normal (A) and 6-OHDA (B) rats. A, modified from Windels et al. (2000). B, modified from Boulet et al. (2006).

Finally, intracerebral microdialysis studies in rats have indicated that extracellular levels of both glutamate and GABA increase in the GPe and SNr during STN-HFS, suggesting a role for excitatory and inhibitory elements of the basal ganglia circuitry in the mode of action of STN-HFS (Windels et al., 2000, 2003). These results confirm the findings of electrophysiological studies showing that in anesthetized rats, the spontaneous firing of SNr cells either increases or decreases in the overall population of SNr cells (Degos et al., 2005). Similarly, almost equal numbers of excitatory and inhibitory responses were found in the SNr in a treadmill-locomotion task under behaviorally effective STN stimulation (Shi et al., 2006). In both cases, STN-HFS regularized the firing pattern of SNr cells (Degos et al., 2005) by subtle effects on both the inhibitory and excitatory BG pathways. STN-HFS preserves the inhibitory influence of the striatonigral pathway and, depending on its intensity, decreases or abolishes the excitatory influence of trans-subthalamic pathways on SNr cells. Thus, by decreasing the relative efficiency of the trans-subthalamic circuits, the STN-HFS introduces a bias between the direct and indirect trans-striatal circuits and restores the balance between the inhibitory and excitatory influences of the striatum and the STN, respectively, on SNr cells.

Given the ability of STN-HFS to stimulate axons, antidromically in particular, and the fact that the STN receives major inputs from the cortex and thalamus (Kita & Kitai, 1994), neuron activation and changes in excitability in deep cortical layers were expected, together with the damping of oscillation in the local field potentials observed during STN-HFS (Butson & McIntyre, 2008; Eusebio et al., 2009; Fraix et al., 2008; Jech et al., 2006; Kuriakose et al., 2009).

However, this cannot entirely account for the relationships between cortical antidromic activation and the impact of STN-HFS on cortical oscillations. This basis of relationships remains to be established, as STN stimulation may also affect the thalamo-cortical oscillators via antidromic activation of the thalamo-STN neurons and orthodromic activation of the subthalamo-cortical projections (Degos et al., 2008).

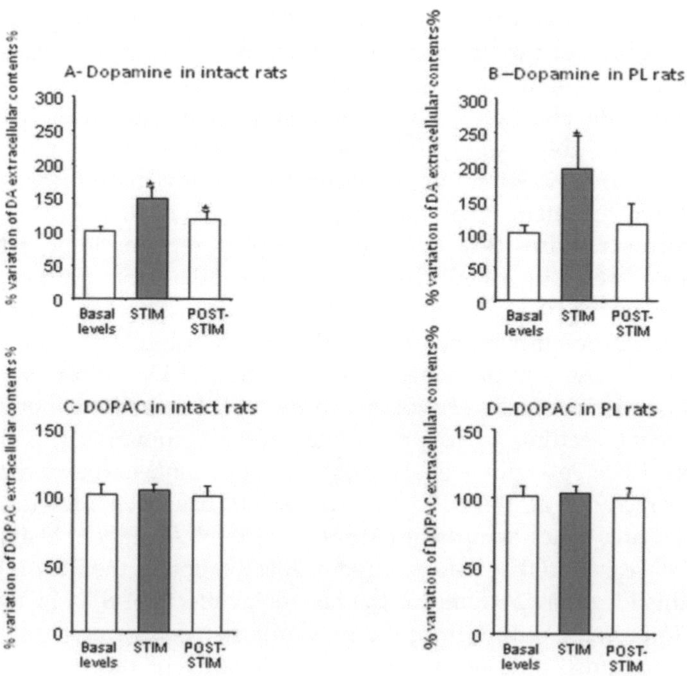

Fig. 5. Extracellular Dopamine (A and B) and DOPAC (C and D) levels determined before, during and after 1 hour STN-HFS in striatum of normal (A and C) and 6-OHDA (B and D) rats. Modified from Bruet et al. (2001).

Finally, variations in the extracellular concentrations of DA and its metabolites have been reported in the striatum of normal (Fig. 5A and C) and parkinsonian animals (Fig. 5B and D) during STN-HFS (Bruet et al., 2001; Meissner et al., 2001, 2002; Zhao et al., 2009). As STN sends direct projections to the striatum (Nakano et al., 1990) and STN-HFS improves all motor symptoms and allows a considerable reduction of dopaminergic medication in parkinsonian patients, it has been suggested that the therapeutic action of STN-HFS may depend partly on changes in striatal DA transmission. Unfortunately, these changes have not been confirmed in PD patients (Abosch et al., 2003; Hilker et al., 2003; Strafella et al., 2003) However, these human studies were carried out on parkinsonian patients on long-term L-Dopa treatment. The effects of this treatment on neuronal plasticity may account for the discrepancies between human and animal studies. The interactions between L-Dopa treatment and STN-SHF will be discussed below.

Over and above the multiple consequences of STN-HFS on distal BG structures, the way in which all these effects contribute to the therapeutic action of STN-HFS remains a key unanswered question.

2.3 Therapeutic effects of STN-HFS and functional considerations

An understanding of the therapeutic mechanisms of STN-HFS requires consideration not only of the local or distal changes in activity in the stimulated area, but also an evaluation of the changes in activity throughout the connected network. A detailed understanding of the neuronal mechanisms underlying the PD motor symptoms corrected by STN-HFS is required to obtain a complete answer to this question. PD is known to be associated with various changes in neuronal activity within the BG network, but the precise role of these changes in the expression of motor symptoms remains a matter of debate. Many possible hypothetical mechanisms of action of therapeutic STN-HFS have been put forward.

In normal conditions, the SNr exerts tonic inhibition on premotor nuclei in the thalamus and brainstem. During the preparation and execution of goal-directed movements (Sato & Hikosaka, 2002), GABAergic striatonigral neurons phasically inhibit SNr neurons, thereby causing disinhibition of their premotor target nuclei (Chevalier & Deniau, 1990). This disinhibition process requires SNr neurons to display regular, tonic activity in resting conditions. It has been suggested that the trans-subthalamic pathway regulates the amplitude of movements and participates in the selection of motor programs through its contribution to the spatiotemporal shaping of the striatal inhibitory signal (Mink & Thach, 1993). Alterations of these two processes by interruption of DA transmission is thought to generate parasitic noise in motor networks and disrupt the spatiotemporal shaping of the disinhibition process, leading to inappropriate motor commands (Boraud et al., 2002; Chesselet & Delfs, 1996; Pessiglione et al., 2005). In PD patients and experimental models of the disease, hyperactivity of the STN and its targets has been identified as a possible mechanism underlying motor symptoms (Albin et al., 1989; Alexander et al., 1990). Together with the clinical observation that the lesioning or inactivation of the STN is effective against PD symptoms, this idea may account for the beneficial effects of STN-HFS in PD, with this treatment first suppressing output from the STN and then counteracting the overactivity of the BG output structures, thus restoring the functionality of the premotor target nuclei. However, STN-HFS also activates the axons of STN cells, and the mean firing rate of GPi neurons has been shown to increase or to remain constant (Hashimoto et al., 2003; Reese et al., 2008). These findings and the observations that the degeneration of SNc dopaminergic neurons primarily affects firing patterns rather than the firing rate of the STN and the BG output neurons (Tai et al., 2003; Wichmann et al., 1999) and that the mean firing rate of STN (Carlson et al., 2010) and thalamic neurons (Pessiglione et al., 2005) is unaffected in PD patients and experimental models of PD, respectively, calls into question the relevance of firing rate per se to the pathophysiology of PD and the mechanism of STN-HFS.

An alternative explanation for the efficacy of STN-HFS is that this procedure reshapes the spatiotemporal structure of neuronal discharge, regularizing the discharge patterns of the STN and BG output nuclei rather than modifying their firing rates. There is experimental evidence to support this view, with the demonstration that the neurons of the STN and basal ganglia output nuclei originally display bursting patterns of firing, with a more regular pattern of pauses imposed by STN-HFS (Carlson et al., 2010; Degos et al., 2005; Dorval et al., 2008; Maltete et al., 2007). Interestingly normalization of the firing pattern of SNr cells was observed whether the cells were inhibited or excited (Degos et al., 2005). This highlights the possible contribution of both inhibitory and excitatory synaptic events to the regularization by STN-HFS of spontaneous discharge and the transmission of cortical information in BG circuits. Local inactivation may decrease the transmission of cortical information via the trans-subthalamic circuits, and this probably helps to restore the balance between the inhibitory striatal input and the excitatory STN input to BG output structures. By reshaping the firing of SNr cells into a tonic and regular pattern and restoring the balance between the trans-striatal and trans-subthalamic pathways, STN-HFS restores the functionality of the disinhibitory mechanisms by which the BG contribute to the organization of movement (Degos et al., 2005; Kravitz et al., 2010).

In conclusion, as a whole, the body of data obtained during STN-HFS does not support the classical view that the therapeutic effects of STN stimulation are mediated by the immediate inhibition of surrounding neurons. Instead, the available data are more consistent with the alternative hypothesis that STN-HFS synchronously activates the surrounding fibers, thereby normalizing or 'jamming' the pathological activity in the BG-thalamocortical network.

3. Possible interactions between STN-HFS and L-DOPA treatment

Until 1960, the only possible approach to the treatment of PD was surgery, because no effective pharmacological treatment was available. The accuracy of this prestereotactic neurosurgery left much to be desired. The discovery in 1960 that dopamine was severely depleted in the basal ganglia of the brains of PD patients provided a springboard for a novel pharmacological concept involving the replacement of a deficient neurotransmitter to treat a degenerative neurological disease. Levodopa, the precursor of dopamine in the catecholamine synthesis pathway, became the practical choice for the development of an oral pharmacological agent, because it crosses the blood brain barrier (for conversion to DA within the brain), whereas DA does not. L-Dopa is a highly effective pharmacological treatment and is now widely used. PD motor symptoms initially respond well to L-Dopa. Subsequently, however, the response to this pharmacological agent declines, mostly due to the occurrence of signs of resistance to treatment and various adverse events, including motor response complications such as wearing-off, 'on-off' fluctuations and L-DOPA-induced dyskinesia (Fahn, 1974; Marsden & Parkes, 1976). The severity of this problem has reignited interest in the surgical approach, which has been rendered all the more interesting by the enormous advances made in recent years in the fields of stereotactic surgery and brain imaging. The discovery that HFS can mimic, in a reversible and adjustable manner, the effects of functional target ablation has revived functional neurosurgery for the treatment of movement disorders, making it possible to target particular areas identified as important through basic neuroscience, such as the STN (Aziz et al., 1991; Benazzouz et al., 1993; Bergman et al., 1990). In the first patients with PD treated by STN-HFS in 1993 (Limousin et al., 1995b), L-Dopa-sensitive symptoms, such as tremor, rigidity and bradykinesia, improved significantly, making it possible to decrease the amount of L-Dopa administered by a mean of 55 % (Krack et al., 2003). Several thousands of patients worldwide have since been fitted with STN-HFS implants and have displayed marked improvements in their symptoms, making this method the reference surgical procedure for advanced PD. Surprisingly, the time course of improvement differs for different cardinal symptoms of PD after the initiation of STN-HFS. Rigidity and resting tremor decrease immediately, within a few seconds after the onset of STN stimulation. By contrast, the amelioration of akinesia and the induction of levodopa-mimicking dyskinesia by STN-HFS generally does not occur until a few minutes, hours or weeks (Krack et al., 2000). These observations, together with clinical observations that the clinical improvement due to STN-HFS is strongly correlated with improvements in parkinsonian signs in a preoperative levodopa challenge test, raise questions about a possible delayed increase in DAergic transmission in the striatum due to the stimulation current. This hypothesis is supported by experimental data from in vivo microdialysis studies showing that STN-HFS increases the amounts of DA and its metabolites in the striatal extracellular compartment in normal and parkinsonian rats (Fig. 5A and B) (Bruet et al., 2001; Meissner et al., 2001, 2002) and monkeys (Zhao et al., 2009), probably through the direct or indirect activation of DAergic SNc neurons. These neurochemical results seem to be consistent with previous electrophysiological and anatomical studies showing a large increase in neural firing in the SNc DAergic neurons of 6-OHDA-treated rats immediately after the start of STN-HFS (Benazzouz et al., 2000) and the existence of moderate numbers of glutamatergic efferents from the STN projecting to the SNc with NMDA receptors located in their dendrites (Groenewegen & Berendse, 1990). Furthermore, the increase in SNc DAergic neuron activity may be induced by the indirect disinhibition of GABAergic SNr neurons. This hypothesis is supported by electrophysiological data demonstrating that SNc neurons are massively under the control of GABAergic collaterals from the SNr (Grace & Bunney, 1979), SNr neurons being inhibited by STN-HFS (Benazzouz et al., 1995; Kita et al., 2005; Maltete et al., 2007; Maurice et al., 2003; Tai et al., 2003).The increase of striatal extracellular concentrations of DA and its metabolites observed in animal models of PD may result from a direct effect of glutamate on SNc DA neurons mediated by NMDA receptors and/or a polysynaptic pathway (Bruet et al., 2001).

Unfortunately, these findings and the hypothesis based on them were not confirmed by clinical studies investigating striatal DA release in PD patients by positron emission tomography (PET) with the ^{11}C-labeled reversible dopamine-D2/3-receptor ligand raclopride. Differences in raclopride binding between "on" and "off" STN-HFS conditions may reflect intervention-induced changes in endogenous transmitter release, because striatal raclopride binding levels are inversely related to DA levels in the synaptic cleft. The use of PET for assessing changes in synaptic DA levels in living humans is now a well established technique (Laruelle et al., 2000; Stoessl & Rivest, 1999). However, although STN-HFS proved highly effective in the patients tested, no significant differences in striatal raclopride binding were observed between the "on" and "off" conditions (Abosch et al., 2003; Hilker et al., 2003; Strafella et al., 2003). There are two probable reasons for the discrepancies between the results obtained for humans and animals: 1) clinical studies were performed on PD patients with chronic exposure to STN-HFS over a number of months whereas STN-HFS in animals reflects more acute effects; 2) the PD patients identified as candidates for STN-HFS have advanced disease and have been on chronic L-Dopa treatment for long periods of time, whereas the animals subjected to stimulation did not receive L-Dopa. Long-term dopatherapy induces a reorganization of the neuronal network, and all PD patients given STN-HFS have previously received L-Dopa treatment. Furthermore, STN-HFS has been reported to decrease motor fluctuations and levodopa-induced-dyskinesia (LID) in PD patients despite the continuation of levodopa treatment in most of these patients (Burchiel et al., 1999; Kumar et al., 1998; Limousin et al., 1998; Moro et al., 1999; Volkmann et al., 2001). It therefore makes more sense to consider the cumulative effects of L-Dopa plus STN-HFS, rather than the effects of STN-HFS alone. LID is thought to result from a combination of additional factors: the severity of dopaminergic brain lesions, as LID is not observed in normal individuals receiving therapeutic doses of levodopa, and the chronic pulsatile administration of high doses of levodopa, as LID is not observed in untreated patients and is more severe in patients treated with high doses of levodopa (Bejjani et al., 2000). As STN-

HFS allows two of these factors – high doses and the pulsatile administration of levodopa and dopaminergic agonists – to be significantly reduced, it would be interesting to determine whether the decrease in LID expression induced by STN-HFS reflects direct and specific functional effects of stimulation on the BG network or an indirect action associated with a decrease in the daily dose of levodopa. Indeed, paradoxically, given the decrease in LID observed after stimulation, STN-HFS may have a dyskinesia-inducing effect in some patients (Krack et al., 2003; Limousin et al., 1996; Volkmann et al., 2001) and in animal models of the disease (Boulet et al., 2006; Oueslati et al., 2007) if the voltage is increased, emphasizing the complex interactions between levodopa treatment and STN-HFS.

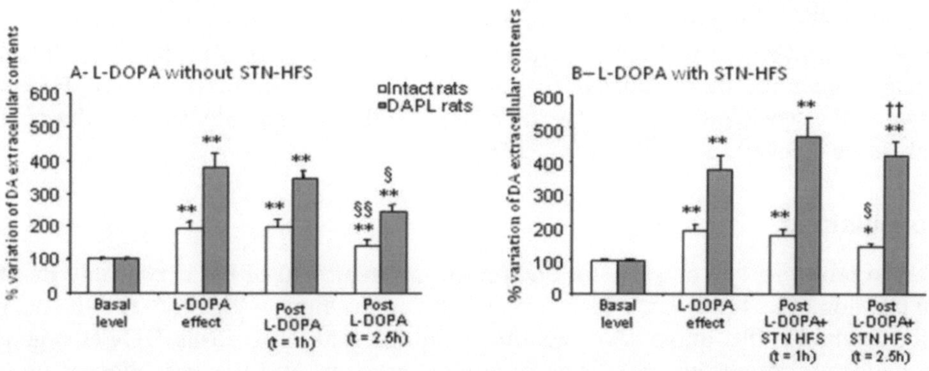

Fig. 6. Effects of L-DOPA alone (A) and L-DOPA plus STN-HFS (B) in extracellular concentration of dopamine in the striatum of normal and partially denervated rats. Modified from Lacombe et al. (2007). *p<0.05, **p<0.001: versus basal values; §: versus L-DOPA effect; †: versus no STN-HFS.

Several recent experimental studies have provided strong evidence that the striatum is a primary site of interaction between levodopa and STN-HFS (Gubellini et al., 2006; Lacombe et al., 2007; Oueslati et al., 2007). A microdialysis study on anesthetized rats with partial DA depletion showed that STN-HFS interacts synergically with levodopa-induced changes in striatal extracellular DA concentration, by stabilizing the levodopa-induced increase in striatal DA levels (Fig. 6A and B) (Lacombe et al., 2007). The authors suggested that this stabilization of striatal DA concentrations may be involved in the alleviation of levodopa-related motor fluctuations, such as the wearing-off phenomenon in particular (Nimura et al., 2005), as De la Fuente-Fernandez et al., (de la Fuente-Fernandez et al., 2001) showed that fluctuations in striatal synaptic DA concentrations precede the clinically apparent wearing-off phenomenon. Another study in 6-OHDA-treated awake rats demonstrated that STN-HFS did not alleviate and might even have prolonged LID and exacerbated LID-associated changes in the levels of several striatal markers, such as preproenkephalin (PPE) and preprodynorphin (PPDyn) mRNA (Oueslati et al., 2007). Despite the apparent difference in these results, STN-HFS potentiates the effects of levodopa rather than counteracting the modifications induced by dopaminergic treatment in both cases. This observation was supported by a behavioral study followed by in vitro patch-clamp electrophysiological recordings in brain slices of 6-OHDA-lesioned rats treated chronically with STN-HFS and dyskinesiogenic doses of L-Dopa. STN-HFS has been shown to abolish the striatal glutamatergic hyperactivity typical of parkinsonian rats and exacerbated by levodopa.

Surprisingly, this effect was paralleled by improvements in akinesia but not in LID (Gubellini et al., 2006). Although these experimental data seem at first sight to be consistent with the indirect improvement of LID by STN-HFS, a direct effect cannot be excluded, given the complexity of LID, which includes a number of phenomena, such as peak dose chorea, the on-off phenomenon, wearing-off fluctuations and off-period dystonia. The mechanisms underlying these types of LID are not well understood and, given the multiple effects of STN-HFS, it would not be surprising to find that STN-HFS has a direct effect on some types of LID, such as off-period dystonia, as suggested in a clinical study (Krack et al., 1999). By contrast, other types of LID, such as on-period dyskinesia, may be decreased essentially by the decrease in the daily dose of levodopa (Guridi et al., 2008) and still others, such as peak dose dyskinesia, may even increase, depending on stimulation status (Nutt et al., 2001). Thus, the improvement in LID mediated by chronic STN-HFS is probably multifactorial, resulting from both the stabilized functioning of the BG induced by STN-HFS and a decrease in the sensitization phenomenon caused by the chronic intermittent administration of high doses of levodopa (Bejjani et al., 2000).

4. Conclusions

The remarkable efficacy of STN stimulation for the treatment of PD is probably due to the nodal position of this nucleus, which concentrates connections with almost all the BG nuclei and the cerebral cortex into a small volume. In addition to local effects, STN-HFS generates system effects through the back-firing of afferent neurons and the activation of projection pathways from the stimulated nucleus. Clearly, when considered in the context of the total BG thalamo-cortical network, the combined effects of STN-HFS partly correct most of the defects in neural discharge thought to be responsible for the motor symptoms of PD. However, this correction is achieved through the imposition, by stimulation, of a particular pattern of activity on the network. The extent to whichsuch a controlled network retains the ability to encode information remains to be determined. Finally, many factors may influence the net effect of STN-HFS: the neurotransmitters released by the fibers stimulated, the intrinsic properties of the neurons, the axonal branching of the network. Thus, in contexts other than PD, an inability to limit the impact of stimulation to the stimulation site may be a disadvantage. This highlights the importance of defining a rationale for the choice of target in the broad range of neurological disorders for which HFS is a potential therapeutic tool.

5. References

Abosch, A., Kapur, S., Lang, A.E., Hussey, D., Sime, E., Miyasaki, J., Houle, S. & Lozano, A.M. (2003) Stimulation of the subthalamic nucleus in Parkinson's disease does not produce striatal dopamine release. Neurosurgery, 53, 1095-1102; discussion 1102-1095.

Albin, R.L., Young, A.B. & Penney, J.B. (1989) The functional anatomy of basal ganglia disorders. Trends Neurosci, 12, 366-375.

Alexander, G.E., Crutcher, M.D. & DeLong, M.R. (1990) Basal ganglia-thalamocortical circuits: parallel substrates for motor, oculomotor, "prefrontal" and "limbic" functions. Prog Brain Res, 85, 119-146.

Aziz, T.Z., Peggs, D., Sambrook, M.A. & Crossman, A.R. (1991) Lesion of the subthalamic nucleus for the alleviation of 1-methyl-4-phenyl-1,2,3,6-tetrahydropyridine (MPTP)-induced parkinsonism in the primate. Mov Disord, 6, 288-292.

Barlas, O., Hanagasi, H.A., Imer, M., Sahin, H.A., Sencer, S. & Emre, M. (2001) Do unilateral ablative lesions of the subthalamic nucleu in parkinsonian patients lead to hemiballism? Mov Disord, 16, 306-310.

Bejjani, B.P., Arnulf, I., Demeret, S., Damier, P., Bonnet, A.M., Houeto, J.L. & Agid, Y. (2000) Levodopa-induced dyskinesias in Parkinson's disease: is sensitization reversible? Ann Neurol, 47, 655-658.

Benabid, A.L., Benazzous, A. & Pollak, P. (2002) Mechanisms of deep brain stimulation. Mov Disord, 17 Suppl 3, S73-74.

Benabid, A.L., Benazzouz, A., Hoffmann, D., Limousin, P., Krack, P. & Pollak, P. (1998) Long-term electrical inhibition of deep brain targets in movement disorders. Mov Disord, 13 Suppl 3, 119-125.

Benabid, A.L., Benazzouz, A., Limousin, P., Koudsie, A., Krack, P., Piallat, B. & Pollak, P. (2000) Dyskinesias and the subthalamic nucleus. Ann Neurol, 47, S189-192.

Benazzouz, A., Gao, D.M., Ni, Z.G., Piallat, B., Bouali-Benazzouz, R. & Benabid, A.L. (2000) Effect of high-frequency stimulation of the subthalamic nucleus on the neuronal activities of the substantia nigra pars reticulata and ventrolateral nucleus of the thalamus in the rat. Neuroscience, 99, 289-295.

Benazzouz, A., Gross, C., Feger, J., Boraud, T. & Bioulac, B. (1993) Reversal of rigidity and improvement in motor performance by subthalamic high-frequency stimulation in MPTP-treated monkeys. Eur J Neurosci, 5, 382-389.

Benazzouz, A., Piallat, B., Pollak, P. & Benabid, A.L. (1995) Responses of substantia nigra pars reticulata and globus pallidus complex to high frequency stimulation of the subthalamic nucleus in rats: electrophysiological data. Neurosci Lett, 189, 77-80.

Bergman, H., Wichmann, T. & DeLong, M.R. (1990) Reversal of experimental parkinsonism by lesions of the subthalamic nucleus. Science, 249, 1436-1438.

Bergman, H., Wichmann, T., Karmon, B. & DeLong, M.R. (1994) The primate subthalamic nucleus. II. Neuronal activity in the MPTP model of parkinsonism. J Neurophysiol, 72, 507-520.

Beurrier, C., Bioulac, B., Audin, J. & Hammond, C. (2001) High-frequency stimulation produces a transient blockade of voltage-gated currents in subthalamic neurons. J Neurophysiol, 85, 1351-1356.

Bevan, M.D. & Wilson, C.J. (1999) Mechanisms underlying spontaneous oscillation and rhythmic firing in rat subthalamic neurons. J Neurosci, 19, 7617-7628.

Blandini, F., Greenamyre, J.T. & Nappi, G. (1996) The role of glutamate in the pathophysiology of Parkinson's disease. Funct Neurol, 11, 3-15.

Blandini, F., Nappi, G., Tassorelli, C. & Martignoni, E. (2000) Functional changes of the basal ganglia circuitry in Parkinson's disease. Prog Neurobiol, 62, 63-88.

Bolam, J.P., Hanley, J.J., Booth, P.A. & Bevan, M.D. (2000) Synaptic organisation of the basal ganglia. J Anat, 196 (Pt 4), 527-542.

Boraud, T., Bezard, E., Bioulac, B. & Gross, C. (1996) High frequency stimulation of the internal Globus Pallidus (GPi) simultaneously improves parkinsonian symptoms and reduces the firing frequency of GPi neurons in the MPTP-treated monkey. Neurosci Lett, 215, 17-20.

Boraud, T., Bezard, E., Bioulac, B. & Gross, C.E. (2002) From single extracellular unit recording in experimental and human Parkinsonism to the development of a functional concept of the role played by the basal ganglia in motor control. Prog Neurobiol, 66, 265-283.

Boulet, S., Lacombe, E., Carcenac, C., Feuerstein, C., Sgambato-Faure, V., Poupard, A. & Savasta, M. (2006) Subthalamic stimulation-induced forelimb dyskinesias are linked to an increase in glutamate levels in the substantia nigra pars reticulata. J Neurosci, 26, 10768-10776.

Bruet, N., Windels, F., Bertrand, A., Feuerstein, C., Poupard, A. & Savasta, M. (2001) High frequency stimulation of the subthalamic nucleus increases the extracellular contents of striatal dopamine in normal and partially dopaminergic denervated rats. J Neuropathol Exp Neurol, 60, 15-24.

Burbaud, P., Gross, C. & Bioulac, B. (1994) Effect of subthalamic high frequency stimulation on substantia nigra pars reticulata and globus pallidus neurons in normal rats. J Physiol Paris, 88, 359-361.

Burchiel, K.J., Anderson, V.C., Favre, J. & Hammerstad, J.P. (1999) Comparison of pallidal and subthalamic nucleus deep brain stimulation for advanced Parkinson's disease: results of a randomized, blinded pilot study. Neurosurgery, 45, 1375-1382; discussion 1382-1374.

Butson, C.R. & McIntyre, C.C. (2006) Role of electrode design on the volume of tissue activated during deep brain stimulation. J Neural Eng, 3, 1-8.

Butson, C.R. & McIntyre, C.C. (2008) Current steering to control the volume of tissue activated during deep brain stimulation. Brain Stimul, 1, 7-15.

Carlson, J.D., Cleary, D.R., Cetas, J.S., Heinricher, M.M. & Burchiel, K.J. (2010) Deep brain stimulation does not silence neurons in subthalamic nucleus in Parkinson's patients. J Neurophysiol, 103, 962-967.

Carlsson, M. & Carlsson, A. (1990) Interactions between glutamatergic and monoaminergic systems within the basal ganglia--implications for schizophrenia and Parkinson's disease. Trends Neurosci, 13, 272-276.

Chesselet, M.F. & Delfs, J.M. (1996) Basal ganglia and movement disorders: an update. Trends Neurosci, 19, 417-422.

Chevalier, G. & Deniau, J.M. (1990) Disinhibition as a basic process in the expression of striatal functions. Trends Neurosci, 13, 277-280.

de la Fuente-Fernandez, R., Lu, J.Q., Sossi, V., Jivan, S., Schulzer, M., Holden, J.E., Lee, C.S., Ruth, T.J., Calne, D.B. & Stoessl, A.J. (2001) Biochemical variations in the synaptic level of dopamine precede motor fluctuations in Parkinson's disease: PET evidence of increased dopamine turnover. Ann Neurol, 49, 298-303.

Degos, B., Deniau, J.M., Le Cam, J., Mailly, P. & Maurice, N. (2008) Evidence for a direct subthalamo-cortical loop circuit in the rat. Eur J Neurosci, 27, 2599-2610.

Degos, B., Deniau, J.M., Thierry, A.M., Glowinski, J., Pezard, L. & Maurice, N. (2005) Neuroleptic-induced catalepsy: electrophysiological mechanisms of functional recovery induced by high-frequency stimulation of the subthalamic nucleus. J Neurosci, 25, 7687-7696.

DeLong, M.R. (1990) Primate models of movement disorders of basal ganglia origin. Trends Neurosci, 13, 281-285.

Dorval, A.D., Russo, G.S., Hashimoto, T., Xu, W., Grill, W.M. & Vitek, J.L. (2008) Deep brain stimulation reduces neuronal entropy in the MPTP-primate model of Parkinson's disease. J Neurophysiol, 100, 2807-2818.

Dostrovsky, J.O. & Lozano, A.M. (2002) Mechanisms of deep brain stimulation. Mov Disord, 17 Suppl 3, S63-68.

Ehringer, H. & Hornykiewicz, O. (1960) [Distribution of noradrenaline and dopamine (3-hydroxytyramine) in the human brain and their behavior in diseases of the extrapyramidal system]. Klin Wochenschr, 38, 1236-1239.

Eusebio, A., Pogosyan, A., Wang, S., Averbeck, B., Gaynor, L.D., Cantiniaux, S., Witjas, T., Limousin, P., Azulay, J.P. & Brown, P. (2009) Resonance in subthalamo-cortical circuits in Parkinson's disease. Brain, 132, 2139-2150.

Fahn, S. (1974) "On-off" phenomenon with levodopa therapy in Parkinsonism. Clinical and pharmacologic correlations and the effect of intramuscular pyridoxine. Neurology, 24, 431-441.

Filali, M., Hutchison, W.D., Palter, V.N., Lozano, A.M. & Dostrovsky, J.O. (2004) Stimulation-induced inhibition of neuronal firing in human subthalamic nucleus. Exp Brain Res, 156, 274-281.

Fraix, V., Pollak, P., Vercueil, L., Benabid, A.L. & Mauguiere, F. (2008) Effects of subthalamic nucleus stimulation on motor cortex excitability in Parkinson's disease. Clin Neurophysiol, 119, 2513-2518.

Galati, S., Mazzone, P., Fedele, E., Pisani, A., Peppe, A., Pierantozzi, M., Brusa, L., Tropepi, D., Moschella, V., Raiteri, M., Stanzione, P., Bernardi, G. & Stefani, A. (2006) Biochemical and electrophysiological changes of substantia nigra pars reticulata driven by subthalamic stimulation in patients with Parkinson's disease. Eur J Neurosci, 23, 2923-2928.

Garcia, L., Audin, J., D'Alessandro, G., Bioulac, B. & Hammond, C. (2003) Dual effect of high-frequency stimulation on subthalamic neuron activity. J Neurosci, 23, 8743-8751.

Gill, S.S. & Heywood, P. (1997) Bilateral dorsolateral subthalamotomy for advanced Parkinson's disease. Lancet, 350, 1224.

Grace, A.A. & Bunney, B.S. (1979) Paradoxical GABA excitation of nigral dopaminergic cells: indirect mediation through reticulata inhibitory neurons. Eur J Pharmacol, 59, 211-218.

Greenamyre, J.T. & O'Brien, C.F. (1991) N-methyl-D-aspartate antagonists in the treatment of Parkinson's disease. Arch Neurol, 48, 977-981.

Groenewegen, H.J. & Berendse, H.W. (1990) Connections of the subthalamic nucleus with ventral striatopallidal parts of the basal ganglia in the rat. J Comp Neurol, 294, 607-622.

Gubellini, P., Eusebio, A., Oueslati, A., Melon, C., Kerkerian-Le Goff, L. & Salin, P. (2006) Chronic high-frequency stimulation of the subthalamic nucleus and L-DOPA treatment in experimental parkinsonism: effects on motor behaviour and striatal glutamate transmission. Eur J Neurosci, 24, 1802-1814.

Guridi, J. & Obeso, J.A. (2001) The subthalamic nucleus, hemiballismus and Parkinson's disease: reappraisal of a neurosurgical dogma. Brain, 124, 5-19.

Guridi, J., Obeso, J.A., Rodriguez-Oroz, M.C., Lozano, A.A. & Manrique, M. (2008) L-dopa-induced dyskinesia and stereotactic surgery for Parkinson's disease. Neurosurgery, 62, 311-323; discussion 323-315.

Hahn, P.J., Russo, G.S., Hashimoto, T., Miocinovic, S., Xu, W., McIntyre, C.C. & Vitek, J.L. (2008) Pallidal burst activity during therapeutic deep brain stimulation. Exp Neurol, 211, 243-251.

Hashimoto, T., Elder, C.M., Okun, M.S., Patrick, S.K. & Vitek, J.L. (2003) Stimulation of the subthalamic nucleus changes the firing pattern of pallidal neurons. J Neurosci, 23, 1916-1923.

Hassani, O.K., Mouroux, M. & Feger, J. (1996) Increased subthalamic neuronal activity after nigral dopaminergic lesion independent of disinhibition via the globus pallidus. Neuroscience, 72, 105-115.

Hershey, T., Revilla, F.J., Wernle, A.R., McGee-Minnich, L., Antenor, J.V., Videen, T.O., Dowling, J.L., Mink, J.W. & Perlmutter, J.S. (2003) Cortical and subcortical blood flow effects of subthalamic nucleus stimulation in PD. Neurology, 61, 816-821.

Hilker, R., Voges, J., Ghaemi, M., Lehrke, R., Rudolf, J., Koulousakis, A., Herholz, K., Wienhard, K., Sturm, V. & Heiss, W.D. (2003) Deep brain stimulation of the subthalamic nucleus does not increase the striatal dopamine concentration in parkinsonian humans. Mov Disord, 18, 41-48.

Hilker, R., Voges, J., Weber, T., Kracht, L.W., Roggendorf, J., Baudrexel, S., Hoevels, M., Sturm, V. & Heiss, W.D. (2008) STN-DBS activates the target area in Parkinson disease: an FDG-PET study. Neurology, 71, 708-713.

Jech, R., Ruzicka, E., Urgosik, D., Serranova, T., Volfova, M., Novakova, O., Roth, J., Dusek, P. & Mecir, P. (2006) Deep brain stimulation of the subthalamic nucleus affects resting EEG and visual evoked potentials in Parkinson's disease. Clin Neurophysiol, 117, 1017-1028.

Kita, H. (2007) Globus pallidus external segment. Prog Brain Res, 160, 111-133.

Kita, H. & Kitai, S.T. (1987) Efferent projections of the subthalamic nucleus in the rat: light and electron microscopic analysis with the PHA-L method. J Comp Neurol, 260, 435-452.

Kita, H. & Kitai, S.T. (1994) The morphology of globus pallidus projection neurons in the rat: an intracellular staining study. Brain Res, 636, 308-319.

Kita, H., Tachibana, Y., Nambu, A. & Chiken, S. (2005) Balance of monosynaptic excitatory and disynaptic inhibitory responses of the globus pallidus induced after stimulation of the subthalamic nucleus in the monkey. J Neurosci, 25, 8611-8619.

Kitai, S.T. & Deniau, J.M. (1981) Cortical inputs to the subthalamus: intracellular analysis. Brain Res, 214, 411-415.

Krack, P., Batir, A., Van Blercom, N., Chabardes, S., Fraix, V., Ardouin, C., Koudsie, A., Limousin, P.D., Benazzouz, A., LeBas, J.F., Benabid, A.L. & Pollak, P. (2003) Five-year follow-up of bilateral stimulation of the subthalamic nucleus in advanced Parkinson's disease. N Engl J Med, 349, 1925-1934.

Krack, P., Poepping, M., Weinert, D., Schrader, B. & Deuschl, G. (2000) Thalamic, pallidal, or subthalamic surgery for Parkinson's disease? J Neurol, 247 Suppl 2, II122-134.

Krack, P., Pollak, P., Limousin, P., Benazzouz, A., Deuschl, G. & Benabid, A.L. (1999) From off-period dystonia to peak-dose chorea. The clinical spectrum of varying subthalamic nucleus activity. Brain, 122 (Pt 6), 1133-1146.

Krack, P., Pollak, P., Limousin, P., Hoffmann, D., Xie, J., Benazzouz, A. & Benabid, A.L. (1998) Subthalamic nucleus or internal pallidal stimulation in young onset Parkinson's disease. Brain, 121 (Pt 3), 451-457.

Kravitz, A.V., Freze, B.S., Parker, P.R.L., Kay, K., Thwin, M.T., Deisseroth, K. & Kreitzer, A.C. (2010) Regulation of parkinsonian motor behaviours by optogenetic control of basal ganglia circuitry. Nature, 466, 622-626.

Krause, M., Fogel, W., Heck, A., Hacke, W., Bonsanto, M., Trenkwalder, C. & Tronnier, V. (2001) Deep brain stimulation for the treatment of Parkinson's disease: subthalamic nucleus versus globus pallidus internus. J Neurol Neurosurg Psychiatry, 70, 464-470.

Kumar, R., Lozano, A.M., Kim, Y.J., Hutchison, W.D., Sime, E., Halket, E. & Lang, A.E. (1998) Double-blind evaluation of subthalamic nucleus deep brain stimulation in advanced Parkinson's disease. Neurology, 51, 850-855.

Kuriakose, R., Saha, U., Castillo, G., Udupa, K., Ni, Z., Gunraj, C., Mazzella, F., Hamani, C., Lang, A.E., Moro, E., Lozano, A.M., Hodaie, M. & Chen, R. (2009) The nature and time course of cortical activation following subthalamic stimulation in Parkinson's disease. Cereb Cortex, 20, 1926-1936.

Lacombe, E., Carcenac, C., Boulet, S., Feuerstein, C., Bertrand, A., Poupard, A. & Savasta, M. (2007) High-frequency stimulation of the subthalamic nucleus prolongs the increase in striatal dopamine induced by acute l-3,4-dihydroxyphenylalanine in dopaminergic denervated rats. Eur J Neurosci, 26, 1670-1680.

Laruelle, M., Abi-Dargham, A., van Dyck, C., Gil, R., D'Souza, D.C., Krystal, J., Seibyl, J., Baldwin, R. & Innis, R. (2000) Dopamine and serotonin transporters in patients with schizophrenia: an imaging study with [(123)I]beta-CIT. Biol Psychiatry, 47, 371-379.

Lee, K.H., Blaha, C.D., Harris, B.T., Cooper, S., Hitti, F.L., Leiter, J.C., Roberts, D.W. & Kim, U. (2006) Dopamine efflux in the rat striatum evoked by electrical stimulation of the subthalamic nucleus: potential mechanism of action in Parkinson's disease. Eur J Neurosci, 23, 1005-1014.

Lee, K.H., Kristic, K., van Hoff, R., Hitti, F.L., Blaha, C., Harris, B., Roberts, D.W. & Leiter, J.C. (2007) High-frequency stimulation of the subthalamic nucleus increases glutamate in the subthalamic nucleus of rats as demonstrated by in vivo enzyme-linked glutamate sensor. Brain Res, 1162, 121-129.

Levy, R., Lang, A.E., Dostrovsky, J.O., Pahapill, P., Romas, J., Saint-Cyr, J., Hutchison, W.D. & Lozano, A.M. (2001) Lidocaine and muscimol microinjections in subthalamic nucleus reverse Parkinsonian symptoms. Brain, 124, 2105-2118.

Li, X.H., Wang, J.Y., Gao, G., Chang, J.Y., Woodward, D.J. & Luo, F. (2010) High-frequency stimulation of the subthalamic nucleus restores neural and behavioral functions during reaction time task in a rat model of Parkinson's disease. J Neurosci Res, 88, 1510-1521.

Limousin, P., Krack, P., Pollak, P., Benazzouz, A., Ardouin, C., Hoffmann, D. & Benabid, A.L. (1998) Electrical stimulation of the subthalamic nucleus in advanced Parkinson's disease. N Engl J Med, 339, 1105-1111.

Limousin, P., Pollak, P., Benazzouz, A., Hoffmann, D., Broussolle, E., Perret, J.E. & Benabid, A.L. (1995a) Bilateral subthalamic nucleus stimulation for severe Parkinson's disease. Mov Disord, 10, 672-674.

Limousin, P., Pollak, P., Benazzouz, A., Hoffmann, D., Le Bas, J.F., Broussolle, E., Perret, J.E. & Benabid, A.L. (1995b) Effect of parkinsonian signs and symptoms of bilateral subthalamic nucleus stimulation. Lancet, 345, 91-95.

Limousin, P., Pollak, P., Hoffmann, D., Benazzouz, A., Perret, J.E. & Benabid, A.L. (1996) Abnormal involuntary movements induced by subthalamic nucleus stimulation in parkinsonian patients. Mov Disord, 11, 231-235.

Magarinos-Ascone, C., Pazo, J.H., Macadar, O. & Buno, W. (2002) High-frequency stimulation of the subthalamic nucleus silences subthalamic neurons: a possible cellular mechanism in Parkinson's disease. Neuroscience, 115, 1109-1117.

Maltete, D., Jodoin, N., Karachi, C., Houeto, J.L., Navarro, S., Cornu, P., Agid, Y. & Welter, M.L. (2007) Subthalamic stimulation and neuronal activity in the substantia nigra in Parkinson's disease. J Neurophysiol, 97, 4017-4022.

Marsden, C.D. & Parkes, J.D. (1976) "On-off" effects in patients with Parkinson's disease on chronic levodopa therapy. Lancet, 1, 292-296.

Maurice, N., Thierry, A.M., Glowinski, J. & Deniau, J.M. (2003) Spontaneous and evoked activity of substantia nigra pars reticulata neurons during high-frequency stimulation of the subthalamic nucleus. J Neurosci, 23, 9929-9936.

McIntyre, C.C., Mori, S., Sherman, D.L., Thakor, N.V. & Vitek, J.L. (2004) Electric field and stimulating influence generated by deep brain stimulation of the subthalamic nucleus. Clin Neurophysiol, 115, 589-595.

Meissner, W., Harnack, D., Paul, G., Reum, T., Sohr, R., Morgenstern, R. & Kupsch, A. (2002) Deep brain stimulation of subthalamic neurons increases striatal dopamine metabolism and induces contralateral circling in freely moving 6-hydroxydopamine-lesioned rats. Neurosci Lett, 328, 105-108.

Meissner, W., Leblois, A., Hansel, D., Bioulac, B., Gross, C.E., Benazzouz, A. & Boraud, T. (2005) Subthalamic high frequency stimulation resets subthalamic firing and reduces abnormal oscillations. Brain, 128, 2372-2382.

Meissner, W., Reum, T., Paul, G., Harnack, D., Sohr, R., Morgenstern, R. & Kupsch, A. (2001) Striatal dopaminergic metabolism is increased by deep brain stimulation of the subthalamic nucleus in 6-hydroxydopamine lesioned rats. Neurosci Lett, 303, 165-168.

Mink, J.W. & Thach, W.T. (1993) Basal ganglia intrinsic circuits and their role in behavior. Curr Opin Neurobiol, 3, 950-957.

Miocinovic, S., Lempka, S.F., Russo, G.S., Maks, C.B., Butson, C.R., Sakaie, K.E., Vitek, J.L. & McIntyre, C.C. (2009) Experimental and theoretical characterization of the voltage distribution generated by deep brain stimulation. Exp Neurol, 216, 166-176.

Moro, E., Scerrati, M., Romito, L.M., Roselli, R., Tonali, P. & Albanese, A. (1999) Chronic subthalamic nucleus stimulation reduces medication requirements in Parkinson's disease. Neurology, 53, 85-90.

Nakano, K., Hasegawa, Y., Tokushige, A., Nakagawa, S., Kayahara, T. & Mizuno, N. (1990) Topographical projections from the thalamus, subthalamic nucleus and pedunculopontine tegmental nucleus to the striatum in the Japanese monkey, Macaca fuscata. Brain Res, 537, 54-68.

Nimura, T., Yamaguchi, K., Ando, T., Shibuya, S., Oikawa, T., Nakagawa, A., Shirane, R., Itoh, M. & Tominaga, T. (2005) Attenuation of fluctuating striatal synaptic dopamine levels in patients with Parkinson disease in response to subthalamic nucleus stimulation: a positron emission tomography study. J Neurosurg, 103, 968-973.

Nutt, J.G., Rufener, S.L., Carter, J.H., Anderson, V.C., Pahwa, R., Hammerstad, J.P. & Burchiel, K.J. (2001) Interactions between deep brain stimulation and levodopa in Parkinson's disease. Neurology, 57, 1835-1842.

Obeso, J.A., Marin, C., Rodriguez-Oroz, C., Blesa, J., Benitez-Temino, B., Mena-Segovia, J., Rodriguez, M. & Olanow, C.W. (2008) The basal ganglia in Parkinson's disease: current concepts and unexplained observations. Ann Neurol, 64 Suppl 2, S30-46.

Oueslati, A., Sgambato-Faure, V., Melon, C., Kachidian, P., Gubellini, P., Amri, M., Kerkerian-Le Goff, L. & Salin, P. (2007) High-frequency stimulation of the subthalamic nucleus potentiates L-DOPA-induced neurochemical changes in the striatum in a rat model of Parkinson's disease. J Neurosci, 27, 2377-2386.

Parent, A. & Hazrati, L.N. (1995a) Functional anatomy of the basal ganglia. I. The cortico-basal ganglia-thalamo-cortical loop. Brain Res Brain Res Rev, 20, 91-127.

Parent, A. & Hazrati, L.N. (1995b) Functional anatomy of the basal ganglia. II. The place of subthalamic nucleus and external pallidum in basal ganglia circuitry. Brain Res Brain Res Rev, 20, 128-154.

Patel, N.K., Heywood, P., O'Sullivan, K., McCarter, R., Love, S. & Gill, S.S. (2003) Unilateral subthalamotomy in the treatment of Parkinson's disease. Brain, 126, 1136-1145.

Perlmutter, J.S., Mink, J.W., Bastian, A.J., Zackowski, K., Hershey, T., Miyawaki, E., Koller, W. & Videen, T.O. (2002) Blood flow responses to deep brain stimulation of thalamus. Neurology, 58, 1388-1394.

Pessiglione, M., Czernecki, V., Pillon, B., Dubois, B., Schupbach, M., Agid, Y. & Tremblay, L. (2005) An effect of dopamine depletion on decision-making: the temporal coupling of deliberation and execution. J Cogn Neurosci, 17, 1886-1896.

Poewe, W.H., Lees, A.J. & Stern, G.M. (1986) Treatment of motor fluctuations in Parkinson's disease with an oral sustained-release preparation of L-dopa: clinical and pharmacokinetic observations. Clin Neuropharmacol, 9, 430-439.

Rascol, O. (2000) The pharmacological therapeutic management of levodopa-induced dyskinesias in patients with Parkinson's disease. J Neurol, 247 Suppl 2, II51-57.

Rattay, F. & Aberham, M. (1993) Modeling axon membranes for functional electrical stimulation. IEEE Trans Biomed Eng, 40, 1201-1209.

Reese, R., Steigerwald, F., Potter, M., Herzog, J., Deuschl, G., Volkmann, J., Pinsker, M.O. & Mehdorn, H.M. (2008) High-frequency stimulation of the subthalamic nucleus increases pallidal neuronal firing rate in a patient with Parkinson's disease. Mov Disord, 23, 1945-1947.

Samii, A., Nutt, J.G. & Ransom, B.R. (2004) Parkinson's disease. Lancet, 363, 1783-1793.

Sato, M. & Hikosaka, O. (2002) Role of primate substantia nigra pars reticulata in reward-oriented saccadic eye movement. J Neurosci, 22, 2363-2373.

Shi, L.H., Luo, F., Woodward, D.J. & Chang, J.Y. (2006) Basal ganglia neural responses during behaviorally effective deep brain stimulation of the subthalamic nucleus in rats performing a treadmill locomotion test. Synapse, 59, 445-457.

Smith, Y., Shink, E. & Sidibe, M. (1998) Neuronal circuitry and synaptic connectivity of the basal ganglia. Neurosurg Clin N Am, 9, 203-222.

Starr, M.S. (1995) Antiparkinsonian actions of glutamate antagonists--alone and with L-DOPA: a review of evidence and suggestions for possible mechanisms. J Neural Transm Park Dis Dement Sect, 10, 141-185.

Stefani, A., Fedele, E., Galati, S., Pepicelli, O., Frasca, S., Pierantozzi, M., Peppe, A., Brusa, L., Orlacchio, A., Hainsworth, A.H., Gattoni, G., Stanzione, P., Bernardi, G., Raiteri, M. & Mazzone, P. (2005) Subthalamic stimulation activates internal pallidus: evidence from cGMP microdialysis in PD patients. Ann Neurol, 57, 448-452.

Stoessl, A.J. & Rivest, J. (1999) Differential diagnosis of parkinsonism. Can J Neurol Sci, 26 Suppl 2, S1-4.

Strafella, A.P., Sadikot, A.F. & Dagher, A. (2003) Subthalamic deep brain stimulation does not induce striatal dopamine release in Parkinson's disease. Neuroreport, 14, 1287-1289.

Tai, C.H., Boraud, T., Bezard, E., Bioulac, B., Gross, C. & Benazzouz, A. (2003) Electrophysiological and metabolic evidence that high-frequency stimulation of the subthalamic nucleus bridles neuronal activity in the subthalamic nucleus and the substantia nigra reticulata. FASEB J, 17, 1820-1830.

Volkmann, J., Allert, N., Voges, J., Weiss, P.H., Freund, H.J. & Sturm, V. (2001) Safety and efficacy of pallidal or subthalamic nucleus stimulation in advanced PD. Neurology, 56, 548-551.

Walker, H.C., Watts, R.L., Schrandt, C.J., Huang, H., Guthrie, S.L., Guthrie, B.L. & Montgomery, E.B., Jr. (2010) Activation of Subthalamic Neurons by Contralateral Subthalamic Deep Brain Stimulation in Parkinson Disease. J Neurophysiol.

Welter, M.L., Houeto, J.L., Bonnet, A.M., Bejjani, P.B., Mesnage, V., Dormont, D., Navarro, S., Cornu, P., Agid, Y. & Pidoux, B. (2004) Effects of high-frequency stimulation on subthalamic neuronal activity in parkinsonian patients. Arch Neurol, 61, 89-96.

Wichmann, T., Bergman, H., Starr, P.A., Subramanian, T., Watts, R.L. & DeLong, M.R. (1999) Comparison of MPTP-induced changes in spontaneous neuronal discharge in the internal pallidal segment and in the substantia nigra pars reticulata in primates. Exp Brain Res, 125, 397-409.

Windels, F., Bruet, N., Poupard, A., Feuerstein, C., Bertrand, A. & Savasta, M. (2003) Influence of the frequency parameter on extracellular glutamate and gamma-aminobutyric acid in substantia nigra and globus pallidus during electrical stimulation of subthalamic nucleus in rats. J Neurosci Res, 72, 259-267.

Windels, F., Bruet, N., Poupard, A., Urbain, N., Chouvet, G., Feuerstein, C. & Savasta, M. (2000) Effects of high frequency stimulation of subthalamic nucleus on extracellular glutamate and GABA in substantia nigra and globus pallidus in the normal rat. Eur J Neurosci, 12, 4141-4146.

Windels, F., Carcenac, C., Poupard, A. & Savasta, M. (2005) Pallidal origin of GABA release within the substantia nigra pars reticulata during high-frequency stimulation of the subthalamic nucleus. J Neurosci, 25, 5079-5086.

Zhao, X.D., Cao, Y.Q., Liu, H.H., Li, F.Q., You, B.M. & Zhou, X.P. (2009) Long term high frequency stimulation of STN increases dopamine in the corpus striatum of hemiparkinsonian rhesus monkey. Brain Res, 1286, 230-238.

13

Thalamic Deep Brain Stimulation for Parkinson's Disease

Ryoma Morigaki[1,2], Shinji Nagahiro[1,2], Ryuji Kaji[1,3] and Satoshi Goto[1,3]
[1]*Parkinson Disease and Dystonia Research Center, Tokushima University Hospital, University of Tokushima*
[2]*Department of Neurosurgery, Institute of Health Biosciences, University of Tokushima*
[3]*Department of Clinical Neuroscience, Institute of Health Biosciences, University of Tokushima, Japan*

1. Introduction

With recent advances in neuroimaging and neurosurgical techniques as well as better understanding of functional motor brain circuits, there is increasing evidence that electrical deep brain stimulation (DBS) can be a powerful and safe therapeutic option for medically intractable movement disorders and neuropsychiatric diseases. For more than half a century, the ventrolateral (VL) nucleus of the thalamus has been an anatomical target for stereotactic surgeries (e.g., ablation surgery and DBS) treating various types of tremors, including Parkinson's disease (PD)-associated tremor. The VL nucleus comprises the nucleus ventralis intermedius (Vim) and the nucleus ventralis oralis (Vo) (Hassler, 1959). Currently, thalamic DBS is widely used because of its reversibility, adjustability, and low level of invasiveness. Thalamic DBS of the Vim nucleus can effectively alleviate parkinsonian tremor; however, it does not provide consistent improvement in parkinsonian symptoms other than tremor. Therefore, its use is limited to patients with tremor-predominant PD, in whom other motor symptoms are not disabling. In this review, we will survey the rationale and current use of thalamic DBS in the treatment of PD.

2. Functional anatomy of the VL thalamic nucleus

The VL thalamic nucleus is a major target for DBS in the treatment of movement disorders. With respect to therapy targeting PD, the Vim nucleus is frequently the site for the treatment of medically intractable tremor. The anatomy and function of the fiber connections of the Vim nucleus (Fig. 1) are important in considering the therapeutic and adverse effects of this surgery. We first present a brief review of anatomical studies based on primate studies of the VL thalamic nucleus.

Cortico-thalamo-basal ganglia loops are suggested to have specialized functions corresponding to the cortical areas participating in each loop (Alexander & Crutcher, 1990). Reciprocal thalamo-cortical connections play a role in maintaining these parallel processing loops. Functionally segregated parallel loops may be integrated via non-reciprocal fiber connections between the thalamus and cortex, terminating in the superficial and deep cortical layers. These terminals could influence various cortical areas that, in turn, project toward the striatum, which sends efferents back to the thalamus. In addition, non-reciprocal corticothalamic projections terminate in thalamic regions that participate in other processing loops (McFarland & Haber, 2002). As a thalamic-level constituent of the motor loop, the VL nucleus mediates movement-related processing.

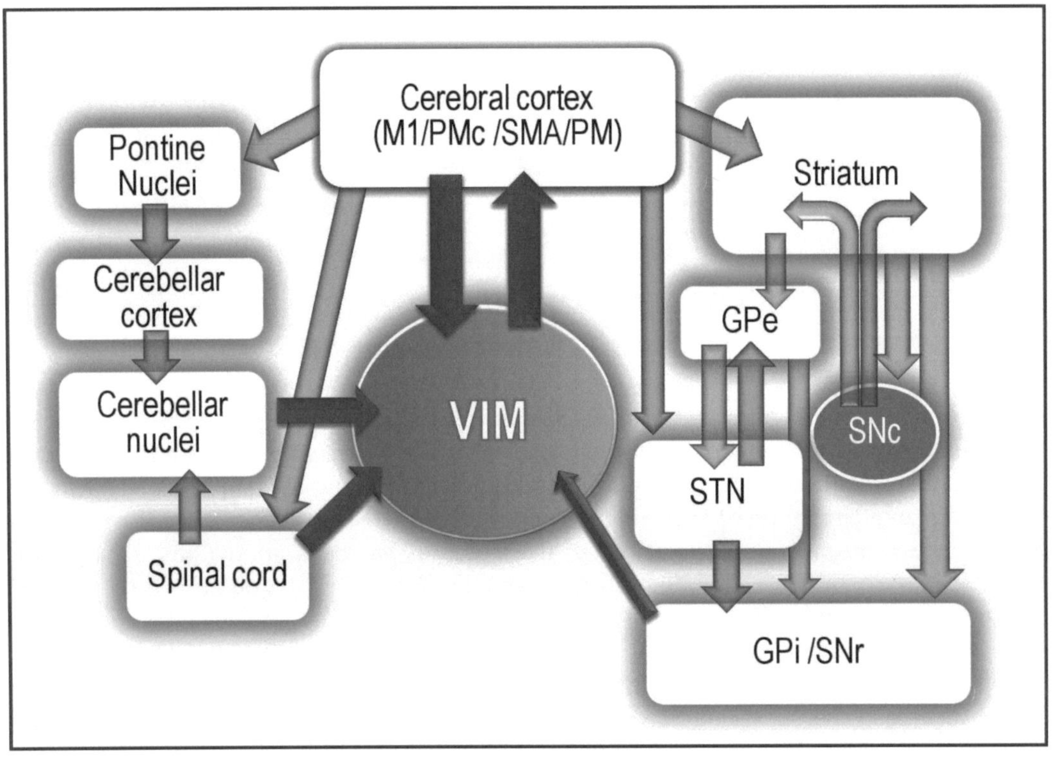

Fig. 1. Major fiber connections of the Vim nucleus in the movement disorders. Abbreviations: PMc, primary motor cortex; SMA, supplementary motor area; PM, premotor cortex; GPe, globus pallidus externa, STN, subthalamic nucleus; GPi, globus pallidus internus; SNr, substantia nigra pars reticulate; SNc, substantia nigra pars compacta.

The VL thalamic nucleus comprises 2 major functional territories (Asanuma et al., 1983a; Kultas-Ilinsky & Ilinski, 1991; Ilinsky & Kultas-Ilinsky, 2002). The cerebellothalamic excitatory afferents terminate predominantly in the contralateral Vim nucleus, creating a posterior-to-anterior gradient of terminal densities through the VL nucleus. In contrast, the pallidothalamic inhibitory afferents terminate preferentially in the ipsilateral Vo nucleus, with an anterior-to-posterior gradient of terminal densities through the VL nucleus (Percheron et al., 1996; Sakai et al., 1996; Gallay et al., 2008). These 2 functional territories thus receive different afferents that interlace and, at least in part, overlap (Rouiller et al., 1994; Sakai et al., 1996). A somatotopic arrangement, i.e., a medial-to-lateral distribution of facial-, forelimb-, and hindlimb-receptive fields, also exists in VL thalamic nucleus (Strick, 1976; Asanuma et al., 1983b; Vitek et al., 1994, 1996; Ohye, 1997). These findings indicate that the Vim and Vo nuclei receive differentially weighted pallidal and cerebellar afferent inputs (Sakai et al., 1996; Gallay et al., 2008) and suggest that they might, at least in part, integrate these inputs in a somatotopic fashion (Sakai et al., 1996). Given that spinothalamic afferents terminate in the posteroventral part of the VL nucleus along a posterior-to-anterior gradient, Craig (2008) suggests that this part of the nucleus is not simply a relay of primary cerebellothalamic inputs, but rather, represents the convergence of the spinothalamic and cerebellothalamic movement-related pathways.

Neurons of the VL nucleus project to the sensorimotor territory of the striatum, preferentially as collaterals of thalamocortical projections via multisynaptic connectivity. Convergence of the thalamic and cortical inputs could occur in this striatal region (McFarland & Haber, 2000, 2001). In a monkey model of PD, corticostriatal and thalamostriatal synapses in the sensorimotor striatum show complex ultrastructural remodeling that might increase synaptic plasticity (Villalba & Smith, 2011). Thus, ventral thalamic motor nuclei might act not only as relay nuclei but also as highly ordered nuclei providing positive feedback to the sensorimotor striatum (Smith et al., 2004) and thus sustaining disinhibition of specific thalamocortical circuits until their goals are achieved. Alternatively, these nuclei might reinforce or facilitate selective basal ganglia circuits, thereby suppressing unwanted movements (McFarland & Haber, 2000).

The thalamic territory innervated by cerebellar afferents sends efferents predominantly to the primary, pre-, and pre-supplementary motor cortices, while the thalamic territory innervated by pallidal afferents sends efferents predominantly to the primary and premotor cortices (Rouiller et al., 1994; Sakai et al., 2002; Morel et al., 2005). This divergence and convergence of projections from pallidal and cerebellar afferent-receiving thalamic areas across multiple areas of motor and premotor cortex is now well accepted (Morel et al., 2005). These pathways seem to directly participate in modulating the nature of motor-related information.

Local GABAergic inhibitory interneurons in the thalamic nuclei receive cerebellar, pallidal, and cortical afferents, and constitute complicated inhibitory and excitatory influences upon thalamocortical projection neurons. The thalamic reticular nucleus also receives excitatory collateral inputs from corticothalamic projections and, in turn, provides inhibitory and excitatory outputs to the thalamocortical projection neurons. The so-called "burst" and "tonic" modes of activity have been observed in thalamic neurons. In the "burst" mode, the transfer of information has a high signal-to-noise ratio that is conveyed in a non-linear manner such that new signals are readily identifiable but not readily analyzed. In the "tonic" mode, there is a linear transfer of the activity of specific afferents, but the signal-to-noise ratio is low (Godwin et al., 1996). Similar patterns of activity have been seen in the lateral thalamus (Tsoukatos et al., 1997; Zirh et al., 1998). The thalamocortical projection plays an important role in the preparation for, and initiation and execution of, the movements in the motor thalamus (Kurata, 2005). Electrical stimulation of corticothalamic fibers causes the thalamic relay neurons to change from "burst" to "tonic" mode (McCormick & Von Krosigk, 1992; Godwin et al., 1996). This switch in the firing patterns of thalamocortical fibers could be mediated by the corticothalamic feedback pathway via reticular neurons (Sherman & Guillery, 2006). Thus, local thalamic circuitry may involve scaling of neural processing, especially by increasing the temporal resolution of afferent information. In addition, these local inhibitory neurons are required for network synchronization (Huguenard, 1999).

3. Pathophysiology of parkinsonian tremor

Accumulating evidence suggests that among parkinsonian symptoms, akinesia/rigidity and tremor may be associated with functional impairments of different motor circuits. It is generally thought that tremor is primarily related to the cerebello-thalamo-cortical pathway, while akinesia/rigidity is rooted in the basal ganglia-thalamo-cortical pathway. Recent results from clinicopathological, electrophysiological, and neuroimaging studies on PD patients are discussed in the following sections.

3.1 Clinicopathological studies

A statistical analysis performed using the Unified Parkinson's Disease Rating Scale (UPDRS) showed that the motor score for tremor is independent of the scores for other motor symptoms in PD patients (Stochl et al., 2008). It was also noted that severity of tremor does not correlate with severity of dopamine loss or clinical disease progression (Zaidel et al., 2009). Rajput et al. (2009) reported that tremor-dominant PD patients showed slower disease progression and less dementia than did akinesia/rigidity-dominant PD patients. A postmortem histopathological study showed that dopaminergic cells in the midbrain retrorubral area, which project to the dorsolateral striatum and ventromedial thalamus, are more severely affected in tremor-dominant PD patients than in akinesia/rigidity-dominant PD patients (Paulus & Jellinger, 1991). Jellinger (1999) also reported that loss of dopaminergic cells is more pronounced in the medial portion of the substantia nigra pars compacta (SNc) in tremor-dominant PD, whereas in akinesia/rigidity-dominant PD, greater cell loss is seen in the ventrolateral portion. These clinicopathological findings suggest that tremor could have a different pathophysiology from akinesia/rigidity in PD patients.

3.2 Magnetoencephalography (MEG)

MEG studies in PD patients suggest a critical role of tremor oscillations in the pathophysiology of akinesia and rigidity (Timmermann et al., 2003). Double tremor oscillations in β range are not coherent with simultaneously recorded tremors (Raz et al., 2000; Lemstra et al., 1999; Hurtado et al., 2005). However, a strong coherence at β range is observed in the primary motor cortex, supplementary motor cortex, premotor cortex, diencephalon (possibly thalamus), and contralateral cerebellum (Timmermann et al., 2003). Interestingly, this coupling can be successfully reduced by dopamine replacement therapy (Salenius et al., 2002; Pollok et al., 2009). Simultaneous recordings using MEG and local field potentials in the subthalamic nucleus (STN) reveal that α and β activities are coupled to temporal brain areas and are involved in a functional separation of basal ganglia-cortex loops with different frequency patterns (Hirschmann et al., 2011). Litvak et al. (2011) reported that in PD patients at rest, α-range activities are coupled with temporoparietal-brainstem areas while β-range activities are coupled with the frontal network. Thus, it is likely that β-range oscillations might correlate with the motor loop and with manifestations of akinesia and rigidity.

3.3 Local field potentials (LFPs)

Intra- and postoperative LFP recordings from DBS electrodes provide further evidence that in patients with PD, synchronized tremor frequency oscillations (α or θ range) are coherent with neuronal oscillations in the motor cortex, as are double tremor frequency oscillations at β range with the globus pallidum internus (GPi) and STN (Levy et al., 2000; 2002). It has been suggested that dopamine depletion could cause neuronal synchronization in basal ganglia circuitry (Liu et al., 2002) and that dopamine therapy could reduce this synchronization (Levy et al., 2002). Gatev et al. (2006) suggested that dopamine activity may play a role in maintaining circuit segregation under normal conditions. STN LFPs in PD patients show synchronized activity with the basal ganglia; these oscillations occur mainly in the β range (15–30 Hz) (Kühn et al., 2004; Hammond et al., 2007). Both STN-DBS and L-dopa administration either ameliorate this β-range oscillation or shift it to a higher (γ range) frequency (Brown et al., 2001; Kühn et al., 2006). The β-range STN stimulation causes further impairment of movement in PD patients (Brown et al., 2001; Fogelson et al., 2005; Chen et al., 2007; Eusebio et al., 2008). These LFP oscillations correlate with akinesia and rigidity but not with tremor (Kühn et al., 2004, 2005, 2006, 2009). In fact, akinesia and rigidity increase when the patients are stimulated at a frequency of 20 Hz (Fogelson et al., 2005; Eusebio et al., 2008). The α-range oscillations in patients with tremor-dominant PD show finely segregated muscle-specific subloops that strongly correlate with the tremor-affected muscles, and tremor suppression can be achieved using STN-DBS in areas with pronounced α oscillations (Reck et al., 2009, 2010). Given that basal ganglia β oscillation correlates with rigidity and akinesia and α oscillation correlates with tremor, these findings further suggest a differential pathophysiology between akinesia-rigidity and tremor.

3.4 Single cell recordings

So-called "kinesthetic" cells receive afferent inputs from muscle spindles and respond to passive joint movements. These cells are located just anterior to the nucleus ventralis caudalis (VC), which receives tactile sensory inputs (Ohye & Narabayashi, 1979; Ohye et al., 1989). Percheron et al. (1996) postulated that the kinesthetic zone is located in the latero-ventral part of the Vim nucleus, a region that sends a majority of its axons to the motor cortex. Vitek et al. (1994) reported that in a monkey model of PD produced using 1-methyl-4-phenyl-1,2,3,6-tetrahydropyridine (MPTP), the kinesthetic zone expands anteriorly into regions that contain the active movement-related neurons. Kiss et al. (2003) reported that in patients with tremor, there is an anterior expansion in representation of the movement-related (kinesthetic) neurons without a change in their receptive field sizes. They suggested that tremor activates receptors responsive to deep sensations and, to a lesser degree, superficial sensations; thereby, repetitive tremor activities could result in a gradual increase in the synaptic efficacy of somatosensory inputs to movement-related neurons. Cells that respond to both somatosensory inputs and active movements are referred to as "combined" cells (Lenz et al., 1990, 1994) and have been identified only in patients with movement disorders.

Cells in the VL thalamic nucleus that demonstrate a discharge pattern with burst frequencies similar to that of tremor are called "tremor cells" (Lenz et al., 1988; Ohye et al., 1974). In a monkey model of resting tremor produced by a lesion of the ventral tegmentum, thalamic activity related to tremor frequency is unchanged following the interruption of sensory inputs (Lamarre & Joffroy, 1979; Ohye et al., 1970). This finding has led to the hypothesis that the tremor cells may represent a central pacemaker of tremor genesis, independent of sensory feedback (Lamarre & Joffroy, 1979; Lee & Stein, 1981). Tremor cells are reportedly located in the Vim nucleus and Vo complex (Lenz et al., 1994; Kobayashi et al., 2003; Brodkey JA, 2004). The distribution of tremor cells is important for thalamic surgery, because tremor has been successfully treated when the radiofrequency lesion was centered within the cluster of tremor cells (Hirai et al., 1979; Nagaseki et al.,1986; Ohye,1979). However, recent studies show that tremor cells are widely distributed in the Vim, Vo, and Vc nuclei, and that they show no apparent differences in proportion within each nucleus (Kobayashi et al., 2003; Brodkey et al., 2004). These findings suggest that the ideal surgical target might not be determined by microelectrode recordings of tremor cells alone (Kobayashi et al., 2003; Katayama et al., 2005). The number of tremor cells in PD patients is much higher than that in patients with other movement disorders, such as essential tremor and multiple sclerosis. This may play a role in the better surgical outcomes seen in PD patients (Brodkey et al., 2004). Based on their experiences, Katayama et al. (2005) postulated that tremor cells might play a predominant role in the lateral portion of the Vim nucleus, which provides the best control of PD-associated tremor, in accordance with previous reports (Atkinson et al., 2002; Hariz & Hirabayashi., 1997).

3.5 Positron emission tomography (PET) and single photon emission computed tomography (SPECT)

PET measurements of local cerebral blood flow (CBF) are used to determine changes in afferent activity onto target synaptic fields or in local neuronal activity, including those of local circuit interneurons, rather than changes in efferent activity. It should be noted that changes in cortical blood flow may not reflect the direct effects of DBS but rather, may reflect sensory feedback from changes in motor activity (Perlmutter & Mink, 2006). The metabolic rate of glucose (CMRglc) measured with (^{18}F)fluoro-2-deoxy-D-glucose PET (FDG-PET) is known as a marker of integrated local synaptic activities and is sensitive to direct neuronal and synaptic damages and to the functional changes in synaptic activity distant from the primary site of pathology (Magistretti et al., 1999).

A recent PET study suggests that the metabolic pattern of tremor-dominant PD is significantly different from that of akinesia/rigidity-dominant PD (Mure et al., 2011). Patients with tremor-dominant PD exhibit better clinical prognoses and slower disease progression with less cognitive decline (Louis et al., 1999; Marras et al., 2002; Rajput et al., 2009). Using FDG-PET, Mure et al. (2011) indicated that these clinical findings correlate with a slow deterioration of the metabolic pattern in patients with tremor-dominant PD. As a significant increase in regional metabolism is found in the rostral cerebellar cortex, dentate nucleus, dorsal pons, putamen, and primary motor cortex, Mure et al. (2011) suggested that both the cerebello-thalamo-cortical pathway and the basal ganglia circuitry are involved in tremor genesis. In patients with PD tremor, high-frequency stimulation of the Vim nucleus reportedly reduces regional metabolism and CBF in the ipsilateral sensorimotor cortex (Parker et al., 1992; Boecker et al., 1997; Wielepp et al., 2001; Mure et al., 2011) and the contralateral dorsal cerebellar nucleus (Parker et al., 1992; Davis et al., 1997; Mure et al., 2011). Interestingly, increases in regional CBF and metabolism are also found in the Vim nucleus ipsilateral to the stimulation site (Rezai et al., 1999; Perlmutter et al., 2002; Haslinger et al., 2003; Fukuda et al., 2004; Mure et al., 2011).

SPECT using Iodine-123 fluoropropyl-carbomethoxy-3 ([^{123}I]FP-CIT SPECT) targets the dopamine transporter and is used to determine ongoing loss of dopaminergic neurons in PD patients (Kaufman & Madras., 1991; Niznik et al., 1991; Seibyl et al., 1998). [^{123}I]FP-CIT SPECT shows significantly higher uptake in the putamen and caudate nucleus in tremor-dominant PD than in akinesia/rigidity-dominant PD (Spiegel et al., 2007; Eggers et al., 2011).

3.6 Functional magnetic resonance imaging (fMRI)

Intrinsic blood oxygen consumption detected by fMRI is correlated with respective low-frequency electrical amplitude fluctuations in classical frequency bands (Logothetis & Wandell, 2004; Laufs et al., 2003; Leopold et al., 2003; He et al., 2008; de Munck et al., 2009). Patients with PD show increased overall activity in networks coupled to the primary motor cortex and cerebellum and reduced functional connections in the supplementary motor area, dorsolateral prefrontal area, and putamen (Wu et al., 2010). Recently, increased functional connections between the STN and cortical motor areas have been found in the resting phase in PD patients (Baudrexel et al., 2011). High-frequency stimulation of the Vim nucleus at an amplitude of 2–4 volts, a frequency of 150 Hz, and a pulse width of 60 µsec reportedly causes metabolic activation of the lateral thalamic wall, GPi, and primary sensorimotor cortex (Rezai et al., 1999).

4. Thalamic deep brain stimulation in Parkinson's disease

The therapeutic mechanism of thalamic DBS remains speculative. With respect to tremor suppression, 4 different hypotheses of Vim-DBS have been proposed. The first proposed mechanism is "conduction block." This hypothesis is supported by the fact that Vim thalamotomy has similar effects to Vim DBS (Benabid et al., 1996). A second possible mechanism involves activation of inhibitory axon terminals that synapse onto and inhibit projection neurons (Wu et al., 2001). A third alternative suggests the superposition of continuous stimuli onto rhythmically oscillating subcortical-cortical loops (Montgomery & Baker, 2000). A final hypothesis is that high-frequency stimulation inhibits neuronal activity near the stimulation site while activating axonal elements that leave the target structure (Vitek, 2002). Recent reports have shown that during high-frequency stimulation, glutamate and adenosine are increased in a calcium-dependent manner, and that these neurotransmitters might be largely derived from astrocytes (Lee et al., 2004; Anderson et al., 2004, 2006; Bekar et al., 2008; Chang et al., 2009; Agnesi et al., 2010; Tawfik et al., 2010). It is hypothesized that this elevated glutamate release excites local interneurons, thereby increasing the production of inhibitory neurotransmitters (e.g., GABA and glycine) and resulting in a decrease in the firing rates of projection neurons (Kang et al., 1998; Fellin & Haydon, 2005; Tian et al., 2005; Fellin et al., 2006; Tawfik VL, 2010). Holsheimer et al. (2000) have suggested that in human brains, the effect of Vim DBS could be mediated through the stimulation of afferent and efferent axons rather than stimulation of cell bodies.

In patients with tremor-dominant PD, tremor suppression can be achieved irrespective of age, disease duration, or baseline disease severity (Benabid et al., 1996; Schuurman et al., 2008). Complete arrest of tremors is usually achieved immediately using continuous stimulation of the Vim nucleus at a high frequency (greater than 100 Hz); these effects are completely reversible (Benabid, 1996).

4.1 Programming challenges in Vim DBS

With stereotactic surgical techniques, the stimulating DBS leads are implanted into the Vim nucleus (Fig. 2). Lesion-like effects of implant are always obtained immediately after the implantation of DBS leads, unless the electrode is misplaced. Initiation of programming is ideally started when the lesion-like effect has almost disappeared. The optimal stimulating parameters are determined using monopolar or bipolar stimulation. For example, first a constant pulse width of 60 μsec and a constant frequency of 130 Hz (or above) is selected. Then the voltage is progressively increased to find the threshold for symptom suppression without adverse effects, using the contact(s) that gives the best effect. As the effect of the stimulation tends to decrease in the weeks or months following surgery and as the threshold for side effects tends to increase, the voltage may have to be further adjusted. Best results are usually obtained at pulse frequencies of 130–185 Hz (no lower than 100 Hz), pulse widths of 60–90 μsec, and amplitudes of 1.5–3.6 volts. Intermittent use of implantable pulse generators is recommended to avoid the development of tolerance (habituation) and to save battery life.

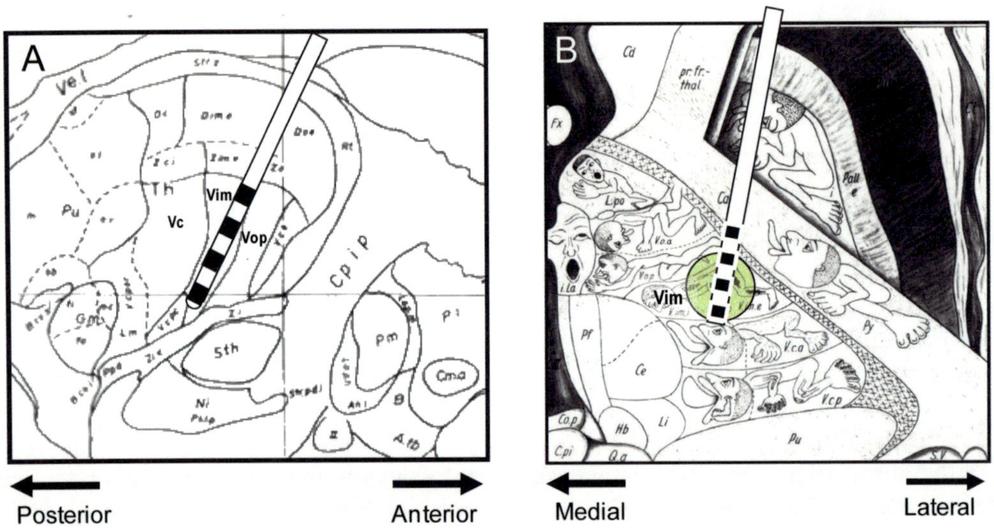

Fig. 2. Schematic drawing of the DBS lead implanted into the Vim nucleus on the the saggital (A) and axial (B) planes of the brain atlas.

4.2 Therapeutic impact of Vim DBS

In early studies with a short-term follow-up (range; 0–40 months), complete or nearly complete tremor resolution was accomplished by Vim DBS in 70–100% of treated patients (Blond et al., 1992; Pollak et al., 1993; Alesch et al., 1995; Benabid et al., 1996; Tasker, 1998; Schuurman et al., 2000; Krauss et al., 2001; Yamamoto et al., 2004). Tremor reduction rate was found to be 71–97% by using the UPDRS Part III motor scale (Hariz et al., 1999; Limousine et al., 1999; Lyons et al., 2001; Kumar et al., 2003; Rehncrona et al., 2003) and 88–93% by using the Tremor Rating Scale (TRS) (Putzke et al., 2003). Based on blind assessments, all the treated patients showed complete or nearly complete relief until at least 2 years after the operation (Schuurman et al., 2000). Assessments with UPDRS Part III revealed tremor reduction rates of 75–83% in the arm and 0–87.9% in the leg (Ondo et al., 1998; Rehncrona et al., 2003). With respect to the long-term efficacy of Vim DBS, Schuurman et al. (2008) reported that 88% of patients showed complete or nearly complete tremor suppression after a mean follow-up period of 5 years, similar to findings of other reports (Kumar et al., 2003; Pahwa et al., 2006; Hariz et al., 2008). Non-tremor parkinsonian symptoms usually remain unchanged at both short- and long-term follow-up points after Vim DBS (Blond et al., 1992; Pollak et al., 1993; Alesch et al., 1995; Benabid et al., 1996; Ondo et al., 1998; Rehncrona et al., 2003; Tarsy et al., 2005; Pahwa et al., 2006; Hariz et al., 2008). However, some reports have shown beneficial effects of Vim DBS on akinesia, rigidity, and L-dopa-induced dyskinesias (Blond, 1992; Tasker, 1998; Limousin et al., 1999; Putzke et al., 2003; Rehncrona et al., 2003; Pahwa, 2006). These additional benefits of Vim stimulation are thought to be due to spreading of the current to the Vo nucleus area that receives pallidal afferents. Additional stereotactic interventions have been used to treat parkinsonian symptoms that could not respond well to thalamic ablation surgery (Goto et al., 2004) or DBS (Nishio et al., 2009)..

Significant improvements in activities of daily living (ADL) scores have been seen after a short-term follow-up (Blond et al., 1992; Alesch et al., 1995; Koller et al., 1997; Hariz et al., 1999; Limousine et al., 1999; Schuurman et al., 2000; Putzke et al., 2003); however, these scores often return to preoperative baseline or even below during long-term follow-ups (Pahwa et al., 2006; Hariz et al., 2008; Schuurman et al., 2008). Putzke et al. (2003) reported that benefits of Vim-DBS on ADL scores persist for the first 24 months after surgery, but disappear after 36 months. It is necessary to increase dosages of anti-parkinsonism drugs in parallel with disease progression, particularly during long-term follow-ups. In addition, the stimulus amplitude often needs to be increased due to progression of disease and/or the so-called "tolerance" phenomenon, which is also known as "habituation" to electrostimulation of the neuronal network (Benabid et al., 1996; Koller et al., 1997; Hariz et al., 1999). This increase in amplitude is undesirable, as it often causes paresthesia and cerebellar adverse effects (Benabid, 1996; Yamamoto et al., 2004). Recurrence of tremor is seen in ~5% of patients several weeks or years after the surgery (Benabid et al., 1996; Tasker, 1998). Neuropsychological assessments have shown that thalamic DBS results in a significant improvement in verbal memory (Tröster et al., 1998; Hugdahl and Wester, 2000; Woods et al., 2001), conceptualization, and emotional adjustment (Woods et al., 2001), while its left-side stimulation is reported to decrease verbal fluency (Schuurman et al., 2002).

4.3 Adverse events related to Vim DBS

Incidences of stimulation-related complications reported at long-term (greater than 5 years) follow-up include paresthesia (4–38%), dysarthria (3–36%), dystonia/hypertonia (3–16%), gait disturbance (11–16%), balance disturbance (5%), and cognitive dysfunction (2%). Among these adverse effects, non-adjustable and long-lasting complications include dysarthria (10–27%), paresthesia (16%), gait disturbance (7%), dystonia (5%), upper limb ataxia (3–4%), and disequilibrium (3–4%) (Rehncrona et al., 2003; Pawha et al., 2006; Tarsy et al., 2006; Hariz et al., 2008). Pahwa et al. (2006) described occurrences of persistent complications including dysarthria, disequilibrium, and gait disturbance after bilateral stimulation, even when the stimulus parameters were optimized.

The incidence of infection appears to be 0–11% during the early follow-up periods and 0–8% throughout the entire postoperative course (Rehncrona et al., 2003; Tarsy et al., 2006; Hariz et al., 2008; Schuurman et al., 2008). Hardware failures are occasionally found in the stimulator (0–3%), the DBS lead (0–8%), or the cable (0–3%), and skin erosion (0–4%) and hematoma requiring evacuation of the stimulator (0–3%) have also been reported (Rehncrona et al., 2003; Tarsy et al., 2006; Hariz et al., 2008; Schuurman et al., 2008).

5. Conclusions

In conclusion, Vim DBS is an appropriate first-line treatment for medically intractable tremor. Although the effect on ADL outcome decreases gradually after the surgery, long-term tremor suppression remains stable. STN DBS is currently considered the preferred surgical procedure in patients with tremor-dominant PD, even when disease progression is taken into consideration (Krack et al., 1997). However, STN DBS carries a potential risk of neuropsychiatric problems, particularly in aged patients. We suggest that Vim DBS is useful for patients with tremor-dominant PD, due to slow progression of disease and good response of non-tremor PD symptoms to dopaminergic therapy. We consider patients with intractable upper tremor to be good candidates for Vim DBS.

6. Acknowledgement

This work was supported by grants from the Ministry of Education, Culture, Sports, Science and Technology of Japan (grant-in-aid for Scientific Research, 23500428, 2139026900).

7. References

Agnesi, F.; Blaha, CD.; Lin, J. & Lee, KH. (2010). Local glutamate release in the rat ventral lateral thalamus evoked by high-frequency stimulation. *J Neural Eng,* Vol.7, No.2, 26009, ISSN 1741-2552.

Alesch, F.; Pinter, MM.; Helscher, RJ.; Fertl, L.; Benabid, AL. & Koos, WT. (1995). Stimulation of the ventral intermediate thalamic nucleus in tremor dominated Parkinson's disease and essential tremor. *Acta Neurochir (Wien),* Vol.136, No.1-2, pp. 75-81, ISSN 0001-6268.

Alexander, GE. & Crutcher, MD. (1990). Functional architecture of basal ganglia circuits: neural substrates of parallel processing. *Trends Neurosci,* Vol.13, No.7, pp. 266-271, ISSN 0166-2236.

Anderson, T.; Hu, B.; Pittman, Q. & Kiss, ZH. (2004). Mechanisms of deep brain stimulation: an intracellular study in rat thalamus. *J Physiol* Vol.15, No.559, pp. 301-313, ISSN 0022-3751.

Anderson, TR.; Hu, B.; Iremonger, K. & Kiss, ZH. (2006). Selective attenuation of afferent synaptic transmission as a mechanism of thalamic deep brain stimulation-induced tremor arrest. *J Neurosci* Vol.26, No.3, pp. 841-850, ISSN 0270-6474.

Asanuma, C.; Thach, WT. & Jones, EG. (1983a). Distribution of cerebellar terminations and their relation to other afferent terminations in the ventral lateral thalamic region of the monkey. *Brain Res Rev,* Vol.5, No.3, pp. 237-265, ISSN 0165-0173.

Asanuma, C.; Thack, WT. & Jones, EG. (1983b). Anatomical evidence for segregated focal groupings of efferent cells and their terminal ramifications in the cerebellothalamic pathway of the monkey. *Brain Res Rev,* Vol.5, No.3, pp. 267-297, ISSN 0165-0173.

Atkinson, JD.; Collins, DL.; Bertrand, G.; Peters, TM.; Pike, GB. & Sadikot, AF. (2002). Optimal location of thalamotomy lesions for tremor associated with Parkinson disease: a probabilistic analysis based on postoperative magnetic resonance imaging and an integrated digital atlas. *J Neurosurg,* Vol.96, No.5, pp. 854-866, ISSN 0022-3085.

Baudrexel, S.; Witte, T.; Seifried, C.; von Wegner, F.; Beissner, F.; Klein, JC.; Steinmetz, H.; Deichmann, R.; Roeper, J. & Hilker, R. (2011). Resting state fMRI reveals increased subthalamic nucleus-motor cortex connectivity in Parkinson's disase. *Neuroimage,* Vol.55, No.4, pp.1728-1738, ISSN 1095-9572.

Bekar, L.; Libionka, W.; Tian, GF.; Xu, Q.; Torres, A.; Wang, X.; Lovatt, D.; Williams, E. Takano, T.; Schnermann, J.; Bakos, R. & Nedergaad, M. (2008). Adenosine is crucial for deep brain stimulation-mediated attenuation of tremor. *Nat Med,* Vol.14, No. 1, pp. 75-80, ISSN 1078-8956.

Benabid, AL.; Pollak, P.; Gao, D.; Hoffmann, D.; Limousin, P.; Gay, E.; Payen, I. & Benazzouz, A. (1996). Chronic electrical stimulation of the ventralis intermedius nucleus of the thalamus as a treatment of movement disorders. *J Neurosurg,* Vol.84, No.2, pp.203-214, ISSN 0022-3085..

Blond, S.; Caparros-Lefebvr, D.; Parker, F.; Assaker, R.; Petit, H.; Guieu, JD. & Christiaens, JL. (1992). Control of tremor and involuntary movement disorders by choronic stereotactic stimulation of the ventral intermediate thalamic nucleus. *J Neurosurg,* Vol.77, No.1, pp. 62-68, ISSN 0022-3085.

Boecker, H.; Wills, AJ.; Ceballos-Baumann, A.; Samuel, M.; Thomas, DG.; Marsden, CD. & Brooks, DJ. (1997). Stereotactic thalamotomy in tremor-dominant Parkinson's disease: An $H_2{}^{15}O$ PET motor activation study. *Ann Neurol,* Vol.41, No.1, pp. 108-111, ISSN 0364-5134.

Brodkey, JA.; Tasker, RR.; Hamani, C.; McAndrews, MP.; Dostrovsky, JO. & Lozano, AM. (2004). Tremor cells in the human thalamus: differences among neurological disorders. *J Neurosurg,* Vol.101, No.1, pp. 43-47, ISSN 0022-3085.

Brown, P.; Oliviero, A.; Mazzone, P.; Insola, A.; Tonali, P. & Di Lazzaro, V. (2001). Dopamine dependency of oscillations between subthalamic nucleus and pallidum in Parkinson's disease. *J Neurosci,* Vol.21, No.3, pp. 1033-1038, ISSN 0270-6474.

Chang, SY.; Shon, YM.; Angesi, F. & Lee, KH. (2009). Microthalamotomy effect during deep brain stimulation: potential involvement of adenosine and glutamate efflux. *Conf Proc IEEE Eng Med Bio Soc,* pp. 3294-3297, ISSN 1557-170X.

Chen, CC.; Litvak, V.; Gilbertson, T.; Kühn A.; Lu, CS.; Lee, ST.; Tsai, CH.; Tisch, S.; Limousin, P.; Hariz, M. & Brown, P. (2007). Excessive synchronization of basal ganglia neurons at 20 Hz slows movement in Parkinson's disease. *Exp Neurol,* Vol.205, No.1, pp. 214-221, ISSN 0014-4886.

Craig, AD. (2008). Retrograde analyses of spinothalamic projections in the macaque monkey: input to the ventral lateral nucleus. *J Comp Neurol,* Vol.508, No.2, pp. 315-328, ISSN 0021-9967.

Davis, KD.; Taub, E.; Houle, S.; Lang, AE.; Dostrovsky, JO.; Tasker, RR. & Lozano, AM. (1997). Globus pallidus stimulation activates the cortical motor system during alleviation of parkinsonian symptoms. *Nat Med,* Vol.3, No.6, pp. 671-674, ISSN 1078-8956.

de Munck, JC.; Gonçalves, SI.; Mammoliti, R.; Heethaar, RM. & Lopes da Silva, FH. (2009). Interactions between different EEG frequency bands and their effect on alpha-fMRI correlations. *Neuroimage,* Vol.47, No.1, pp. 69-76, ISSN 1053-8119.

Eggers, C.; Kahraman, D.; Fink, GR.; Schmidt, M. & Timmermann, L. (2011). Akinetic-rigid and tremor-dominant Parkinson's disease patients show different patterns of FP-CIT single photon emission computed tomography. *Mov Disord,* Vol.26, No.3, pp.416-423, ISSN 1531-8257.

Eusebio, A.; Chen, CC.; Lu, CS.; Lee, SR., Tsai, CH.; Limousin, P.; Hariz, M. & Brown, P. (2008). Effects of low-frequency stimulation of the subthalamic nucleus on movement in Parkinson's disease. *Exp Neurol,* Vol. 209, No.1, pp. 125-130, ISSN 0014-4886.

Fellin, T. & Haydon, PG. (2005). Do astrocytes contribute to excitation underlying seizures? *Trends Mol Med,* Vol.11, No.12, pp. 530-533, ISSN 1471-4914.

Fellin, T.; Pascual, O. & Haydon, PG. (2006). Astrocytes coordinate synaptic networks: balanced excitation and inhibition. *Physiology (Bethesda),* Vol.21, pp. 208-215, ISSN 1548-9213.

Fogelson, N.; Kühn, AA.; Silberstein, P.; Limousin, PD.; Hariz, M.; Trottenberg, T.; Kupsch, A & Brown, P. (2005). Frequency dependent effects of subthalamic nucleus stimulation in Parkinson's disease. *Neurosci Lett,* Vol.382, No.1-2, pp. 5-9, ISSN 1872-7972.

Fukuda, M.; Barnes, A.; Simon, ES.; Holmes, A.; Dhawan, V.; Giladi, N.; Fodstad, H.; Ma, Y. & Eidelberg, D. (2004). Thalamic stimulation for parkinsonian tremor: correlation between regional cerebral blood flow and physiological tremor characteristics. *Neuroimage,* Vol.21, No.2, pp. 608-615, ISSN 1053-8119.

Gallay, MN.; Jeanmonod, D.; Liu, J. & Morel, A. (2008). Human pallidothalamic and cerebellothalamic tracts: anatomical basis for functional stereotactic neurosurgery. *Brain Struct Funct,* Vol.212, No.6, pp. 443-463, ISSN 1863-2653.

Gatev, P.; Darbin, O. & Wichmann, T. (2006). Oscillations in the basal ganglia under normal conditions and in movement disorders. *Mov Disord,* Vol.21, No.10, pp. 1566-1577, ISSN 1863-2653.

Godwin, DW.; Vaughan, JW. & Sherman, SM. (1996). Metabotropic glutamate receptors switch visual response mode of lateral geniculate nucleus cells from burst to tonic. *J Neurophysiol,* Vol.76, No.3, pp. 1800-1816, ISSN 0022-3077.

Goto, S.; Yamada, K. & Ushio, Y. (2004). Subthalamic nucleus stimulation in a parkinsonian patient with previous bilateral thalamotomy. *J Neurol Neurosurg Psychiatry,* Vol.75, No.1, pp. 164-165, ISSN 0022-3050.

Hammond, C.; Bergman, H. & Brown, P. (2007). Pathological synchronization in Parkinson's disease: networks, models and treatments. *Trends Neurosci,* Vol.30, No.7, pp. 357-364, ISSN 0166-2236.

Hariz, MI. & Hirabayashi, H. (1997). Is there a relationship between size and site of the stereotactic lesion and symptomatic results of pallidotomy and thalamotomy? *Stereotact Funct Neurosurg,* Vol.69, No. 1-4, pp. 28-45, ISSN 1011-6125.

Hariz, MI.; Shamsgovara, P.; Johansson, F.; Hariz, G. & Fodstad, H. (1999). Tolerance and tremor rebound following long-term chronic thalamic stimulation for Parkinsonian and essential tremor. *Stereotact Funct Neurosurg,* Vol.72, No.2-4, pp. 208-218, ISSN 1011-6125.

Hariz, MI.; Krack, P.; Alesch, F.; Augustinsson, LE.; Bosch, A.; Ekberg, R.; Johansson, F.; Johnels, B.; Meyerson, BA.; N'Guyen, JP.; Pinter, M.; Pollak, P.; von Raison, F.; Rehncrona, S.; Speelman, JD.; Sydow, O. & Benabid, AL. (2008). Multicentre European study of thalamic stimulation for parkinsonian tremor: a 6 year follow-up. *J Neurol Neurosurg Psychiatry,* Vol.79, No.6, pp. 694-699, ISSN 0022-3050.

Haslinger, B.; Boecker, H.; Büchel, C.; Vesper, J.; Tronnier, VM.; Pfister, R.; Alesch, F.; Moringlane, JR.; Krauss, JK.; Conrad, B.; Schwaiger, M. & Ceballos-Baumann, AO. (2003). Differential modulation of subcortical target and cortex during deep brain stimulation. *Neuroimage,* Vol.18, No.2, pp. 517-524, ISSN 1053-8119.

Hassler, R. (1959). Introduction to stereotaxis with an atlas of the human brain, In: *Anatomy of the thalamus,* G. Schaltenbrand & P. Bailey, (Eds.), pp. 230-290, Thieme, Stuttgart.

He, BJ.; Snyder, AZ.; Zempel, JM.; Smyth, MD. & Raichle, ME. (2008). Electrophysiological correlates of the brain's intrinsic large-scale functional architecture. *Proc Natl Acad Sci USA,* Vol.105, No.41, pp. 16039-16044, ISSN 0027-8424.

Hirai, T.; Shibazaki, T.; Nakajima, H.; Imai, S. & Ohye, C. (1979). Minimal effective lesion in the stereotactic treatment of tremor [proceedings]. *Appl Neurophysiol,* Vol.42, No.5, pp. 307-308, ISSN 0302-2773.

Hirschmann, J.; Özkurt, TE.; Butz, M.; Homburger, M.; Elben, S.; Hartmann, CJ.; Vesper, J.; Wojtecki, L. & Schnitzler, A. (2011). Distinct oscillatory STN-cortical loops revealed by simultaneous MEG and local field potential recordings in patients with Parkinson's disease. *Neuroimage,* Vol.55, No.3, pp. 1159-1168, ISSN 1053-8119.

Holsheimer, J.; Demeulemeester, H.; Nuttin, B. & de Sutter, P. (2000). Identification of the target neuronal elements in electrical deep brain stimulation. *Eur J Neurosci,* Vol.12, No.12, pp. 4573-4577, ISSN 0953-816X.

Hugdahl, K. & Wester, K. (2000). Neurocognitive correlates of stereotactic thalamotomy and thalamic stimulation in Parkinsonian patients. *Brain Cogn,* Vol.42, No.2, pp. 231-252, ISSN 0278-2626.

Huguenard, JR. (1999). Neuronal circuitry of thalamocortical epilepsy and mechanisms of antiabsence drug action. *Adv Neurol,* Vol.79, pp. 991-999, ISSN 0091-3952.

Hurtado, JM.; Rubchinsky, LL.; Sigvardt, KA.; Wheelock, VL. & Pappas, CT. (2005). Temporal evolution of oscillations and synchrony in GPi/muscle pairs in Parkinson's disease. *J Neurophyiol,* Vol.93, No. 3, pp. 1569-1584,ISSN 0022-3077.

Ilinsky, IA, & Kultas-Ilinsky, K. (2002). Motor thalamic circuits in primates with emphasis on the area targeted in treatment of movement disorders. *Mov Disord,* Vol.17, suppl 3, pp. s9-s14, ISSN 0885-3185.

Jellinger, KA. (1999). Post mortem studies in Parkinson's disease - is it possible to detect brain areas for specific symptoms? *J Neural Transm Suppl,* Vol.56, pp. 1-29, ISSN 0303-6995.

Kang, J.; Jiang, L.; Goldman, SA. & Nedergaard, M. (1998). Astrocyte-mediated potentiation of inhibitory synaptic transmission. *Nat Neurosci,* Vol.1, No.8, pp. 683-692, ISSN 1097-6256.

Katayama, Y.; Kano, T.; Kobayashi, K.; Oshima, H.; Fukaya, C. & Yamamoto, T. (2005). Difference in surgical strategies between thalamotomy and thalamic deep brain stimulation for tremor control. *J Neurol,* Vol.252, suppl 4, pp.17-22, ISSN 0340-5354.

Kaufman, MJ. & Madras, BK. (1991). Severe depletion of cocaine recognition sites associated with the dopamine transporter in Parkinson's-diseased striatum. *Synapse,* Vol.9, No.1, pp. 43-49, ISSN 0887-4476.

Kiss, ZH.; Davis, KD.; Tasker, RR.; Lozano, AM.; Hu, B. & Dostrovsky, JO. (2003). Kinaesthetic neurons in thalamus of humans with and without tremor. *Exp Brain Res,* Vol.150, No.1, pp. 85-94, ISSN 0014-4819..

Kobayashi, K.; Katayama, Y.; Kasai, M.; Oshima, H.; Fukaya, C. & Yamamoto, T. (2003) Localization of thalamic cells with tremor-frequency activity in Parkinson's disease and essential tremor. *Acta Neurochir Suppl,* Vol.87, pp. 137-139, ISSN 0065-1419.

Koller, W.; Pahwa, R.; Busenbark, K.; Hubble, J.; Wilkinson, S.; Lang, A.; Tuite, P.; Sime, E.; Lazano, A.; Hauser, R.; Malapira, T.; Smith, D.; Tarsy, D.; Miyawaki, E.;

Norregaard, T.; Kormos, T. & Olanow CW. (1997). High-frequency unilateral thalamic stimulation in the treatment of essential and parkinsonian tremor. *Ann Neurol.* Vol.42, No.3, pp.292-299, ISSN 0364-5134.

Krack, P.; Pollak, P.; Limousin, P.; Benazzouz, A. & Benabid, AL. (1997). Stimulation of subthalamic nucleus alleviates tremor in Parkinson's disease. *Lancet,* Vol.350, Issue.9092, p.1675, ISSN 0140-6736.

Krauss, JK.; Simpson, RK Jr.; Ondo, WG.; Pohle, T.; Burgunder, JM. & Jankovic, J. (2001). Concepts and methods in chronic thalamic stimulation for treatment of tremor: technique and application. *Neurosurgery* Vol.48, No.3, pp. 535-543, ISSN 0148-396X.

Kultas-Ilinsky, K. & Ilinsky, IA. (1991). Fine structure of the ventral lateral nucleus (VL) of the Macaca mulatta thalamus: cell types and synaptology. *J Comp Neurol,* Vol.314, No.2, pp. 319-349, ISSN 0021-9967.

Kumar, R.; Lozano, AM.; Sime, E. & Lang, AE. (2003). Long-term follow-up of thalamic deep brain stimulation for essential and parkinsonian tremor. *Neurology.* Vol.61, No.11, pp. 1601-1604, ISSN 0028-3878.

Kurata, K. (2005). Activity properties and location of neurons in the motor thalamus that project to the cortical motor areas in monkeys. *J Neurophysiol,* Vol.94, No.1, pp. 550-566, ISSN 0022-3077.

Kühn, AA.; Williams, D.; Kupsch, A.; Limousin, P.; Hariz, M.; Schneider, GH.; Yarrow, K. & Brown P. (2004). Event-related beta desynchronization in human subthalamic nucleus correlates with motor performance. *Brain,* Vol.127, pp. 735-746, ISSN 0006-8950.

Kühn, AA.; Trottenberg, T.; Kivi, A.; Kupsch, A.; Schneider, GH. & Brown, P. (2005). The relationship between local field potential and neuronal discharge in the subthalamic nucleus of patients with Parkinson's disease. *Exp Neurol,* Vol.194, No.1 pp.212-220, ISSN 0014-4886.

Kühn, AA.; Kupsch, A.; Scheider, GH. & Brown, P. (2006). Reduction in subthalamic 8-35 Hz oscillatory activity correlates with clinical improvement in Parkinson's disease. *Eur J Neurosci,* Vol.23, No.7, pp.1956-1960, ISSN 0953-816X.

Kühn, AA.; Tsui, A.; Aziz, T.; Ray, N.; Brücke, C.; Kupsch, A.; Schneider, GH. & Brown, P. (2009). Pathological synchronization in the subthalamic nucleus of patients with Parkinson's disease relates to both bradykinesia and rigidity. *Exp Neurol,* Vol.215, No.2, 380-387, ISSN 0014-4886.

Lamarre, Y. & Joffroy, AJ. (1979). Experimental tremor in monkey: activity of thalamic and precentral cortical neurons in the absence of peripheral feedback, In: *Advances in Neurology,* L.J. Poirier, T.I. Sourkes & P. Bedard, (Eds), Vol.24, pp. 109-122, Raven Press, New York, ISBN 0-89004-369-8.

Laufs, H.; Kleinschmidt, A.; Beyerle, A.; Eger, E.; Salek-Haddadi, A.; Preibisch, C. & Krakow, K. (2003). EEG-correlated fMRI of human alpha activity. Neuroimage, Vol.19, No.4, pp.1463-1476, ISSN 1053-8119.

Lee, KH.; Chang, SY.; Roberts, DW. & Kim, U. (2004). Neurotransmitter release from high-frequency stimulation of the subthalamic nucleus. J Neurosurg, Vol.101, No.3, pp.511-517, ISSN 0022-3085.

Lee, RG. & Stein, RB. (1981). Resetting of tremor by mechanical perturbations: a comparison of essential tremor and parkinsonian tremor. *Ann Neurol*, Vol.10, No.6, pp. 523-531, ISSN 0364-5134.

Lemstra, AW.; Verhagen Metman, L.; Lee, JI.; Dougherty, PM. & Lenz, FA. (1999). Tremor-frequency (3-6 Hz) activity in the sensorimotor arm representation of the internal segment of the globus pallidus in patients with Parkinson's disease. Neurosci Lett, Vol.267,No.2, pp. 129-132, ISSN 0304-3940.

Lenz, FA.; Tasker, RR.; Kwan, HC.; Schnider, S.; Kwong, R.; Murayama, Y.;, Dostrovsky, JO. & Murphy, JT. (1988). Single unit analysis of the human ventral thalamic nuclear group: correlation of thalamic "tremor cells" with the 3-6 Hz component of parkinsonian tremor. *J Neurosci*, Vol.8, No.3, pp. 754-764, ISSN 0270-6474.

Lenz, FA.; Kwan, HC.; Dostrovsky, JO.; Tasker, RR.; Murphy, JT. & Lenz, YE. (1990). Single unit analysis of the human ventral thalamic nuclear group: activity correlated with movement. *Brain*, Vol.113, pp. 1795-1821, ISSN 0006-8950.

Lenz, FA.; Kwan, HC.; Martin, RL.; Tasker, RR.; Dostrovsky, JO. & Lenz, YE. (1994). Single unit analysis of the human ventral thalamic nuclear group: tremor-related activity in functionally identified cells. *Brain*, Vol.117, pp. 531-543, ISSN 0006-8950.

Leopold, DA.; Murayama, Y. & Logothetis, NK. (2003). Very slow activity fluctuations in monkey visual cortex: implications for functional brain imaging. Cereb Cortex, Vol. 13, No.4, pp. 422-433, ISSN 1047-3211.

Levy, R.; Hutchison, WD.; Lozano, AM. & Dostrovsky, JO. (2000). High-frequency synchronization of neuronal activity in the subthalamic nucleus of parkinsonian patients with limb tremor. *J Neurosci*, Vol.20, No.20, pp. 7766-7775, ISSN 0270-6474.

Levy, R.; Hutchison, WD.; Lozano, AM. & Dostrovsky, JO. (2002). Synchronized neuronal discharge in the basal ganglia of parkinsonian patients is limited to oscillatory activity. *J Neurosci*, Vol.22, No.7, pp. 2855-2861, ISSN 0270-6474.

Limousin, P.; Speelman, JD.; Gielen, F. & Janssens, M. (1999). Multicenter European study of thalamic stimulation in parkinsonian and essential tremor. *J Neurol Neurosurg Psychiatry*, Vol.66, No.3, pp. 289-296, ISSN 0022-3050.

Litvak, V.; Jha, A.; Eusebio, A.; Oostenveld, R.; Foltynie, T.; Limousin, P.; Zrinzo, L.; Hariz, MI.; Friston, K. & Brown, P. (2011). Resting oscillatory cortico-subthalamic connectivity in patients with Parkinson's disease. *Brain*, Vol.134, 359-374, ISSN 1460-2156.

Liu, X.; Ford-Dunn, HL.; Hayward, GN.; Nandi, D.; Miall, RC.; Aziz, TZ. & Stein, JF. (2002). The oscillatory activity in the Parkinsonian subthalamic nucleus investigated using the macro-electrodes for deep brain stimulation. Clin Neurophysiol, Vol.113, No.11, pp. 1667-1672, ISSN 1388-2457.

Logothetis, NK. & Wandell, BA. (2004). Interpreting the BOLD signal. *Annu Rev Physiol*, Vol. 66, pp. 735-769, ISSN 0066-4278.

Louis, ED.; Tang, MX.; Cote, L.; Alfaro, B.; Mejia, H. & Marder, K. (1999). Progression of parkinsonian signs in Parkinson disease. *Arch Neurol*, Vol.56, No.3, pp. 334-337, ISSN 0003-9942.

Lyons, KE.; Koller, WC.; Wilkinson, SB. & Pahwa, R. (2001). Long term safery and efficacy of unilateral deep brain stimulation of the thalamus for parkinsonian tremor. *J Neurol Neurosurg Psychiatry*, Vol.71, No.5, pp. 682-684, ISSN 0022-3050.

Magistretti, PJ.; Pellerin, L.; Rothman, DL. & Shulman, RG. (1999). Energy on demand. *Science*, Vol.283, pp. 496-497, ISSN 0193-4511,.

Marras, C.; Rochon, P. & Lang, AE. (2002). Predicting motor decline and disability in Parkinson disease: a systemic review. Arch Neurol, Vol.59, No.11, pp. 1724-1728, ISSN 0003-9942.

McCormick, DA. & von Krosigk, M. (1992). Corticothalamic activation modulates thalamic firing through glutamate "metabotropic" receptors. *Proc Natl Acad Sci USA*, Vol. 89, No.7, pp. 2774-2778, ISSN 0027-8424.

McFarland, NR. & Haber, SN. (2000). Convergent inputs from thalamic motor nuclei and frontal cortical areas to the dorsal striatum in the primate. *J Neurosci*, Vol.20, No.10, pp. 3798-3813, ISSN 0270-6474.

McFarland, NR. & Haber, SN. (2001). Organization of thalamostriatal terminals from the ventral motor nuclei in the macaque. *J Comp Neurol*, Vol.429, No.2, pp. 321-336, ISSN 0021-9967.

McFarland, NR. & Haber, SN. (2002). Thalamic relay nuclei of the basal ganglia form both reciprocal and nonreciprocal cortical connections, linking multiple frontal cortical areas. *J Neurosci*, Vol.22, No.18, pp. 8117-8132, ISSN 0270-6474.

Montgomery, EB Jr. & Baker, KB. (2000). Mechanisms of deep brain stimulation and future technical developments. *Neurol Res*, Vol.22, No.3, pp. 259-266, ISSN 0161-6412.

Morel, A.; Liu, J.; Wannier, T.; Jeanmonod, D. & Rouiller, EM. (2005). Divergence and convergence of thalamocortical projections to premotor and supplementary motor cortex: a multiple tarcing study in the macaque monkey. *Eur J Neurosci*, Vol.21, No.4, pp.1007-1029, ISSN 0953-816X.

Mure, H.; Hirano, S.; Tang, CC.; Isaias, IU.; Antonini, A.; Ma, Y.; Dhawan, V. & Eidelberg, D. (2011). Parkinson's disease tremor-related metabolic network: characterization, progression, and treatment effects. *Neuroimage*, Vol.54, No.2, pp. 1244-1253, ISSN 1053-8119.

Nagaseki, Y.; Shibazaki, T.; Hirai, T.; Kawashima, Y.; Hirato, M.; Wada, H.; Miyazaki, M. & Ohye, C. (1986). Long-term follow-up results of selective VIM-thalamotomy. *J Neurosurg*, Vol.65, No.3, pp. 296-302, ISSN 0022-3085.

Nishio, M.; Korematsu, K.; Yoshida, S.; Nagai, Y.; Maruo, T.; Ushio, Y.; Kaji, R. & Goto, S. (2009). Long-term suppression of tremor by deep brain stimulation of the ventral intermediate nucleus of the thalamus combined with pallidotomy in hemiparkinsonian patients. *J Clin Neurosci*, Vol.16, No.11, pp. 1489-1491, ISSN 0967-5868.

Niznik, HB.; Fogel, EF.; Fassos, FF. & Seeman, P. (1991). The dopamine transporter is absent in parkinsonian putamen and reduced in the caudate nucleus. *J Neurochem*, Vol.56, No.1, pp. 192-198, ISSN 0022-3042.

Ohye, C.; Bouchard, R.; Larochelle, L.; Bédard, P.; Boucher, R.; Raphy, B. & Poirier, LJ. (1970). Effect of dorsal rhizotomy on postural tremor in the monkey. *Exp Brain Res*, Vol.10, No.2, pp. 140-150, ISSN 0014-4819.

Ohye, C.; Saito, U.; Fukamachi, A. & Narabayashi, H. (1974). An analysis of the spontaneous rhythmic and non-rhythmic burst discharges in the human thalamus. *J Neurol Sci*, Vol.22, No.2, pp. 245-259, ISSN 0022-510X.

Ohye, C. & Narabayashi, H. (1979). Physiological study of presumed ventralis intermedius neurons in the human thalamus. *J Neurosurg*. Vol.50, No.3, pp. 290-297, ISSN 0022-3085.

Ohye, C.; Shibazaki, T.; Hirai, T.; Wada, H.; Hirato, M. & Kawashima, Y. (1989). Further physiological observations on the ventralis intermedius neurons in the human thalamus. *J Neurophysiol*, Vol.61, No.3, pp. 488-500, ISSN 0022-3077.

Ohye, C. (1997). Functional organization of the human thalamus, stereotactic interventions, In: *Thalamus vol II Experimental and clinical aspects,* M. Sterade, E.G. Jones & D.A. McCormick, (Eds.), 517-542, Elsevier, ISBN 0-08-042507-0, Amsterdam.

Ondo, WG.; Jankovic, J.; Schwartz, K.; Almaguer, M. & Simpson, RK. (1998). Unilateral thalamic deep brain stimulation for refractory essential tremor and Parkinson's disease tremor. *Neurology*, Vol.51,No.4, pp. 1063-1069, ISSN 0028-3878.

Pahwa, R.; Lyons, KE.; Wilkinson, SB.; Simpson, RK Jr.; Ondo, WG.; Tarsy, D.; Norregaard, T.; Hubble, JP.; Smith, DA.; Hauser, RA. & Jankovic, J. (2006). Long-term evaluation of deep brain stimulation of the thalamus. *J Neurosurg*. Vol.104, No.4, pp. 506-512, ISSN 0022-3085.

Parker, F.; Tzourio, N.; Blond, S.; Petit, H. & Mazoyer, B. (1992). Evidence for a common network of brain structures involved in parkinsonian tremor and voluntary repetitive movement. *Brain Res,* Vol.584, No.1-2, pp. 11-17, ISSN 0006-8993.

Paulus, W. & Jellinger, K. (1991). The neuropathologic basis of different clinical subgroups of Parkinson's disease. *J Neuropathol Exp Neurol*, Vol.50, No.6, 743-755, ISSN 0022-3069.

Percheron, G.; François, C.; Talbi, B.; Yelnik, J. & Fénelon, G. (1996). The primate motor thalamus. Brain Res Brain Rev, Vol.22, No.2, pp. 93-181, ISSN 0165-0173.

Perlmutter, JS.; Mink, JW.; Bastian, AJ.; Zackowski, K.; Hershey, T.; Miyawaki, E.; Koller, W. & Videen, TO. (2002). Blood flow responses to deep brain stimulation of thalamus. *Neurology,* Vol.58, No.9, pp. 1388-1394, ISSN 0028-3878.

Perlmutter, JS. & Mink, JW. (2006). Deep brain stimulation. *Annu Rev Neurosci,* Vol.29, pp. 229-257, ISSN 0147-006X.

Pollak, P.; Benabid, AL.; Gervason, CL.; Hoffmann, D.; Seigneuret, E. & Perret, J. (1993). Long-term effects of chronic stimulation of the ventral intermediate thalamic nucleus in different types of tremor. *Adv Neurol*. Vol.60, pp. 408-413, ISSN 0091-3952.

Pollok, B.; Makhloufi, H.; Butz, M.; Gross, J.; Timmermann, L.; Wojtecki, L. & Schnitzler, A. (2009). Levodopa affects functional brain networks in parkinsonian resting tremor. *Mov Disord,* Vol.24, No.1, pp. 91-98, ISSN 0885-3185.

Putzke, JD.; Wharen, RE Jr.; Wszolek, ZK.; Turk, MF.; Strongosky, AJ. & Uitti, RJ. (2003). Thalamic deep brain stimulation for tremor-predominant Parkinson's disease. *Parkinsonism Relat Disord,* Vol.10, No.2, pp. 81-88, ISSN 1353-8020.

Rajput, AH.; Voll, A.; Rajput, ML.; Robinson, CA. & Rajput, A. (2009). Course in Parkinson disease subtypes. A 39-year clinicopathologic study. *Neurology,* Vol.73, No.3, pp. 206-212, ISSN 0028-3878.

Raz, A.; Vaadia, E. & Bergman, H. (2000). Firing patterns and correlations of spontaneous discharge of pallidal neurons in the normal and the tremulous 1-methyl-4-phenyl-1,2,3,6-tetrahydropyridine vervet model of parkinsonism. *J Neurosci*. Vol.20, No. 22, pp. 8559-8571, ISSN 0270-6474.

Reck, C.; Florin, E.; Wojtecki, L.; Krause, H.; Groiss, S.; Voges, J.; Maarouf, M.; Sturm, V.; Schnitzler, A. & Timmermann, L. (2009). Characterisation of tremor-associated local field potentials in the subthalamic nucleus in Parkinson's disease. *Eur J Neurosci*, Vol.29, No.3, pp. 599-612, ISSN 0953-816X.

Reck, C.; Himmel, M.; Florin, E.; Maarouf, M.; Sturm, V.; Wojtecki, L.; Schnitzler, A.; Fink, GR. & Timmermann, L. (2010). Coherence analysis of local field potentials in the subthalamic nucleus: differences in parkinsonian rest and postural tremor. *Eur J Neurosci*, Vol.32, No.7, pp. 1202-1214, ISSN 0953-816X.

Rehncrona, S.; Johnels, B.; Widner, H.; Törnqvist, AL.; Hariz,M. & Sydow,O.(2003). Long-term efficacy of thalamic deep brain stimulation for tremor: double-blind assessments. *Mov Disord*, Vol.18, No.2, pp. 163-170, ISSN 0885-3185.

Rezai, AR.; Lozano, AM.; Crawley, AP.; Joy, ML.; Davis, KD.; Kwan, CL.; Dostrovsky, JO.; Tasker, RR. & Mikulis, DJ. (1999). Thalamic stimulation and functional magnetic resonance imaging: localization of cortical and subcortical activation with implanted electrodes. Technical note. *J Neurosurg*, Vol.90, No.3, pp. 583-590, ISSN 0022-3085.

Rouiller, EM.; Liang, F.; Babalian, A.; Moret, V. & Wiesendanger, M. (1994). Cerebellothalamocortical and pallidothalamocortical projections to the primary and supplementary motor cortical areas: a multiple tracing study in macaque monkeys. *J Comp Neurol*, Vol. 345, No.2, pp. 185-213, ISSN 0021-9967.

Sakai, ST.; Inase, M. & Tanji, J. (1996). Comparison of cerebellothalamic and pallidothalamic projections in the monkey (Macaca fuscata): a double anterograde labeling study. *J Comp Neurol*, Vol.368, No.2, pp. 215-228, ISSN 0021-9967.

Sakai, ST.; Inase, M. & Tanji, J. (2002). The relationship between MI and SMA afferents and cerebellar and pallidal efferents in the macaque monkey. *Somatosens Mot Res*, Vol.19, No.2, pp. 139-148, ISSN 0899-0220.

Salenius, S.; Avikainen, S.; Kaakkola, S.; Hari, R. & Brown, P. (2002). Defective cortical drive to muscle in Pakinson's disease and its improvement with levodopa. *Brain*, Vol.125, pp. 491-500, ISSN 0006-8950.

Seibyl, JP.; Marek, K.; Sheff, K.; Zoghbi, S.; Baldwin, RM.; Charney, DS.; van Dyck, CH. & Innis, RB. (1998). Iodine-123-beta-CIT and iodine-123-FPCIT SPECT measurement of dopamine transporters in healthy subjects and Parkinson's patients. *J Nucl Med*, Vol.39, No.9, pp. 1500-1508, ISSN 0161-5505.

Schuurman, PR.; Bosch, DA.; Bossuyt, PM.; Bonsel, GJ.; van Someren, EJ.; de Bie, RM.; Merkus, MP. & Speelman, JD. (2000). A comparison of continuous thalamic stimulation and thalamotomy for suppression of severe tremor. *N Engl J Med*, Vol.342, No.7, pp.461-468, ISSN 0028-4793.

Schuurman, PR.; Bruins, J.; Merkus, MP., Bosch, DA. & Speelman, JD. (2002). A comparison of neuropsychological effects of thalamotomy and thalamic stimulation. *Neurology*, Vol.59, No.8, pp. 1232-1239, ISSN 0028-3878.

Schuurman, PR.; Bosch, DA.; Merkus, MP. & Speelman, JD. (2008). Long-term follow-up of thalamic stimulation versus thalamotomy for tremor suppression. *Mov Disord*, Vol.23, No.8, pp. 1146-1153, ISSN 0885-3185.

Sherman, SM. & Guillery, RW. (2006). Function of burst and tonic response modes in the thalamocortical relay, In: *Exploring the thalamus and its role in cortical function (second edition)*, The MIT Press, ISBN 0-262-19532-1, Cambridge.

Smith, Y.; Raju, DV.; Pare, JF. & Sidibe, M. (2004). The thalamostriatal system: a highly specific network of the basal ganglia circuitry. *Trends Neurosci*, Vol.27, No.9, pp. 520-527, ISSN 0166-2236.

Spiegel, J.; Hellwig, D.; Samnick, S.; Jost, W., Möllers, MO.; Fassbender, K.; Kirsch, CM. & Dillmann, U. (2007). Striatal FP-CIT uptake differs in the subtypes of early Parkinson's disease. *J Neural Transm*, Vol.114, No.3, pp. 331-335, ISSN 0300-9564.

Stochl, J.; Boomsma, A.; Ruzicka, E.; Brozova, H. & Blahus, P. (2008). On the structure of motor symptoms of Parkinson's disease. *Mov Disord*, Vol.23, No.9, pp. 1307-1312, ISSN 0885-3185.

Strick, PL. (1976). Activity of ventrolateral thalamic neurons during arm movement. *J Neurophysiol*, Vol.39, No.5, pp.1032-1044, ISSN 0022-3077.

Tasker, RR. (1998). Deep brain stimulation is preferable to thalamotomy for tremor suppression. *Surg Neurol*, Vol.49, No.2, pp. 145-153, ISSN 0090-3019.

Tarsy, D.; Scollins, L.; Corapi, K.; O'Herron, S.; Apetauerova, D. & Norregaard, T. (2005). Progression of Parkinson's disease following thalamic deep brain stimulation for tremor. *Stereotact Funct Neurosurg*, Vol.83, No.5-6, pp. 222-227, ISSN 1011-6125.

Tawfik, VL.; Chang, SY.; Hitti, FL.; Roberts, DW.; Leiter, JC.; Jovanovic, S. & Lee, KH. (2010). Deep brain stimulation results in local glutamate and adenosine release: investigation into the role of astrocytes. *Neurosurgery*, Vol.67, No.2, pp. 367-375, ISSN 0148-396X.

Tian, GF.; Azmi, H.; Takano, T.; Xu, Q.; Peng, W.; Lin, J.; Oberheim, N.; Lou, N.; Wang, X.; Zielke, HR.; Kang, J. & Nedergaard, M. (2005). An astrocytic basis of epilepsy. *Nat Med*, Vol.11, No.9, pp. 973-981, ISSN 1078-8956.

Timmermann, L.; Gross, J.; Dirks, M.; Volkmann, J.; Freund, HJ. & Schnitzler, A. (2003). The cerebral oscillatory network of parkinsonian resting tremor. *Brain*, Vol. 126, No.1, pp. 199-212, ISSN 0006-8950.

Tröster, AI.; Wilkinson, SB.; Fields, JA.; Miyawaki, K. & Koller, WC. (1998). Chronic electrical stimulation of the left ventrointermediate (Vim) thalamic nucleus for the treatment of pharmacotherapy-resistant Parkinson's disease: a differential impact on access to semantic and episodic memory? *Brain Cogn*, Vol.38, No.2, pp. 125-149, ISSN 0278-2626.

Tsoukatos, J.; Kiss, ZH.; Davis, KD.; Tasker, RR. & Dostrovsky, JO. (1997). Patterns of neuronal firing in the human lateral thalamus during sleep and wakefulness. *Exp Brain Res*, Vol.113, No.2, pp. 273-282, ISSN 0014-4819.

Villalba, RM. & Smith, Y. (2011). Differential structural plasticity of corticostriatal and thalamostriatal axo-spinous synapses in MPTP-treated parkinsonian monkeys. *J Comp Neurol*, Vol.519, No.5, pp. 989-1005, ISSN 0021-9967.

Vitek, JL.; Ashe, J.; DeLong, MR. & Alexander, GE. (1994). Physiologic properties and somatotopic organization of the primate motor thalamus. *J Neurophysiol*, Vol.71, No.4, pp.1498-1513, 0022-3077.

Vitek, JL.; Ashe, J.; DeLong, MR. & Kaneoke, Y. (1996). Mircostimulation of primate motor thalamus: somatotopic organization and differential distribution of evoked motor responses among subnuclei. *J Neurophysiol*, Vol.75, No.6, pp. 2486-2495, 0022-3077.

Vitek, JL. (2002). Mechanisms of deep brain stimulation: excitation or inhibition. *Mov Disord*, Vol.17, suppl 3, pp. s69-s72, ISSN 0885-3185.

Wielepp, JP.; Burgunder, JM.; Pohle, T.; Ritter, EP.; Kinser, JA. & Krauss, JK. (2001). Deactivation of thalamocortical activity is responsible for suppressin of parkinsonian tremor by thalamic stimulation: a ^{99m}Tc-ECD SPECT study. *Clin Neurol Neurosurg,* Vol.103, No.4, pp. 228-231, ISSN 0303-8467.

Wu, YR.; Levy, R.; Ashby, P.; Tasker, RR. & Dostrovsky, JO. (2001). Does stimulation of the GPi control dyskinesia by activating inhibitory axons? *Mov Disord,* Vol.16, No.2, pp. 208-216, ISSN 0885-3185.

Wu, T.; Chan, P. & Hallett M (2010). Effective connectivity of neural networks in automatic movements in Parkinson's disease. Neuroimage, Vol.49, No.3, pp. 2581-2587, ISSN 1053-8119.

Woods, SP.; Fields, JA.; Lyons, KE.; Koller, WC.; Wilkinson, SB.; Pahwa, R. & Tröster, AI. (2001). Neuropsychological and quality of life changes following unilateral thalamic deep brain stimulation in Parkinson's disease: a one-year follow-up. *Acta Neurochir (Wien),* Vol.143, No.12, pp. 1273-1277, ISSN 0001-6268.

Yamamoto, T.; Katayama, Y.; Kano, T.; Kobayashi, K.; Oshima, H. & Fukaya, C. (2004). Deep brain stimulation for the treatment of parkinsonian, essential, and poststroke tremor: a suitable stimulation method and changes in effective stimulation intensity. *J Neurosurg,* Vol.101, No.2, pp. 201-209, ISSN 0022-3085.

Zaidel, A.; Arkadir, D.; Israel, Z. & Bergman, H. (2009). Akineto-rigid vs. tremor syndromes in parkinsonism. *Curr Opin Neurol,* Vol. 22, No.4, pp. 387-393, ISSN 1350-7540.

Zirh, TA.; Lenz, FA.; Reich, SG. & Dougherty, PM. (1998). Patterns of bursting occurring in thalamic cells during parkinsonian tremor. *Neuroscience,* Vol.83, No.1, pp. 107-121, ISSN 0306-4522.

14

Post-Operative Management of Parkinson Patients with Deep Brain Stimulation

Niels Allert[1] and Volker Arnd Coenen[2]
[1]*Neurological Rehabilitation Center Godeshoehe, Bonn*
[2]*Stereotaxy and MR-based OR-techniques/Department of Neurosurgery, University of Bonn, Germany*

1. Introduction

Oral medication still remains the mainstay for treating Parkinson's disease (PD). Since the introduction in the late 60ies levodopa is regarded as the gold standard because of the best efficacy on akinesia and rigidity compared to other drugs like dopamine agonists or anticholinergics (Poewe et al., 2010). However, oral dopaminergic treatment of motor symptoms is complicated by the development of motor fluctuations and dyskinesias. These complications can be observed in 40 % after 5 years and 80 % after 10 years PD duration. Moreover, tremor can be refractory to oral medication. During the past 15 years deep brain stimulation (DBS) has become an important therapeutic option for patients with these motor complications. DBS has been approved in Europe for the treatment of tremor in 1995 and for advanced PD in 1998. Approval by the Food and Drug Administration (FDA) was given for tremor in 1997 and for advanced PD in 2002. The main targets for DBS are the subthalamic nucleus (STN), the internal globus pallidus (GPi) and the ventral intermediate (Vim) thalamic nucleus. DBS is a symptomatic treatment and does not influence the progression of the disease (Hilker et al., 2005). Therefore, the number of patients eligible for DBS is limited. Experts estimate that some 10 to 15 % of PD patients are suitable candidates. The implantation of stimulation electrodes is not therapeutic in itself. Apart from the precise electrode localization the subsequent programming of optimal stimulation parameters and adjustment of medication is mandatory (Deuschl et al., 2006). An increasing number of PD patients are treated by DBS so that more and more doctors and care givers involved in the treatment of PD patients are regularly concerned with the special demands of these patients. The following chapter gives an overview on specific issues in the post-operative management of PD patients with DBS.

2. Post-operative management of PD patients with DBS

One of the reasons for the resurgence of surgical therapies in the treatment of PD is that DBS surgery is associated with a limited risk of permanent morbidity of 1 % (Voges et al., 2007). Furthermore, DBS is adjustable and reversible concerning efficacy as well as side effects. This is in contrast to earlier neurosurgical techniques which used permanent lesions of the GPi (pallidotomy) or Vim (thalamotomy). The implantation of electrodes alone does not result in a permanent clinical benefit but requires optimal programming of stimulation parameters and adjustment of medication. However, the surgical procedure often results in a transient microlesion effect already mimicking some of the benefits of chronic DBS (Mann et al., 2009). This microlesion effect implies that motor symptoms like tremor or akinesia are improved immediately after surgery although DBS has not been started. A microlesion effect is usually observed for a couple of days but can last even longer up to weeks. A significant microlesion effect can make the evaluation of stimulation effects on motor symptoms difficult. Therefore, some DBS centers routinely release patients after electrode implantation and admit them a couple of weeks later to start DBS programming. In other centers, DBS programming is started shortly after electrode implantation.

2.1 Surgical issues – Follow-up of wound healing and proper technical function

Proper technical function of the DBS system should be ascertained after surgery. Most notably, the impedances of all stimulation contacts of the commonly used quadripolar stimulation electrodes should be checked. A disconnection of a single or more electrode contacts is characterized by high impedances (depending on the impulse generator model measurements of >2.000 Ohm, >4.000 Ohm or >40.000 Ohm) when measured in a monopolar stimulation mode with the respective contact as cathode and the impulse generator case as anode. Moreover, in this case increasing the voltage will not result in stimulation effects of the central nervous system and will not increase the baseline current of the impulse generator. A short circuit on the other hand is characterized by very low impedances (< 100 Ohm) of the respective contacts when measured in a bipolar stimulation mode with one contact as cathode and the other contact as anode. Detecting a disconnection of single contacts or a short circuit does not necessarily imply a surgical revision. If stimulation of alternative contacts is effective and satisfying the dysfunction should only be regularly controlled in the course of time to exclude extension of technical problems to other leads. In contrast, complete fractures of electrodes or extension leads necessitate surgical revision. Lead fractures have been reported in up to 5 % of the patients in earlier reports (Hamani & Lozano, 2006). In most of these cases the connection between stimulation electrode and extension lead was located below the mastoid. This risk can be significantly reduced if the connection is located at the calvarium (Blomstedt & Hariz, 2005).

Wound healing should be carefully controlled during the first weeks after surgery but also at control visits thereafter. A sterile seroma can occur around the impulse generator but resolves spontaneously in most cases. However, bacterial infections can develop requiring surgical and antibiotic treatment. Bacterial infections are most often found at the impulse generator site within 4 to 6 weeks after implantation but can also occur at other parts of the DBS system (extension lead, electrode). They are exceptionally rare intracranially (Sillay et al., 2008). In most cases of a bacterial infection at the DBS system mere antibiotic treatment does not eradicate bacteria completely so that the system or part of the system needs to be explanted and replaced after a period of consolidation (Bhatia et al., 2010). Apart from infections, skin erosions can be a problem (Sixel-Döring et al., 2010). Such skin erosions can even occur after months and need surgical revision to prevent secondary bacterial infection (Lanotte et al., 2009).

2.2 Determination of optimal stimulation parameters

DBS for PD is a chronic high frequency stimulation of central nervous tissue without feedback mechanisms like the sensing of intrinsic electric activity by cardiac pacemakers. Telemetric programming allows adjusting the stimulation frequency (in Hz), the impulse width (in µs) and the stimulation amplitude (in V in case of constant voltage stimulation and in µA in case of constant current stimulation). Furthermore, quadripolar stimulation electrodes allow variable activation of single or more electrode contacts for either monopolar DBS with the impulse generator serving as anode or bipolar DBS with anode and cathode both being located at the electrode. The principle of DBS programming in PD is to systematically evaluate the clinical responses to stimulation in order to obtain maximal benefit on motor symptoms without or with minimized side effects. This process has to encounter variable latencies of stimulation effects at the different DBS targets which range from seconds to weeks.

2.2.1 Subthalamic nucleus - STN

The subthalamic nucleus has become the primary DBS target in PD during the last 10 to 15 years (Benabid et al., 2009). The sub-target for PD motor symptoms is the dorsolateral hence sensorimotor STN better referred to as the anterior lateral and superior STN (Coenen et al., 2008). The main reasons for this preference are that all PD motor symptoms including tremor, akinesia and rigidity are improved allowing a reduction of dopaminergic medication by some 60 %. The latter also results in a significant reduction of dyskinesias. Recent studies, however, have questioned whether GPi DBS may be equally effective or even superior in individual patients (Follett et al., 2010).

STN DBS directly improves PD off symptoms. Therefore, stimulation effects are best evaluated in the medication off state. The influence of the different stimulation parameters on motor symptoms has been evaluated more systematically in several studies (e.g. Moro et al., 2002). Stimulation frequency has to be above 60 Hz. An increase of the frequency to more than 100 Hz improves DBS efficacy whereas the further benefit of frequencies above 130 Hz is usually limited. To prevent unnecessary current drainage a frequency of 130 Hz can be recommended as the preferred frequency for STN DBS. The impulse width is commonly set at the lowest technical option of 60 µs. Increasing the impulse width does usually not result in specific advantages but results in a negative relationship of DBS efficacy and current drainage. Activation of different contacts of the commonly used quadripolar stimulation electrodes allows to further modify the volume of tissue activated. Initially, efficacy of DBS as well as side effects is evaluated for all contacts separately to determine the contact(s) with the best short term efficacy within seconds to minutes.

Rigidity has been found to be a particularly valuable symptom because of a short latency response. Moreover, rigidity can be reliably evaluated when using reinforcing manoeuvres like voluntary movements of the contralateral hand (Froment's manoeuvre). Akinesia often responds within short time as well but full anti-akinetic effect of DBS may take hours to days. Whereas tremor in DBS of the Vim usually responds within seconds, variable latencies can be observed in STN DBS which range from seconds to weeks. Stimulation-induced dyskinesias are another important motor phenomenon to evaluate DBS efficacy. Stimulation-induced dyskinesias have been demonstrated to be a predictor of good long-term outcome of DBS (Gago et al., 2008). Most importantly, dyskinesias often develop or increase in severity with a latency of minutes to hours so that careful observation of patients after initiation of DBS is recommended. In case of persistent stimulation induced dyskinesias or if the therapeutic window of sufficient symptom control and the induction of dyskinesias is narrow a more dorsal stimulation contact often offers a beneficial alternative.

Apart from motor symptoms DBS can induce psychiatric and behavioural changes. Most of these changes are transient but can be observed during periods of days to weeks and even a couple of months (Temel et al., 2006). The origin of such changes still needs further exploration. Both, direct stimulation of nervous tissue involved in the processing of emotions as well as changes in dopaminergic medication seem to play a role. Although direct stimulation-induced depression has been observed in PD patients with STN DBS (Bejjani et al., 1999), depression seems to be more often due to the reduction of dopaminergic medication and can be improved by increasing this medication (Thobois et al., 2010). In contrast, hypomania seems to be more directly related to stimulation effects. Stimulation of the inferior and medial STN corresponding to the limbic subnucleus of the STN has been proposed as a likely structure. Our own studies also suggest the medial forebrain bundle as a candidate (Coenen et al., 2009). Clinically, stimulation induced hypomania can usually be improved by either reducing the volume of tissue activated or by stimulating a more dorsal contact.

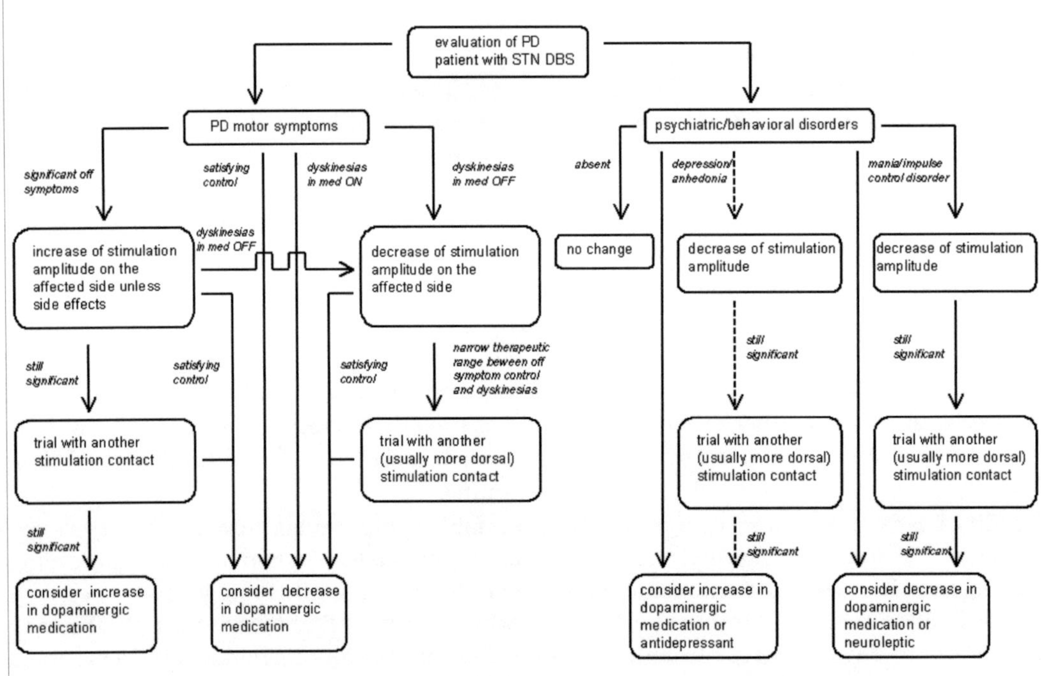

Fig. 1. Algorithm for stimulator and medication adjustments in PD patients with STN DBS (dotted arrows: rare) (adapted from Allert et al., 2011)

Due to the different latencies of stimulation effects as well as adaptive changes with chronic stimulation patients need to be observed and stimulation parameters as well as medication continuously adapted during the first days to weeks. Figure 1 depicts a clinical algorithm for this process of stimulator and medication adjustments.

2.2.2 Globus pallidus internus - GPi

Stimulation of the GPi also improves the major PD motor symptoms, i. e. tremor, akinesia and rigidity. However, initial studies suggested a less profound effect on akinesia corresponding to only little changes in dopaminergic medication. Moreover, failure of GPi DBS has been reported within the first years as well as after longer periods up to 10 years (Durif et al., 2002; Allert et al., 2010). More recent studies, in contrast, have demonstrated similar motor outcome after STN DBS and GPi DBS with more favourable effects on non-motor symptoms like depression in patients with GPi DBS (Follett et al., 2010). Further studies are certainly needed to evaluate the differential effects of GPi DBS and STN DBS on motor and non-motor symptoms in PD.

DBS of the GPi differs in some aspects from DBS of the STN. Anatomically, the sensorimotor area of the GPi is larger than the sensorimotor area of the subthalamic nucleus. To increase the volume of tissue activated higher amplitudes and impulse widths are used. Correspondingly, the higher energy consumption results in a shorter battery longevity of impulse generators. A differential effect of variable impulse widths has not been demonstrated. Historically, longer impulse widths were often used for pallidal stimulation in the 90ies, because the most common impulse generators at that time doubled energy consumption above amplitudes of 3.6 V so that the combination of an amplitude below 3.7 V and a longer impulse width resulted in improved battery longevity. Newer generations of impulse generators have a linear relationship of stimulation amplitude and current consumption so that the initial use of short impulse widths (60 μs) is justified and probably preferable.

Another important difference is that GPi DBS reduces levodopa-induced dyskinesias directly. Hence, stimulation effects have to be evaluated in the medication on and off state separately. This is even more important because DBS of different parts of the GPi can have opposite motor effects. Thus, a more ventral target in the GPi may result in suppression of levodopa induced dyskinesias but increase in akinesia whereas a more dorsal target may even elicit dyskinesias while improving OFF akinesia (Krack et al., 1998).

As mentioned above, changes of dopaminergic medication are less profound in GPi DBS than in STN DBS (Follett et al., 2010). Adjustment of medication after GPi DBS is, therefore, less likely to induce dopaminergic withdrawal symptoms like apathy and anhedonia and probably contributes to the more favorable outcome on non-motor symptoms like depression (Follett et al., 2010).

2.2.3 Ventral intermediate thalamic nucleus - Vim

Whereas in the late 80ies the ventral intermediate thalamic nucleus has been the first target for DBS in patients with medically refractory tremor it's role in PD has diminished with the demonstration that DBS of the GPi and STN not only improves tremor but also reduces akinesia and rigidity. Vim DBS is very effective in reducing PD tremor but has no impact on akinesia and rigidity. Stimulation effects can be observed within seconds making DBS programming easier than that in STN and GPi DBS. Stimulation parameters are comparable to those for GPi and STN DBS, i. e. a frequency of 130 Hz and short impulse widths of 60 µs can be recommended for initial programming. In case of unsatisfactory tremor control higher stimulation frequencies can be helpful although a significant benefit of higher stimulation frequencies for tremor suppression has not been systematically demonstrated. The most important side effects of Vim DBS, particularly in the case of bilateral DBS are impairment of speech and gait/balance. These side effects are reversible and depend on the volume of tissue activated. If tremor is incompletely suppressed the aim of DBS programming is to find an optimal compromise between tremor control and acceptable side effects.

2.3 Adjustment of medication

Adjustment of dopaminergic medication is primarily necessary in PD patients with STN DBS. A reduction of some 60 % of the levodopa equivalent dosage has been reported in a number of studies (Benabid et al., 2009) whereas little changes are observed in PD patients with GPi DBS (Follett et al., 2010; Deep brain stimulation for Parkinson's disease study group, 2001). Since Vim DBS only improves tremor but not akinesia and rigidity, the possibility to reduce dopaminergic medication depends on the tremor control by DBS and prevalence of akinesia and rigidity in the individual patient.

Adjustment of dopaminergic medication is very important in patients undergoing STN surgery. In most DBS centers test stimulation is used during electrode implantation to evaluate neurophysiologically the localization of the electrode. Patients are awake and examined for characteristic side effects like muscle contractions from stimulation of the pyramidal tract, dysaesthesias from stimulation of the medial lemniscus, oculomotor disorders from stimulation of the oculomotor nerve or the pyramidal tract (gaze palsy). Moreover, test stimulation is used to evaluate the effect on PD motor symptoms. The latter can best be evaluated in the medication off state so that dopaminergic medication is not given on the day of surgery. To prevent unforeseen long-term effects of dopamine agonists with a long half-life some DBS centers routinely reduce or even discontinue dopamine agonists for a couple of days before surgery. A reduction of dopaminergic medication may also be necessary immediately after electrode implantation because of a microlesion effect with an increase in dyskinesias. Many DBS centers favour a levodopa monotherapy during the first weeks of DBS programming because of the short half-life which allows better adjustments in response to the DBS effect. A mean reduction of 60 % of the levodopa equivalent dosage can be observed in STN DBS with complete withdrawal in 10 to 30 %. If the DBS effects consolidate and the need for further dopaminergic medication can be better evaluated dopamine agonists can be initiated and adjusted following the same principles as in PD patients without DBS. Apart from the effects on motor symptoms the effects of dopaminergic medication on non-motor symptoms have to be evaluated. Most notably, apathy and anhedonia/depression have been associated with a treatable dopaminergic deficit (Thobois et al., 2010; Czernecki et al., 2008). The goal of DBS and medication adjustment, therefore, should be optimal control of both, motor as well as non-motor symptoms but not a drastic reduction or even withdrawal of dopaminergic medication.

2.4 Management of symptom deterioration

DBS of neither target prevents further disease progression (Hilker et al., 2005). All patients with successful DBS therapy will experience worsening of symptoms and development of new symptoms during the following years.

In case of acute onset of symptoms a technical dysfunction of the DBS system should be excluded. This check should include determination of battery function and a control of the impedances to detect a possible lead fracture/disconnection or a short circuit. Battery failure or a disconnection of the active stimulation contact(s) can result in a sudden increase in PD motor symptoms. A short circuit, in contrast, can result in sudden spread of electrical current to adjacent nervous tissue like the pyramidal tract or the oculomotor nerve with consequent tetanic muscle contraction or eye deviation. A secondary dislocation of stimulation electrodes has been reported in early studies of hardware complications (Blomstedt & Hariz, 2005; Hamani & Lozano, 2006). However, with improved surgical techniques it has become very uncommon in our own experience. In the first step, test stimulation can be helpful to detect a dislocation since either no centrally elicited stimulation effects will be observed or the thresholds for stimulation effects and side-effects will have changed significantly compared to previous stimulation protocols. As a second step, X-ray and computertomography can be used to further evaluate a probable dislocation. In case of disconnections of only single contacts of an electrode or short circuits between contacts the first step should be to evaluate DBS efficacy after reprogramming. In our experience this approach often results in satisfactory symptom control, thereby avoiding surgical revision. Moreover, it is of note, that the individual leads for the 4 contacts of a quadripolar stimulation electrode cannot be sufficiently visualized radiologically so that in case of a disconnection or a short circuit of single contacts X-ray can only demonstrate abnormal loops or sharp bends as possible loci minoris resistentiae.

Battery failure requires immediate impulse generator replacement particularly in patients with STN DBS because of the often dramatic increase in PD motor symptoms and the increased demand of dopaminergic medication. In fact, sudden battery failure should be avoided by regularly checking the remaining battery capacity to anticipate the appropriate time for impulse generator replacement. It is noteworthy that a reduction of symptom control after replacement of impulse generators can be observed (Allert et al., 2009). The origin of such deterioration can be an erroneous change of stimulation parameters or an erroneous connection of the stimulation electrodes to the 2 channels of a double channel impulse generator resulting in a change of the laterality. However, even if such iatrogenic errors are avoided, some patients may need DBS reprogramming for optimal symptom control (Allert et al., 2009).

In case of a rather slow symptom worsening three possibilities have to be encountered. Firstly, DBS efficacy has deteriorated but can be improved by reprogramming (Okun et al., 2005; Moro et al., 2006). Secondly, PD medication needs to be adjusted to obtain the full therapeutic potential. Thirdly, symptom worsening is due to the natural course of the disease. Optimization of stimulation parameters is particularly important during the first months of DBS. In many patients a slow reduction of DBS efficacy after the initial programming is observed which can be compensated by increasing the stimulation amplitude. In more complex clinical situations reprogramming with changes of the active stimulation contacts can be helpful. If stimulation parameters have been optimized but symptoms continue to be worsened the response to dopaminergic medication needs to be evaluated. Particularly in the case of STN DBS dopaminergic medication may have been decreased too much.

2.5 Counseling of patients and care givers

The selection of appropriate candidates for DBS surgery is a work-up of the individual risk and benefit relationship. It is important to identify those symptoms that will most probably respond to DBS, but also those symptoms that are likely to persist or even take a risk of deterioration. Comorbidities have to be evaluated in the same way as psychosocial risk factors. Moreover, the patient has to be informed on the mere symptomatic nature of the therapy which cannot prevent disease progression (Hilker et al., 2005).

The success of DBS as perceived by the patient strongly depends on the own expectations and it is an important goal of the pre-operative counseling to ensure that these expectations are realistic. Apart from the limitations of the prognostic benefit, complications of DBS surgery (most notably infection rate and risk of haemorrhage) should be discussed. Furthermore, the time course of stabilization should be outlined. Although many patients experience significant improvements within a short time after surgery, the stabilization period for motor control and side effects can take 3 to 6 months. Particularly after STN DBS the possibility of behavioural and psychiatric changes has to be discussed with patients and care givers. Hypomania is often rather perceived and complained about by family and friends than by the patient. Important decisions on social and financial issues, e. g. divorce, selling or buying expensive goods etc. should not be planned shortly after DBS surgery.

Another issue to be discussed before surgery are limitations to drive a motor vehicle. Depending on the country's legal regulations driving may be restricted for a certain time period because of the neurosurgical intervention itself. Apart from that, the ability to drive a motor vehicle should be evaluated during the stabilization period after DBS surgery by examining both significant motor impairments as well as cognitive/behavioural limitations.

After surgery patients with DBS and their care givers require counseling on how to behave in daily life. Issues of concern are limitations for medical diagnostics and therapies as described in 2.6. Furthermore, the risk of interference of DBS with environmental electromagnetic waves has to be discussed. The main models of impulse generators in the 90ies had a magnetic reed switch that could not be switched off. Strong electromagnetic waves for example from an electric drill or other sources could result in sudden discontinuation of DBS with reoccurrence of motor symptoms. In newer generations of impulse generator a magnetic reed switch has been omitted or can be telemetrically disabled by the clinician programmer. The risk of interference with environmental electromagnetic waves in these impulse generators appears to be very low.

A handheld patient programmer is an optional device to have limited control of impulse generator functions. In our experience many but not all DBS centers provide patients with such a patient programmer to enable them on the one hand to make sure that DBS is on in case of symptom worsening and on the other hand to allow them checking the impulse generator battery. In some patients the patient programmer may even be helpful to further adjust and optimize stimulation parameters within predefined limits. In any case, the patient and/or patient care giver requires sufficient and often repeated education on the use of such a patient programmer. In fact, if the patient programmer is not used in daily life there is a significant risk of erroneous use which can for example result in accidentally switching off DBS.

Another area of concern for patients is limitations for physical activities particularly sports. Damage of either the stimulation electrode or the extension lead seems feasible if they are hit by high energy so that activities with a likelihood of such events should be avoided. Falls also seem to bear a risk. However, in our own experience technical damage related to physical activity or falls is exceptionally rare although patients may ask for a confirmation of normal function after such events. Heat, exposure to sunlight or the use of a sauna do not bear a particular risk for patients with DBS. In summary, physical activities are not substantially restricted in patients with DBS.

2.6 Implications of DBS on medical diagnostics/therapies

Chronic DBS has implications for several medical diagnostics and therapies. A surface electrocardiogram (ECG) can show electrical artefacts particularly in the monopolar stimulation mode when the impulse generator serves as the anode (Martin et al., 2003). The artefact can be reduced or prevented by either switching off DBS during the ECG or by programming a bipolar stimulation mode when both cathode and anode are located intracranially (Frysinger et al., 2006). The latter also allows for longer ECG monitoring like ambulatory 24 hours Holter ECG.

Similarly, DBS artefacts can interfere with other electrodiagnostics like electroencephalography (EEG), electromyography and evaluation of evoked potentials. If DBS cannot be switched off during the examination, a bipolar DBS mode is advised to reduce or eliminate these artefacts. The use of transcranial magnetic stimulation (TMS) has not been sufficiently investigated. In vitro experiments indicate that TMS can induce currents of charge densities that can induce tissue damage so that routine application should be avoided (Shimojima et al., 2010; Deng et al., 2010).

A cardiac pacemaker or defibrillator is not a contraindication for DBS. A major concern is that the high frequency stimuli of the impulse generator are sensed by the pacemaker and interfere with proper function. Therefore, a bipolar DBS mode is recommended and has been found safe in such patients (Capelle et al., 2005).

X-ray examinations including computertomography (CT) can be safely performed in patients with DBS. In contrast, magnetic resonance imaging (MRI) should only be performed within important limitations. A full body radiofrequency coil cannot be used in patients with DBS because of the risk of electrode heating and tissue damage (Henderson et al., 2005). The use of head transmit coils has been found to be safe and helpful by many groups (Chhabra et al., 2010; Nazarro et al., 2010, Tagliati et al., 2009) but is only recommended according to the manufacturer's guidelines in experienced centers. One study of the effects of 1.5 Tesla MRI in 570 patients did not report any local cutaneous nor neurological disorders during or after the MRI. Moreover, no change of the impulse generator settings occurred in impulse generators without magnetic reed switch or when the magnetic reed switch remained disabled during the procedure (Fraix et al., 2010).

Diathermy (e.g. shortwave diathermy, microwave diathermy or therapeutic ultrasound diathermy) is contraindicated because it can result in tissue damage or damage of parts of the neurostimulation system (Nutt et al., 2001).

3. Conclusion

DBS has become an important therapeutic option for PD patients. DBS is a symptomatic treatment of motor complications requiring not only expertise for the precise implantation of stimulation electrodes but also for the post-operative patient management. Optimal stimulation parameters are determined by clinical evaluation of short and long-term responses. Apart from motor symptoms, stimulation induced non motor symptoms have to be observed, most notably psychiatric and behavioural changes. Similarly, medication has to be adjusted in response to the DBS motor and non-motor effects. Impedance measurements along with the clinical evaluation of stimulation effects are helpful to evaluate proper technical function. Regular follow-up visits are recommended to ensure optimal DBS efficacy. Impulse generators should be replaced before complete battery failure to prevent sudden recurrence of motor symptoms particularly in the case of STN DBS. DBS systems have implications on other medical therapies and diagnostics. Most notably, MRI with full body radiofrequency coils and diathermy are contraindicated because of possible tissue damage or damage of parts of the DBS system.

4. References

Allert, N.; Kirsch, H.; Weirich, W. & Karbe, H. (2009) Stability of symptom control after replacement of impulse generators for deep brain stimulation. *Journal of Neurosurgery,* Vol.110, No.6, pp. 1274-1277

Allert, N.; Lehrke, R.; Sturm, V. & Volkmann J. (2010) Secondary failure after ten years of pallidal neurostimulation in a patient with advanced Parkinson's disease. *Journal of Neural Transmission,* Vol.117, No.3, pp. 349-351

Allert, N.; Dohle, C.; Horn, J. W.; Kelm, S.; Kirsch, H.; Nolte, P. N.; Weirich, W. & Karbe, H. (2011) Rehabilitation of Parkinson's patients with deep brain stimulation – Experiences of the Neurological Rehabilitation Center Godeshoehe. *Nervenarzt* Vol.82, No.4, pp. 462-467

Bejjani, B. P.; Damier, P.; Arnulf, I.; Thivard, L.; Bonnet, A. M.; Dormont, D.; Cornu, P.; Pidoux, B.; Samson, Y. & Agid, Y. (1999) Transient acute depression induced by high-frequency deep-brain stimulation. *New England Journal of Medicine,* Vol.340, No.19, pp. 1476-1480

Benabid, A. L.; Chabardes, S. ; Mitrofanis, J. & Pollak, P. (2009) Deep brain stimulation of the subthalamic nucleus for the treatment of Parkinson's disease. *Lancet Neurology,* Vol.8, No.1, pp. 67 – 81

Bhatia, S.; Zhang, K.; Oh, M.; Angle C. & Whiting, D. (2010) Infections and hardware salvage after deep brain stimulation surgery: a single-center study and review of the literature. *Stereotactic and Functional Neurosurgery,* Vol.88, No.3, pp. 147-155

Blomstedt, P. & Hariz, M. I. (2005) Hardware-related complications of deep brain stimulation: a ten year experience. *Acta Neurochirurgica,* Vol.147, pp. 1061–1064

Capelle, H. H.; Simpson, R. K. Jr; Kronenbuerger, M.; Michaelsen, J.; Tronnier, V. & Krauss, J. K. (2005). Long-term deep brain stimulation in elderly patients with cardiac pacemakers. J *Neurosurgery,* Vol.102, No.1, pp.53-59

Chhabra, V.; Sung, E.; Mewes K.; Bakay R. A.; Abosch A. & Gross R. E. (2010) Safety of magnetic resonance imaging of deep brain stimulator systems: a serial imaging and clinical retrospective study. *Journal of Neurosurgery,* Vol.112, No.3, pp. 497-502

Coenen, V. A.; Honey, C. R.; Hurwitz, T.; Rahman, A. A.; McMaster, J; Bürgel, U. & Mädler, B. (2009) Medial Forebrain bundle stimulation as a pathophysiological mechanism for hypmania in subthalamic nucleus deep brain stimluation for Parkinson's disease. *Neurosurgery,* Vol.64,No.6, pp. 1106-1115

Coenen, V. A.; Prescher, A.; Schmidt, T.; Picozzi, P. & Gielen, F. L. (2008) What is dorso-lateral in the subthalamic nucleus (STN)?—a topographic and anatomical consideration on the ambiguous description of today's primary target for deep brain stimulation (DBS) surgery. Acta Neurochir (Wien), Vol.150, No.11, pp. 1163-1165

Czernecki, V.; Schüpbach, M.; Yaici, S.; Lévy, R.; Bardinet, E.; Yelnik, J.; Dubois, B. & Agid, Y. (2008) Apathy following subthalamic stimulation in Parkinson disease: a dopamine responsive symptom. *Movement Disorders,* Vol.23, No.7, pp. 964-969

Deep brain stimulation for Parkinson's disease study group (2001) Deep-brain stimulation of the subthalamic nucleus or the pars interna of the globus pallidus in Parkinson's disease. *New England Journal of Medicine,* Vol.345, No.13, pp. 956-963

Deng, Z. D.; Lisanby, S. H. & Peterchev, A. V. (2010) Transcranial magnetic stimulation in the presence of deep brain stimulation implants: Induced electrode currents. *Conf Proc IEEE Eng Med Biol Soc,* Vol.1, pp. 6821-6824

Deuschl, G.; Herzog, J.; Kleiner-Fisman, G.; Kubu, C.; Lozano, A. M.; Lyons, K. E.; Rodriguez-Oroz, M. C.; Tamma, F.; Tröster, A. I.; Vitek, J. L.; Volkmann, J. & Voon, V. (2006) Deep brain stimulation: postoperative issues. *Movement Disorders,* Vol.21, Suppl. 14, pp. S219-237

Durif, F.; Lemaire, J. J.; Debilly, B. & Dordain, G. (2002) Long-term follow-up of globus pallidus chronic stimulation in advanced Parkinson's disease. *Movement Disorders,* Vol.17, No.4, pp. 803-807

Follett, K. A.; Weaver, F. M.; Stern, M.; Hur, K.; Harris, C.L.; Luo, P.; Marks, W. J. Jr; Rothlind, J.; Sagher, O.; Moy, C.; Pahwa, R.; Burchiel, K.; Hogarth, P.; Lai, E. C.; Duda, J. E.; Holloway, K.; Samii, A.; Horn, S.; Bronstein, J. M.; Stoner, G.; Starr, P. A.; Simpson, R.; Baltuch, G.; De Salles, A.; Huang, G. D.; Reda, D. J.; CSP 468 Study Group. (2010) Pallidal versus subthalamic deep-brain stimulation for Parkinson's disease. *New England Journal of Medicine,* Vol.362, No.22, pp. 2077–2091

Fraix V.; Chabardes S.; Krainik A.; Seigneuret E.; Grand S.; Le Bas J. F. ; Krack P.; Benabid A. L. & Pollak P. (2010) Effects of magnetic resonance imaging in patients with implanted deep brain stimulation systems. *Journal of Neurosurgery,* Vol.113, No.6, pp. 1242-1245

Frysinger, R. C.; Quigg, M. & Elias, W. J. (2006) Bipolar deep brain stimulation permits routine ECG, EEG, and polysomnography. Neurology, Vol.66, No.2, pp. 268-270

Gago, M. F.; Rosas, M. J.; Linhares, P.; Ayres-Basto, M.; Sousa, G. & Vaz, R. (2008) Transient Disabling Dyskinesias: A Predictor of Good Outcome in Subthalamic Nucleus Deep Brain Stimulation in Parkinson's Disease. *European Neurology,* Vol.61, No.2, pp. 94-99

Hamani, C. & Lozano, A. M. (2006) Hardware-related complications of deep brain stimulation: a review of the published literature. *Stereotactic and Functional Neurosurgery,* Vol. 84, pp. 248–251

Henderson, J. M.; Tkach, J.; Phillips, M.; Baker, K; Shellock, F. G. & Rezai, A. R. (2005) Permanent neurological deficit related to magnetic resonance imaging in a patient with implanted deep brain stimulation electrodes for Parkinson's disease: case report. *Neurosurgery,* Vol.57, No.5, p. E1063

Hilker, R.; Portman, A. T.; Voges, J.; Staal, M. J.; Burghaus, L.; van Laar, T.; Koulousakis, A.; Maguire, R. P.; Pruim, J.; de Jong, B. M.; Herholz, K.; Sturm, V.; Heiss, W. D. & Leenders, K. L. (2005) Disease progression continues in patients with advanced Parkinson's disease and effective subthalamic nucleus stimulation. *Journal of Neurology, Neurosurgery and Psychiatry, Vol.*76, No.9, pp. 1217-1221

Krack, P.; Pollak, P.; Limousin, P.; Hoffmann, D.; Benazzouz, A.; Le Bas, J. J.; Koudsie, A. & Benabid, A. L. (1998) Opposite motor effects of pallidal stimulation in Parkinson's disease. *Annals of Neurology, Vol.*43, No.2, pp. 180-192

Lanotte, M.; Verna, G.; Panciani, P. P.; Taveggia, A.; Zibetti, M.; Lopiano, L. & Ducati, A. (2009) Management of skin erosion following deep brain stimulation. *Neurosurgical Review,* Vol.32, No.1, pp. 111-114

Mann, J. M.; Foote, K. D.; Garvan, C. W.; Fernandez, H. H.; Jacobson, C. E. 4th; Rodriguez, R. L.; Haq, I. U.; Siddiqui, M. S.; Malaty, I. A.; Morishita, T.; Hass, C. J. & Okun, M. S.

(2009) Brain penetration effects of microelectrodes and DBS leads in STN or GPi. *Journal of Neurology, Neurosurgery and Psychiatry*, Vol.80, No.7, pp. 794-797

Martin, W. A.; Camenzind E. & Burkhard P. R. (2003) ECG artifact due to deep brain stimulation. *Lancet* Vol.361, p. 1431

Moro, E.; Esselink, R. J.; Xie, J.; Hommel, M.; Benabid, A. L. & Pollak, P. (2002) The impact on Parkinson's disease of electrical parameter settings in STN stimulation. *Neurology*, Vol.59, No.5, pp. 706-713

Moro, E.; Poon, Y. Y.; Lozano, A. M.; Saint-Cyr, J. A. & Lang, A. E. (2006) Subthalamic nucleus stimulation: improvements in outcome with reprogramming. *Archives of Neurology*, Vol.63, No.9, pp. 1266-1272

Nazzaro, J. M.; Lyons K. E.; Wetzel L. H. & Pahwa R. (2010) Use of brain MRI after deep brain stimulation hardware implantation. *International Journal of Neurosciences*, Vol.120, No.3, pp. 176-183

Nutt, J. G.; Anderson, V. C.; Peacock, J. H.; Hammerstad, J. P. & Burchiel, K. J. (2001) DBS and diathermy interaction induces severe CNS damage. *Neurology*, Vol.56, No.10, pp. 1384-1386

Okun, M. S.; Tagliati, M.; Pourfar, M.; Fernandez, H. H.; Rodriguez, R. L.; Alterman, R. L. & Foote, K. D. (2005) Management of referred deep brain stimulation failures: a retrospective analysis from 2 movement disorders centers. *Archives of Neurology*, Vol.62, No.8, pp. 1250-1255

Poewe, W.; Antonini, A.; Zijlmans J. C.; Burkhard, P. R. & Vingerhoets, F. (2010) Levodopa in the treatment of Parkinson's disease: an old drug still going strong. *Journal of Clinical Interventions in Aging*, Vol.5, pp. 229-238

Shimojima, Y.; Morita, H.; Nishikawa, N.; Kodaira, M.; Hashimoto, T. & Ikeda, S. (2010) The safety of transcranial magnetic stimulation with deep brain stimulation instruments. *Parkinsonism & Related Disorders*, Vol.16, No.2, pp. 127-131

Sillay, K. A.; Larson, P. S. & Starr P. A. (2008) Deep brain stimulator hardware-related infections: incidence and management in a large series. *Neurosurgery*, Vol.62, No.2, pp. 366-367

Sixel-Döring, F.; Trenkwalder, C.; Kappus, C. & Hellwig, D. (2010) Skin complications in deep brain stimulation for Parkinson's disease: frequency, time course, and risk factors. *Acta Neurochirurgica (Wien)*, Vol.152, No.2, pp. 195-200

Tagliati, M.; Jankovic, J.; Pagan, F.; Susatia, F.; Isaias, I. U. & Okun, M. S., National Parkinson Foundation DBS Working Group (2009) Safety of MRI in patients with implanted deep brain stimulation devices. *Neuroimage*, Vol.47, Suppl. 2, pp. T53-57

Temel, Y; Kessels, A.; Tan, S. ; Topdag, A. ; Boon, P. & Visser-Vandewalle V. (2006) Behavioural changes after bilateral subthalamic stimulation in advanced Parkinson disease: a systematic review. *Parkinsonism & Related Disorders*, Vol.12, No.5, pp. 265-272

Thobois, S.; Ardouin, C.; Lhommée, E.; Klinger, H.; Lagrange, C.; Xie, J.; Fraix, V.; Coelho Braga, M. C.; Hassani, R.; Kistner, A.; Juphard, A.; Seigneuret, E.; Chabardes, S.; Mertens, P.; Polo, G.; Reilhac, A.; Costes, N.; LeBars, D.; Savasta, M.; Tremblay, L.; Quesada, J. L.; Bosson, J. L.; Benabid, A. L.; Broussolle, E.; Pollak, P. & Krack, P. (2010) Non-motor dopamine withdrawal syndrome after surgery for Parkinson's disease: predictors and underlying mesolimbic denervation. *Brain*, Vol.133, No.4, pp. 1111-1127

Voges, J.; Hilker, R.; Bötzel, K.; Kiening, K. L.; Kloss, M.; Kupsch, A.; Schnitzler, A.; Schneider, G. H.; Steude, U.; Deuschl, G. & Pinsker, M. O. (2007) Thirty days complication rate following surgery performed for deep-brain-stimulation. *Movement Disorders*, Vol.22, No.10, pp. 1486-1489